Assessment and management
of developmental changes
and problems in children

Assessment and management of developmental changes and problems in children

MARCENE LEE POWELL, R.N., B.S.N., M.N.

Associate Professor, College of Nursing, University of Utah;
Doctoral Candidate, The Graduate School of Social Work,
University of Utah, Salt Lake City, Utah; formerly
Associate Professor, University of Washington School of Nursing,
Child Development and Mental Retardation Center,
Seattle, Washington

Chapter 9 contributed by
PEGGY L. PIPES, M.A., M.P.H.

SECOND EDITION

With 159 *illustrations*
Original photographs by **Janis K. Smith**
Original drawings by **Mary K. Shrader**
Original cover by **Greg Owen**

The C. V. Mosby Company

ST. LOUIS • TORONTO • LONDON   1981

MOSBY

1906 **75** 1981
YEARS

A TRADITION OF PUBLISHING EXCELLENCE

SECOND EDITION

Previous edition copyrighted 1976

Printed in the United States of America

The C. V. Mosby Company
11830 Westline Industrial Drive, St. Louis, Missouri 63141

Library of Congress Cataloging in Publication Data

Powell, Marcene Lee, 1938-
 Assessment and management of developmental changes and problems in children.

 First ed. published in 1976 under title: Assessment and management of developmental changes in children.
 Includes bibliographies and index.
 1. Child development—Testing. 2. Children—Care and hygiene. 3. Children—Management. 4. Pediatric nursing. I. Title.
RJ51.D48P68 1981 618.92′0075 80-27040
ISBN 0-8016-1520-8

GW/M/M 9 8 7 6 5 4 3 2 1 03/D/330

With love and affection to my parents
George Bingham Powell, Sr. and **Gretchen Spencer Powell**
and to my brothers and their wives
George Bingham, Jr. and **Linda Powell**
C. Spencer and **Joan Powell**
Frank Neff and **Dorothy Powell**
and
Keith II and **Janet Powell**

PREFACE

The second edition of this book emphasizes the crucial changes in the practice of
assessment and management of developmental
changes and problems in children. The major
purpose of the book is to underscore the dramatic need for child care professionals to be
more sensitive and develop a heightened responsiveness to the ever-changing needs and
concerns of both parents and children.

An important focus of the book is the emphasis on the urgent need for child care professionals to abandon outmoded concepts of
assessment, screening, and child-parent management practices. This edition specifically up-
dates models and approaches that have been observed to assist professionals to respond in more
appropriate ways to the needs of infants, children, parents, and members of the nuclear and
extended family.

This edition does not depart from the book's
original goal of providing child care professionals with standardized assessment and screening
tools. It essentially represents an effort to
update current knowledge of assessment and
screening tools to enhance the management
skills of child care professionals. In a larger
sense topics are presented so that professionals
in child care can be in a more optimal position
to deliver the quality of child and parent care
services so urgently needed today.

I have elected to add an important and needed
section on assessment and management of the
child with developmental problems or delays,
such as occur with the child with mental retardation. In doing so, I have included the
Washington Guide to Promoting Development
in the Young Child, as one more useful tool
that practitioners can use not only in screening
but also to enhance and facilitate development
in children with and without developmental delays. A unique and beneficial aspect of the guide
is the suggestions offered to parents and child
care professionals to foster the young child's
development.

One of the most salient features of the second
edition is the emphasis on promoting a problem-
solving and mutual participation interaction
model for the solution of parents, children, and
professional care providers' concerns, needs,
and commonly encountered dilemmas.

In accordance with the aims of the first edition, I have closely and precisely adhered to the
philosophy that assessment and management
skills with infants, children, and parents are essential if not paramount for professionals in the
field of child care.

Assessment, hand in hand with newly emerging ideologies of management practices with
children and their parents, is continuously
viewed and kept in perspective as a multifaceted, complex, and dynamic process that presents demanding challenges to the professional
child care provider. Thus, within this context,
assessment, screening, and management practices call for a variety of skills on the part
of health care professionals ranging from the

ability to have rapport with infants and children to developing sensitive, supportive approaches with parents before, during, and after screening or assessment of a child.

Developmental assessments of infants and children do not end with administering test items, recording and scoring a child's response, and assigning a score. The process involves communicating the assessment results to parents and other members of health care disciplines and interpreting these results and their implications for parents and other caregivers. It also requires the ability to participate in a decision-making process with others.

The content of this book is presented to provide those involved in child care with the necessary knowledge to use a variety of developmental screening and assessment tools. The book is not meant to be a substitute for assessment manuals. It supplements some of the material contained in test manuals and other assessment tools. It goes further, however, in considering many important management implications that can be derived from developmental assessment of infants and children. Mastery of the assessment process requires supervised experiences and proficiency testing. Supervision is particularly necessary for those just beginning to use new assessment tools. Assistance in the early phases can help the beginner reduce subjectivity and increase independent reliability.

A major feature of this book is the discussion of assessment tools that serve to detect and prevent developmental problems. A unique aspect of the book is the focus on assessment tools to predict children's future outcomes.

Systematic approaches to assessing infants, their subtle interactions with the environment, and their neurological status are included, as are assessment tools to measure maternal perception of infant behavior. Assessment methods that measure infant temperament are also incorporated. Screening tools for determining a child's functional levels are integrated into the text as well.

Methods and guides for assessing the adequacy of the home environment as the child develops are a unique facet of the book. An important focus is on assessing readiness of children for developmental changes and readiness of parents to respond to these changes. Methods for observing and documenting behavioral interactions are also a major focus so as to enable parents and child care professionals to achieve mutual child management goals.

The various assessment tools contained in the text are discussed to enable child care professionals to promote early quality care for infants and children. The book underscores the importance of making parent-child interactions as rewarding as possible. By using numerous assessment tools, professionals in child care can help parents to gain a confidence and mastery in childrearing that they otherwise might not have. The material has been written so that professionals in early child care can become more sensitive to the needs of infants, children, and parents. With this knowledge of assessment and management of developmental changes in children, the professional in child care no longer has to be a passive caregiver but can be an accountable, responsible, and visible care provider.

I would like to extend my appreciation to all the individuals who gave me permission to incorporate their screening and assessment tools into this book. Also, I would like to give special thanks to the mothers and fathers who allowed me to include photographs of their children and themselves.

Marcene Lee Powell

CONTENTS

Assessment and management of developmental changes and problems in children

1

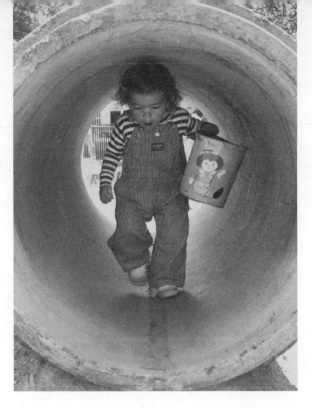

CHANGING TRENDS IN ASSESSMENT AND MANAGEMENT PRACTICE

The major goals of all professionals providing care to newborns, infants, and children are to assess the functional abilities and adaptive behaviors of the child within his environment. Child care professionals need to screen infants for the possibility of developmental delays so that if they are present, more realistic goals can be set to keep the child functioning optionally, to increase his independent functioning, and to promote an increase in adaptive behaviors but not to promote greater dependency or more maladaptive interactions. Professionals also need to screen for the child's developmental progress in all areas of functioning.

OBSTACLES TO ASSESSMENT AND CARE

Several obstacles have stood in the way of child care professionals assisting newborns, infants, and children to master their developmental tasks. If outmoded concepts or attitudes about children are used, they tend to be reflected in assessment practices or care approaches that professionals choose. Before outmoded concepts of screening and assessment can be rejected, they must be examined and

identified. Child care professionals need to think about emerging and improved practices in screening, assessment, and care practices with children and their parents.

In the past, professionals have used and relied on the pediatric pathological model for screening and assessment of infants and children, awaiting the presence of gross clinical manifestations before a diagnosis was made or treatment plans could be initiated and carried out. However, now the developmental and educational models for assessment and child care practices are available. The developmental model helps child care professionals to take a more optimistic view of the child and his potential for change and to look for developmental changes in children, no matter how small these changes are. The educational model can also be used, whereby principles of teaching and learning are applied so that the child can master small segments of behavior and successfully perform developmental tasks. By using both the educational and developmental model, child care professionals reject simple physical and custodial models of care for children.

Instead of waiting for gross clinical mani-

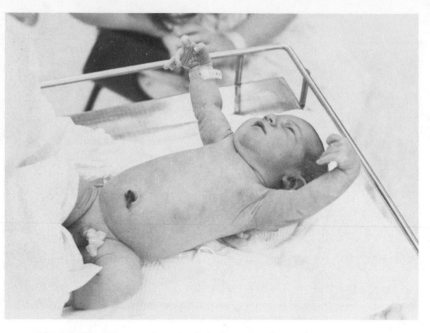

Fig. 1-1. The Moro response is elicited as part of a newborn assessment.

festations to be present, professionals need to begin as early as the neonatal period to observe infant behavior. In the past too much attention has been paid to the functions of the infant's gastrointestinal tract. Nurses, physicians, and parents have been oriented to how much formula the infant drank, how many stools he had, and how many times he voided in a 24-hour period. These are important considerations. However, professionals in child care can also learn to observe and record specific behavior about the infant, for example, his levels of consciousness, or "states," activity levels, adaptive behaviors, interactions with others in his environment, purposeful behaviors, alertness, ways he consoles himself, and ability to attend to both animate and inanimate stimuli. This information is extremely important for parents so that they can view their infant as a person and learn about his strengths and appealing traits. This will enable them to become better acquainted with their infant, to develop feelings of closeness, and to discover his individual differences and unique traits.

Labeling

In the past, health professionals have generalized about newborns, infants, children, and their parents, tending to view most infants and children as being alike and having the same needs. If they get into the habit of generalizing about children and parents, they become caught in a trap that interferes with optimal child care approaches. Some of the common statements that are made or written down about a child or infant include "slow," "backward," "fussy," "unmanageable," "passive," "apathetic," "floppy infant," "minimal brain dysfunction," "he's behind," "she's stubborn," or "he's untestable." Labels or comments about parents may include "rejecting," "hostile," "resistant," "unaccepting," "poor mothering," "angry," "neurotic," "overprotective," or "inadequate." Child care professionals have been inclined to formulate many generalizations about children, parents, and their behavior, thereby coming to some dangerous conclusions about them.

What are some of the hazards of labeling children and parents? If professionals routinely stereotype or rely on labeling, it becomes difficult, if not impossible, for them to plan individualized intervention for a child or parent. It is difficult for a child or parent to lose the label once it is applied. No matter how much children progress developmentally, they are subject to being stigmatized because of a label. Label-

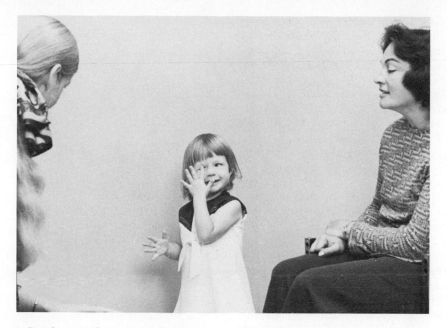

Fig. 1-2. Developmental screening of receptive language abilities. The child correctly points to her eye when asked.

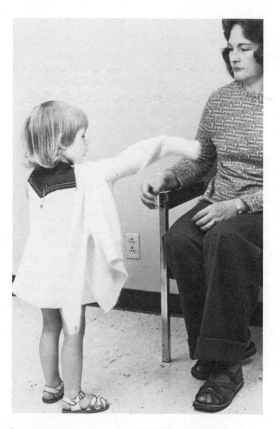

Fig. 1-3. Developmental screening of personal-social abilities. The child demonstrates the ability to put on a sweater independently.

ing can bias a professional who will interact with a child or parent. If a child care professional hears that the parent is "angry" or "hostile," an expectation is set up. The professional may be prepared to deal with anger and may become defensive, instead of making a personal interpretation of the client's behavior after meeting him. The label may interfere with rapport between a professional and a client. Labeling may perpetuate a negative view of an individual, and this may tend to diminish his strengths.

Reliance on labeling leads to a narrow view and inappropriate treatment or care approaches. Professionals may even be confused by labels and what they should do. Once a label is applied, it seems to slow down, interfere with, or even stop intervention. Labeling can serve practical purposes, such as obtaining services that people need, but the label tells little about the child's current functional abilities, adaptive behaviors, and strengths and tells nothing about the child's future. Child care professionals need to be sensitive when they hear parents using labels in front of children, since the parents may not be aware of the devastating effects that labels have on a child. Labels may generate a self-fulfilling prophecy; that is, the parent or child may act the way he thinks people expect him to behave.

Child care professionals also must remember that labels lead to a circular definition, such as "the child is hyperactive; he is always out of his chair; if he weren't out of his chair, he wouldn't be hyperactive; if he weren't hyperactive, he wouldn't be out of his chair." One of the worst aspects of labeling is that when dealing with global descriptions of behavior, parents and child care professionals alike tend to become confused about what they should be doing for a child. How can you plan goals for a "temperamental child"? How can you speed up a "slow learner"? How can you firm up a "floppy infant"? How can you decrease a baby's "fussiness"? There are alternatives to labeling, including careful observations and documentation of specific behaviors before any plan of care is implemented. Child care professionals must become accustomed to clarifying and differentiating behaviors that need to be increased, decreased, or left alone.

Negative observations

In general, professionals in child care as well as others have become stuck in habits of focus-

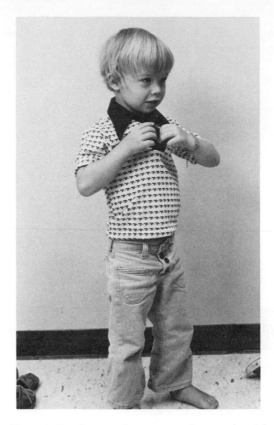

Fig. 1-4. Developmental screening of personal-social abilities. The child demonstrates the ability to unbutton without assistance.

ing on and listening and watching for what the child or parent *cannot do*. It is easy to look for negative traits because usually they are highly conspicuous.

Child care professionals must consider emphasizing the assets and positive features of an infant, child, or parent. They must pay more attention to what the child or parent *can do*. This is far more important. During the screening or assessment process it is important to be oriented to a strengths model instead of a deficit model and to share observations of the child's assets and appealing traits with the parents before presenting the child's weaknesses. Child care professionals also need to remember that parents are sensitive; they make valid observations of children. They can problem solve and can actively participate in crucial decisions about their infant or child. The professional needs to comment on the parents' obvious abilities to interact appropriately with their child, acknowledging their observation skills and

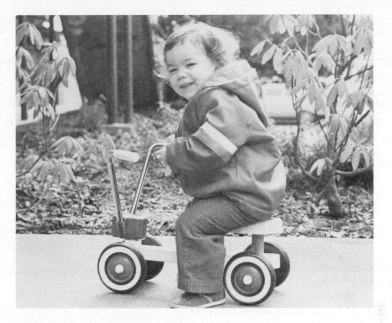

Fig. 1-5. Play equipment available in a child's environment is assessed

ability to problem solve. As the strengths of an infant or child are presented to the parents, they must also be asked what they see as strengths in their child.

Subjective methods

Child care professionals have also tended to rely on highly subjective methods in obtaining assessment data about a child's developmental or functional status, including considerable use of guessing and hunches about children's and parents' behavior. Instead of saying, I think he's doing better, or he has made some progress, or he's really coming along, or he's catching up, specific clarification about the child's behavioral progress is needed. Instead of guessing, the professional has the means to collect data in an objective way. Instead of saying that the child is always looking around, the professional can count the child's attending behavior and state that he looked at the toy twenty times, reached for the spoon four times, reached for a block seven times, attended to the picture for 20 seconds, initiated a task five times, and complied with a simple request four times. There is no question that child care professionals need to get into the habit of keeping records and counting behaviors and also to orient parents to the need for keeping records. Parents should be encouraged to be future problem solvers, not perpetual and future help seekers.

Inadequate data

Child care professionals have been inclined to obtain developmental assessment data on a one-shot basis and, worse, have planned care based on fragmentary and incomplete information. This dangerous practice should be avoided at all costs. Obtaining data on a child only once does not give anyone sufficient behavior samples to permit interpretations or conclusions about care planning. Data should be gathered on a serial basis to note specific progress or lack of it and to give feedback to a child's care providers. Longitudinal data are needed to make comparisons with a child's earlier performance, or baseline behaviors. It is necessary to remember that children change in their behavior. Intervention can no longer be planned in haphazard ways because the child's needs will not be met, the parents may end up more frustrated, and the child care professional will be unable to achieve successful outcomes.

Reliance on numbers

There has been a tendency to interpret screening results to parents by giving them numbers, for example, telling parents that their child is functioning at the 4-month level or the 2-year 2-month level. What can parents learn about their children by the use of numbers? Do they learn the child's strengths or weaknesses or steps they should take in promoting the child's functional levels in his environment? Can you, as a child care professional, plan intervention based on a number? Professionals need to accustom themselves to telling parents about specific behaviors that they observed in the child at a given time. No one can benefit from hearing a number, including the child care professional who is responsible for promoting the child's development. Most screening and assessment tools were not designed with the idea of simply presenting a number to a parent because it is not sufficient information and will never substitute for specific behavioral observations.

PARENTAL PARTICIPATION

Parents live with their child on a moment-to-moment, hour-by-hour, day-by-day, month-to-month, year-in and year-out basis, and are therefore important in the screening and assessment process. However, child care professionals have tended to neglect them in this role and have overlooked their needs, contributions, and concerns. By omitting parents in the assessment and care process, what does the professional unintentionally do? Basically, the professional may increase fears that they are inadequate in their parenting roles; they may view themselves as chronic failures. They may continue to pursue unrealistic goals for a child and for themselves.

Their goals for helping a child accomplish developmental tasks may be too high or too low according to the child's actual level of functioning. Child care professionals have somehow fallen short in acknowledging parental competencies, giving parents the message that they really do not know what is going on and cannot help their child. This, in turn, makes them dependent on health care professionals in the process. Essentially, if parents are omitted, they may become more anxious about what they are doing or are not doing, and they may feel more inadequate and even incompetent as persons. Child care professionals inadvertently reinforce the *powerlessness* that parents may feel. Parents may lack role models, standards, precedents, or role referents in their child-rearing practices. We, as child care professionals, are in a position to help reduce the chaos, confusion, and frustration that some parents may experience. Parents can be included in the assessment process by making comments on their concerns, observations, and problem-solving abilities. It is helpful to follow an assessment process whereby the child care profes-

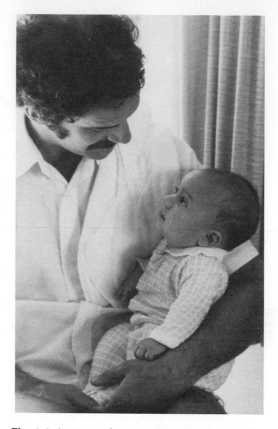

Fig. 1-6. Assessing the interactions between a father and his infant.

sional uses a mutual participation interaction model, in which the parents' views are elicited and the parents are active participants in decision making and care planning; the parents should not be encouraged to remain passive recipients of care.

It is well to recall that the screening process is a series of steps whereby the child care professional observes, records, analyzes, and describes a child's performance outcomes with a screening tool or procedure. In this model the parent and child are prepared for the screening process, developmental items are presented to the child so that he can perform at his best, and then the child care professional scores or rates the child's performance according to the screening tool scoring criteria. Next is the interpretative phase, when the parents receive information about the child's performance in a systematic and objective way.

It is important to follow a model whereby the child care professional explains the purpose of the screening tool to the parents and then

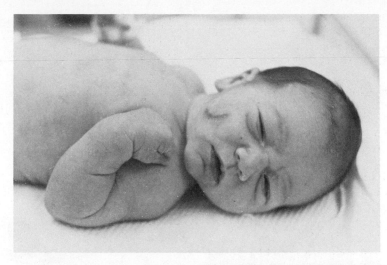

Fig. 1-7. Assessing an infant's ability to quiet herself.

asks them how well they think their child will do in all the areas in which he will be screened, such as social performance, fine motor skills, gross motor skills, and language skills. After the screening items have been administered to the child and the screening test has been scored, it is important to ask the mother or father how well they thought the child did in all the areas screened. Then the professional presents observations of the child's performance by emphasizing the child's strengths first and the areas that were "not as easy" for him last. The parents should be asked if they agree with the professional's observations. Did they notice something different? This approach of including the parents should begin in early infancy, even during the newborn period, with an emphasis on pointing out and underscoring the child's strengths, then discussing what was more difficult for the child and what the parents intend to do about their concern, once they have defined it for the child care professional.

From the neonatal period on, parents need to participate in observations about their infant or child and in planning and evaluating care practices, whether the child is in an inpatient or home setting. Child care professionals must stop perpetuating the view of parents and children as passive recipients. They must not be treated as if they do not matter or cannot act appropriately. Do not do things *to* parents or children. Invite their input and their comment and acknowledge their strengths, abilities, and efforts. *Interact with* the parent and child rather than *react to* them. In addition, studies show

that parents are more accurate in estimating their child's developmental status than health care professionals have given them credit for. If they do make errors in estimating their child's performance, this tends to be in an upward direction, giving the child more credit than he deserves. In the main, however, parents are highly accurate in perceiving their children's developmental status, and professionals must convey to parents that their observations and estimates of their child's performance are valuable.

Another study shows the importance of observing the parents' teaching interactions with their children. Steward and Steward[1] showed that an examination of the "teaching loop" which the parent uses can be advantageous to both parent and child. The child care professional should observe how the parent gets the child's attention, what and how the parent feels, how the parent clarifies what the child is to do, how the parent observes the child performing at his own rate, and how, when, and the appropriateness with which the parent acknowledges the child's performance. It is important for any child care professional to observe a parent's teaching loop before expecting a parent to carry out a program of teaching at home. It is also significant that the child care professional examine his own style of teaching and interacting with a child in appropriate and effective ways.

Once it has been determined that parents are concerned about a child's behavior or performance and have requested help with chang-

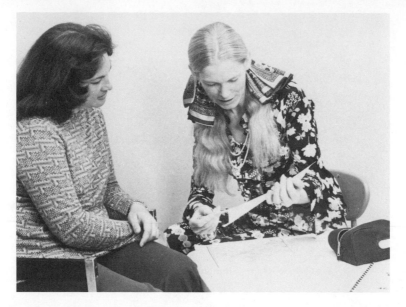

Fig. 1-8. A mother is learning the results of the screening assessment of her child's abilities in fine motor tasks, gross motor skills, and language skills.

ing that behavior, it is important for the child care professional to check with the parents' perceptions of the child's behavior once change begins. How do the parents react to this change and what does it mean to them? A child care professional should never change a child's behavior without *always* planning to check the parents' perceptions of what the child's change means to them. This should be done throughout a program that has been planned with consideration of the parents' priorities.

Collecting and sharing data

Somehow we, as child care professionals, have perpetuated a mystique about data collection. We convey that we have a corner on developmental data and do not automatically share information about a child with his parents. Maybe we did not know what to share or were insecure about what to say. We can reverse this and answer parents' questions about children's development.

In the past, child care professionals have lacked standardized tools that would assist them in screening children's developmental changes in a systematic, objective way. There still is no perfect tool that will screen or assess children of different ages, ethnic origins, and cultural settings. Most standardized tools today have both advantages and disadvantages in helping

the professional to determine children's functional abilities and adaptive behaviors. In addition, professionals have failed to use standardized tools correctly when they were available. Child care professionals can no longer just screen a child's gross motor abilities and be satisfied that they have used a screening tool satisfactorily. They must screen for fine motor skills, language abilities, personal-social behaviors, and preacademic skills as well. A number of standardized screening tools are available for use and are presented throughout this book. Each requires attention to the standardized procedure, which is carefully spelled out. Substitutions for testing cannot be made, or the screening results will be invalidated and jeopardized. Most screening tools are not intended for diagnosis, prediction of future outcomes, or estimation of a child's IQ. Specially designed, standardized IQ tests, administered by professionally trained persons who know how to administer, score, and interpret what these scores mean statistically, are the only safe measures professionals can rely on for IQ scores.

Somehow professionals in child care are obsessed with the need to give instant advice to parents when they ask a question, present a concern, or request help with children's developmental tasks. Traditionally much advice is immediately offered and given in a haphazard

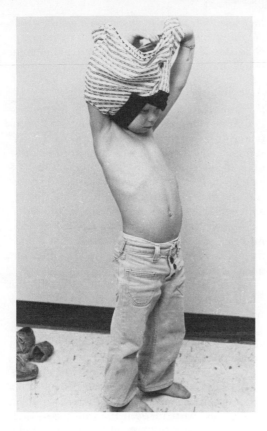

Fig. 1-9. Developmental screening of personal-social abilities. The child demonstrates the ability to undress without assistance.

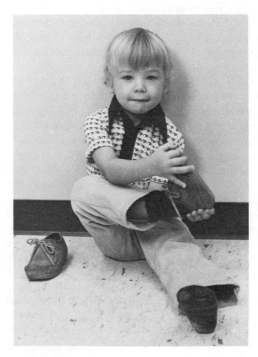

Fig. 1-10. Developmental screening of personal-social abilities. The child demonstrates the ability to remove shoes without help.

manner. Whose needs are being met when the professional tells a mother twenty different things to do? If instant advice is the choice, the professional fails to interact in a mutual problem-solving way with a parent. The parent may be overwhelmed and unable to carry out the recommended steps. With this approach the parent invariably feels more of a failure, and the child gets frustrated and is doomed to failure also.

Instead of giving instant advice, the professional can think immediately of ways to collect data. What has the parent tried? What is her definition of her problem? What has worked? What has failed? What are the parents' expectations of the child's performance?

Professionals in child care need to feel comfortable, relaxed, and successful with the counseling, advice, and reassurance they give parents. Most of us in child care need to give ourselves permission to stop acting quickly, being busy, being all things to all people, and having the right answer immediately. There are ways child care professionals can experience success, however. It calls for adhering to a systematic and objective approach that can be carried out in a nurturing, humanistic framework. Professionals can be successful in teaching parents and children independence in feeding, toileting, play, socialization, and better ways to communicate. This can be achieved only after adequate data are collected, the concern has been carefully defined, and both the parent and professional in child care have committed themselves to work together from the beginning for the successful outcomes that are anticipated. Once behaviors are documented and priorities are determined by parents and child care professionals, there is the existing possibility of change and successful experiences in the change process. Both parents and child care professionals need to remember that ten behaviors cannot be changed at once, and it is recommended that concerns which parents express as being the most important should be examined first.

In the past, child care professionals have been oriented to focusing on one symptom or one behavior. A number of studies suggest the need to look at clusters of minor anomalies that may suggest the presence of a more serious defect. It is important that professionals be more sensitive in examining one minor anomaly and observing it carefully while simultaneously searching for other signs that may signal the presence of something more serious. They must increase their index of suspicion once they note anything unusual or different in an infant or child and be prepared to be vigilant and monitor behavioral changes in a child.

Assessing the parents

Formerly, child care professionals were satisfied in focusing on the child alone. This orientation does not guarantee success with intervention. They need to assess parents' readiness to be involved in teaching or promoting behavioral change. They also need to assess the interactions of others with a child, including siblings and members of the extended family. In a situation where one family member may be stuck, hurting, delayed, or in distress, other family members may be hurting too, and approaches must be considered.

Parents may already be doing a number of significant activities but need feedback on how well they are managing. Parents should be acknowledged when they keep records of their children's behavior, do therapy, and carry out programs in the home. Health care professionals also need to respond to parents in more sensitive ways. They sometimes need to inject a hope for change and help parents to ease up on themselves, particularly if they are too self-critical for not starting something earlier. If the professional watches and listens, parents will relate their concerns, strengths, and worries. The professional is at an advantage because he can hear better and be more objective and thus acknowledge their efforts to help themselves and their child.

A child care professional must never discount what parents say about themselves or their child.

NEW APPROACHES TO ASSESSMENT

A new trend is emerging that is exciting because of its implications for assessing developmental changes in children. Professionals no longer merely determine a child's developmental status. They must be prepared to use newly developed tools that help them assess and measure certain aspects of the environment in which a child is growing and developing. Does the environment offer the physical, social, and cognitive support that a child needs as he changes in his development?

Formerly, the numbers of diagnosed cases of mental retardation increased dramatically at the age of school entrance. This may be correlated with the fact that this was the first time

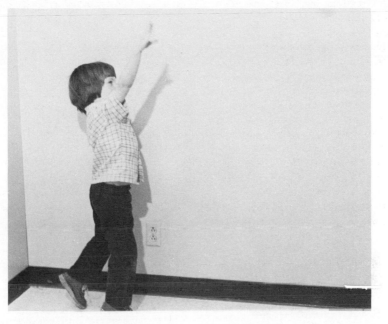

Fig. 1-11. Developmental screening of gross motor skills. The child demonstrates the ability to throw the ball to the examiner, using an overhand throw.

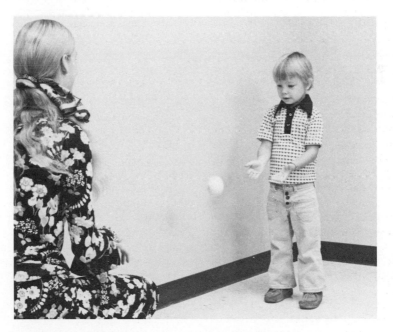

Fig. 1-12. Developmental screening of gross motor skills. The child is getting ready to catch the ball with his two hands.

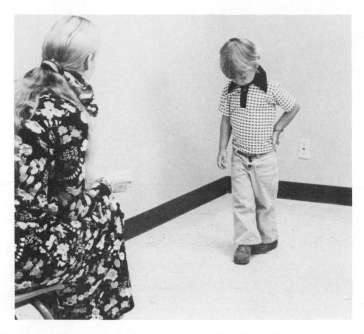

Fig. 1-13. Developmental screening of gross motor skills. The child demonstrates the ability to walk by placing the heel of one foot in front of and touching the toe of the other foot.

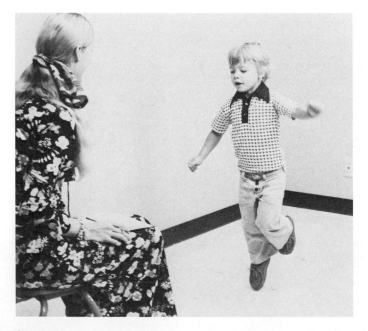

Fig. 1-14. Developmental screening of gross motor skills. The child shows the ability to hop on one foot two or more times in a row without holding on to anything.

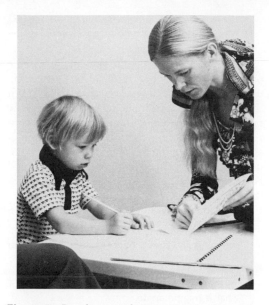

Fig. 1-15. Developmental screening for fine motor skills. The child is concentrating on drawing a square that he is copying from a picture.

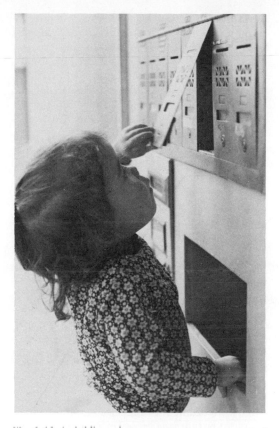

Fig. 1-16. A child's exploratory behaviors are assessed.

a child's development was screened objectively and systematically. All professionals in child care have a tremendous responsibility in early case finding so that treatment and intervention can be implemented earlier. They can no longer say they do not have the time. The tools and technology to improve case finding in many significant ways are available and are discussed in this book.

It used to be the role of the physician to assess a child, gather other child care team members together, and present the assessment findings to the parents.

Now there is evidence of nurses, occupational therapists, physical therapists, nutritionists, social workers, and physicians trading roles in being the case manager for a young child. The use of the interdisciplinary approach is emerging today as the best way to meet the needs of children and their parents.

It is also recognized that the physician is not the only individual responsible for conducting a parent-informing interview if the child has been assessed by an interdisciplinary team.

Another new trend is emerging that holds promise for presenting assessment findings to parents. This is the practice of abandoning the virtuoso model and substituting an interaction model with parents. Child care professionals no

longer need to impress and intimidate parents with their findings. Rather, they are becoming committed to conducting an informing interview with a heightened sense of awareness and sensitivity to the needs of parents. Instead of meeting the parents with a long list of medical, biochemical, and microscopic findings, child care professionals can give and pace the information to allow parents to ask questions in their own time and style.

Parents obviously want answers, but instead of continuing with traditional styles of interacting with them, professionals should listen to what parents are saying and asking. Never underestimate what parents say about themselves or their children. Child care professionals should learn to respond comfortably to the parents' needs and not simply to impose their needs or views on parents. They definitely have their own ideas. Professionals need to reinforce parents' efforts when they seek help and to reinforce their critiquing the quality of care they and their children receive without becoming defensive. Above all else, *professionals must stop* telling parents how to feel.

Rather than thinking in terms of limited goals, child care professionals need to consider lifetime goals and include both the parent and child in achieving objectives in the most realistic, comfortable way possible. They must automatically obtain their input and not rely solely on observations or assumptions.

Instead of intervening during a crisis, child care professionals should concentrate on giving anticipatory guidance.

It is unequivocal that professionals cannot plan a developmental program for a child until they observe and document the functional levels of his behavior within many environments.

In the not too distant past, child care professionals tended to give attention to the concerns only of the mother and shared important information about the child with her. Now professionals must actively seek out fathers, acknowledge their concerns, and be prepared to give them the same kinds of support and information offered to mothers and children.

INTERACTING WITH PARENTS

It is important for child health professionals to *define parenting behaviors* so that they can be identified and to be so specific that it is possible to *individualize* the parent. Often, professionals mistakenly deal with global concerns, misconceptions, or perceptions about parents. There is no global prescription for parenting. Child care professionals have to assess where they are, where the parents are, what they want from professionals, what their strengths are, what they feel they need help with, and what is bothering them.

Child care professionals need to:

- Be attuned to what (1) parents are saying to them, (2) parents are acting out for them, and (3) parents are saying to each other
- Be available on a long-term rather than sporadic basis, so that parents can lean on them when they need to be dependent
- Be consistent
- Listen to what *parents are saying*—as well as listen to themselves
- Let parents define their own needs and never intervene until they have clarified what their concern is; it is dangerous to operate on *assumptions* rather than facts about individual parents
- Avoid stereotypes and the pathological framework

- Become sensitive in viewing parents as persons who are resourceful rather than passive recipients.

Child care professionals usually reinforce parents for disowning themselves, giving up their powers, and alienating themselves from themselves. Professionals usually respond by taking over, becoming omnipotent, and conveying the message that the parents are not adequate and not in charge of themselves. What do the parents want to do next? Parents should be talked to separately and together to see that they both agree on the best way to go.

Professionals need to:

- Become sensitive to parents' strengths and competencies and comment about them, rather than emphasizing their weaknesses or problems
- *Always* acknowledge the appropriate things parents are doing, not what they *are failing to do* or what is inappropriate
- Become attuned to themselves, their own pain and dilemmas, before they can be responsive to the pain of others
- Give parents the credit they deserve

The main goal of child care professionals is to help parents believe that they are in charge of themselves and their children and are most capable of making decisions and problem solving.

SCREENING AND ASSESSMENT TOOLS

Counseling, guidance, and approaches to successful management are strictly dependent on documented data from parents, child care professionals, and assessment tools. Planning for change is based on corroborative evidence that a problem exists before collaborative strategies or interventions can be planned with parents. Accurate use of assessment tools is particularly important because of the emerging responsibilities that exist for educating others who will assist nurses and physicians in the ambulatory care of well children.

Child care professionals now rely on a number and variety of standardized screening tools designed to help do a better, more accurate job of developmental assessment than ever before. For each tool, the assessment protocol is carefully spelled out, the directions for administering developmental items are clear, and the criteria for passing or failing a child are readily available for reference. Carrying out each screening procedure in a standardized way results in valid information about a child's behaviors and removes confusion and guessing about how well the child is doing.

Screening tools are intended for assessment of a child's developmental status prior to intervention and at periodic intervals during intervention. Developmental screening tools should not be misused. They are not intended to represent or be a substitute for a full psychometric evaluation. They do not diagnose children. Until carefully conducted longitudinal studies of normal children of different racial, socioeconomic, and educational backgrounds have been completed, the majority of developmental screening inventories popular today cannot be used for predicting a child's future. Furthermore, no single standardized developmental screening test will satisfy the needs of all professional disciplines; certain tools have benefits for one discipline but only limited usefulness for others.

A number of assessment tools have been developed that are particularly helpful in evaluating successful changes that occur in an infant's or child's life over a period of time.

The Denver Developmental Screening Test (DDST), for example, is administered periodically from birth to 6 years of age. The Developmental Profile, a newer tool, can be used from birth to beginning adolescence to assess an individual's level of functioning. These screening tools make it easier to gather, accumulate, and monitor continuous developmental change and organize these data into efficient record systems. As mentioned before, effective documentation enhances planning, implementing, evaluating, and changing approaches as an individual child responds to intervention designed for his optimal and maximal growth and development.

Since one or two tools by themselves are not considered sufficient for evaluating a child's developmental status, increased emphasis is placed on using a variety of tools at different times that are designed to assess different facets of a child's development. The Neonatal Behavioral Assessment Scale, for example, is used to assess an infant's adaptation to the external environment and is used from the first week of life to the first month. The Carey Infant Temperament Questionnaire is designed to measure temperament and responses of infants from 4 to 8 months of age. The Home Observation for Measurement of the Environment (HOME) is designed to assess the environment in which developmental change is occurring. This particular scale is useful with infants from birth to 3 years of age and for children 3 to 6 years of age.

The most reliable assessment tools are designed to observe the infant or child directly under uniform conditions. Some tools such as the DDST, the HOME, and the Developmental Profile combine reports of the child's performance with direct observation, whereas other screening tools may rely more heavily and more exclusively on descriptions about the child's behaviors and abilities. The Carey Infant Temperament Questionnaire relies more heavily on the mother's answers; observations are encouraged.

The Washington Guide to Promoting Development in the Young Child was constructed and revised in 1969 by Dr. Kathryn Barnard and Marcene Powell to assist child care professionals, particularly nurses, to be more effective in assessing and preventing handicapping conditions in children. The tool is used by a variety of nurse clinicians in a number of settings: community health nurses; nurses in day care centers, residential schools, maternity and infant care projects, and institutions for children with handicapping conditions; and nurses in general pediatric settings.

There is increasing use of assessment tools that have been found to be reliable and valid with large numbers of similar-aged infants and children whose responses to test items are observed in exact or similar conditions. A standardized assessment tool requires that those who present assessment items to children follow the same format for presenting tasks, to use exactly the same format for instructing children to follow directions or for prompting, to follow the same criteria in scoring whether the child passes or fails, and to uniformly use the same methods of interpreting data to others.

When used by an individual well trained in procedures for administering, scoring, and interpreting results, assessment tools can produce narrative descriptions that are useful in planning for the needs of a child. An individual becomes proficient in using assessment tools and maintains proficiency by practicing with a number of children of different ages and levels of development, trying out a variety of assessment tools in different environments, and talking with parents who have concerns about their

Outmoded concepts of care	Emerging practices in assessment and management
Use the pediatric pathological model	Use the developmental and educational model
Wait for gross clinical manifestations before making a diagnosis	Begin to observe infants early
Generalize, stereotype, and label children	Observe for individual differences
Look for the negative features or traits	Emphasize the assets and positive features of an infant, child, or parent
Guess about how well a child is doing	Collect objective data in the decision-making process
Gather data only once	Gather data on a serial basis
Omit parents in the assessment and care process	Elicit the parents' perceptions of the child's development and behavior
Fail to share assessment and care progress data with parents	Use the mutal participation model for problem solving
Lack of standardized assessment tools	Use current standardized screening and assessment tools
Give instant advice	Think of ways to collect data and problem solve with the child's parents or caregivers
Use a trial-and-error approach	Document behavioral change and its evaluation
Focus on one symptom	Look for clusters of minor anomalies that may signal the presence of a major defect
Focus on the child alone	Consider the needs of siblings and parents
Screen at school entrance	Conduct early case finding during newborn period; screen periodically
Make physician responsible for diagnosis, informing interview, and management	Use an interdisciplinary approach
Plan short-term goals	Consider lifetime goals
Intervene during crisis	Anticipate guidance before stress and crisis
Use physical evaluation	Use developmental screening
Conduct once-a-year checks	Conduct ongoing, repeated assessments
Tell parents what to do	Ask parents what their concerns are and what they want to do
Emphasize the abnormalities in a child	Look for the child's similarities with others
View the handicap first	See the child as an individual first; emphasize handicaps secondarily
Include only the mother in assessment and management	Emphasize the father's full participation in the child's assessment and care
Use a trial-and-error approach in teaching parents and children	Stress an individualized approach to teaching and learning

children. Practicing with a new tool in the presence of someone who is already proficient in its use increases systematic objectivity and lessens subjective errors in interpretation.

Information about a child's development no longer needs to be fragmented or guessed at, but rather data can be gathered, monitored, and organized in a systematic framework over an extended period of time. As the subjectivity, guessing, confusion, and error in evaluating a child's ability are reduced, the probability of planning successful approaches for developmental change drastically increases.

Success in assessment and preventive management is to a large degree influenced by the ability and discipline of the individual applying the principles and systematic knowledge of multiple measures and a variety of assessment tools, gathering early baseline information, and relying on multiphasic screening assessment methods. No single person, approach, assessment tool, sign or symptom, observation of a child, or explanation of the results of an assessment will provide sufficient information to determine the progress that has been made, is being made, or will likely be made. The following chapters present a number of assessment methods and tools that are effective in determining the overall developmental status of a child at any given time. By using the appropriate developmental screening tool at the proper time, objective data can be made available for planning effective anticipatory and preventive guidance.

REFERENCE

1. Steward, Margaret and Steward, David: The observation of Anglo, Mexican, and Chinese mothers teaching their young sons, Child Dev. **44:**329-337, 1975.

SUGGESTED READINGS

Alpern, Gerald D., and Boll, Thomas J.: Developmental profile, Indianapolis, 1972, Psychological Development Publications.

Anderson, Frederick P.: Evaluation of the routine physical examination of infants in the first year of life, Pediatrics **45:**950-960, 1970.

Ashton, R.: The state variable in neonatal research: a review, Merrill-Palmer Q. Behav. Dev. **19:**3-20, Jan., 1973.

Barnard, Kathryn E., and Bee, Helen: Child health assessment. Part I: a literature review, DHEW publication no. HRA 75-30, Washington, D.C., 1974, U.S. Government Printing Office.

Barnard, Kathryn E., and Erickson, Marcene L.: Teaching children with developmental problems: a family care approach, ed. 2, St. Louis, 1976, The C. V. Mosby Co.

Barness, Lewis A.: Manual of pediatric physical diagnosis, Chicago, 1971, Year Book Medical Publishers, Inc.

Battle, Constance: Sleep and sleep disturbances in young children, Clin. Pediatr. **9:**675-683, 1970.

Bee, Helen: The developing child, New York, 1975, Harper & Row, Publishers.

Brazelton, T. Berry: Infants and mothers, New York, 1972, Dell Publishing Co., Inc.

Brazelton, T. Berry: The Neonatal Behavioral Assessment Scale, London, 1973, William Heinemann Ltd., and Philadelphia, 1973, J. B. Lippincott Co.

Broussard, Elsie R., and Hartner, Miriam Sergay Sturgeon: Maternal perception of the neonate as related to development, Child Psychiatry Hum. Dev. **1:**16-25, Fall, 1970.

Broussard, Elsie R., and Hartner, Miriam Sergay Sturgeon: Further considerations regarding maternal perception of the first born. In Hellmuth, Jerome, editor: Exceptional infant: studies in abnormalities, vol. 2, New York, 1971, Brunner/Mazel, Inc.

Caldwell, Bettye M.: Descriptive evaluations of child development and of developmental settings, Pediatrics **40:**46-54, 1967.

Caldwell, Bettye M.: What is the optimal learning environment for the young child, Am. J. Orthopsychiatry **37:**8-21, 1967.

Caldwell, Bettye M.: Home Observation for Measurement of the Environment, birth to three, unpublished, 1975.

Caldwell, Bettye M., and Drachman, R. H.: Comparability of three methods of assessing the developmental level of young infants, Pediatrics **34:**51-57, 1964.

Camp, Bonnie W., Frankenburg, William, and Goldstein, Arnold: The revised Denver Developmental Screening Test: its accuracy as a screening instrument, J. Pediatr. **79:**988-995, 1971.

Capute, Arnold J., and Biehl, Robert F.: Functional developmental evaluation: prerequisite to habilitation, Pediatr. Clin. North Am. **20:**3-26, 1973.

Carey, William B.: Clinical applications of infant temperament measurements, J. Pediatr. **81:**823-828, 1972.

Chinn, Peggy L., and Leitch, Cynthia J.: Child health maintenance: a guide to clinical assessment, ed. 2, St. Louis, 1979, The C. V. Mosby Co.

Comparetti-Milani, A., and Gidoni, E. A.: Routine developmental examination in normal and retarded children, Dev. Med. Child Neurol. **9:**631-638, 1967.

Dargassies, S. Saint-Anne: Neurodevelopmental symptoms during the first year of life, Dev. Med. Child Neurol. **14:**235-246, 1972.

DeMeyer, M. K., and others: A comparison of five diagnostic systems of childhood schizophrenia and infantile autism, J. Autism Child Schizo. **1:**175-189, 1971.

Dittman, Laura L.: Early child care: the new perspectives, New York, 1968, Atherton Press.

Drage, J. S., Kennedy, C., Berendes, H., and others: The Apgar score as an index of infant morbidity, Dev. Med. Child Neurol. **8:**141-148, 1966.

Dubowitz, Lilly, Dubowitz, Victor, and Goldberg, Cissie: Clinical assessment of gestational age in the newborn infant, J. Pediatr. **77:**1-10, 1970.

Falkner, Frank: Human development, Philadelphia, 1966, W. B. Saunders Co.

Farr, V., Mitchell, R. G., Neligan, G. A., and others: The definition of some external characteristics used in the assessment of gestational age in the newborn infant, Dev. Med. Child Neurol. **8:**507-511, 1966.

Forfar, J. O.: At risk registers, Dev. Med. Child Neurol. **10:**384-395, 1968.

Frankenburg, William K., Camp, Bonnie W., and Van Natta, P.: Validity of the Denver Developmental Screening Test, Child Dev. **42:**475-485, 1971.

Frankenburg, William K., and Dodds, Josiah B.: The Denver Developmental Screening Test, J. Pediatr. **71:**181-191, Aug., 1967.

Frankenburg, William K., and North, Frederick A.: A guide to screening for the early and periodic screening, diagnosis, and treatment program (EPSDT), American Academy of Pediatrics, Social and Rehabilitation Service, Washington, D.C., 1974, U.S. Department of Health, Education, and Welfare.

Guthrie, John: Educational assessment of the handicapped child, Pediatr. Clin. North Am. **20:**89-103, 1973.

Haslam, Robert A.: Physical examination and clinical investigation of the handicapped child, Pediatr. Clin. North Am. **20:**27-44, 1973.

Haynes, Una: A developmental approach to case findings, Children's Bureau Publication No. 449, Washington, D.C., 1967, Superintendent of Documents, U.S. Government Printing Office.

Hellmuth, Jerome, editor: Exceptional infant: the normal infant, vol. 1, Seattle, 1967, Special Child Publications, Bernie Traub and Jerome Hellmuth Co., Publishers.

Hellmuth, Jerome, editor: Exceptional infant: studies in abnormalities, vol. 2, New York, 1971, Brunner/Mazel, Inc.

Ingram, T. T. S.: The new approach to early diagnosis of handicaps in childhood, Dev. Med. Child Neurol. **11:**279-290, 1969.

James, L. Stanley, editor: Symposium on the newborn I, Pediatr. Clin. North Am. **13:**573-942, 1966.

James, L. Stanley, editor: Symposium on the newborn II, Pediatr. Clin. North Am. **13:**941-1301, 1966.

Knoblock, Hilda, and Pasamanick, B.: The developmental behavioral approach to the neurologic examination in infancy, Child Dev. **33:**181-192, 1962.

Korsch, Barbara: Practical techniques of observing, interviewing, and advising parents in pediatric practice as demonstrated in an attitude study project, Pediatrics **18:**467-490, 1956.

Korsch, Barbara: Pediatricians' appraisals of patients' intelligence, Pediatrics **27:**990-1003, 1961.

Korsch, Barbara, Negrete, Vida Francis, Mercer, Ann S., and Freeman, Barbara: How comprehensive are well child visits? Am. J. Dis. Child **122:**483-488, 1971.

Laestadius, Nancy D., Aase, Jon M., and Smith, David W.: Normal inner canthal and outer orbital dimensions, J. Pediatr. **74:**465-468, 1969.

Mackeith, Ronald: Developmental pediatrics (editorial), Dev. Med. Child Neurol. **8:**127-218, 1966.

Maier, John: Screening and assessment of young children at development risk, Washington, D.C., 1973, U.S. Department of Health, Education, and Welfare.

McClelland, Charles Q., Staples, William I., Wiesberg, Israel, and Bergen, Mary E.: The practitioner's role in behavioral pediatrics, J. Pediatr. **82:**325-331, 1973.

Moriarty, A. E.: Review of the Denver Developmental Screening Test. In Buros, O. K., editor: The seventh mental measurements yearbook, New Jersey, 1972, Cryphon Press.

Murphy, Lois Barclay: Assessments of infants and young children. In Dittman, Laura L., editor: Early child care: the new perspectives, New York, 1968, Atherton Press.

Nellhaus, Gerhard: Head circumference from birth to eighteen years, Pediatrics **41:**106-114, 1968.

Neubauer, Peter B.: The third year of life: the two year old. In Dittman, Laura L., editor: Early child care: the new perspectives, New York, 1968, Atherton Press.

Paine, R. S.: Neurologic examination of infants and children, Pediatr. Clin. North Am. **7:**471-510, 1960.

Paine, R. S., and Oppe, I. E.: Neurological examination of children, Clinics in Developmental Medicine 20/21, Suffolk, England, 1966, National Spastic Society in association with William Heinemann Ltd.

Parmelee, A. H.: Sleep cycles in infants, Dev. Med. Child Neurol. **2:**794-795, 1969.

Parmelee, A. H., Wnner, W. H., and Schulz, H. R.: Infant sleep patterns: from birth to 16 weeks of age, J. Pediatr. **65:**576-582, 1964.

Pavenstedt, Eleanor: Development during the second year: the one year old. In Dittman, Laura L., editor: early child care: the new perspectives, New York, 1968, Atherton Press.

Peiper, A.: Cerebral function in infancy and childhood, New York, 1963, Consultants Bureau.

Prechtl, H. R.: Neurological sequelae of prenatal and perinatal complications, Br. Med. J. **4:**763-766, 1967.

Prechtl, Heinz, and Beintema, David L.: The neurological examination of the full-term newborn infant, London, 1964, The Spastics International Medical Publications in association with William Heinemann Ltd.

Provence, Sally: The first year of life: the infant. In Dittman, Laura L., editor: Early child care: the new perspectives, New York, 1968, Atherton Press.

Ragins, N., and Schacter, J.: A study of sleep behavior in two-year-old children, Am. Acad. Child Psychiatry **10:**464-480, 1971.

Raynor, Elizabeth Ann: A study of teacher assessment practices of pre-school age children, unpublished master's thesis, University of Washington, 1973.

Robinson, Roger: Cerebral function in the newborn, Dev. Med. Child Neurol. **8:**561-567, 1966.

Rogers, Michael G. H.: Risk registers and early detection of handicaps, Dev. Med. Child Neurol. **10:**651-661, 1968.

Sheridan, Mary P.: Infants at risk of handicapping conditions, Monthly Bull. Minist. Health **70:**238-245, 1962.

Smith, David W.: Recognizable patterns of human malformations, vol. 7, Philadelphia, 1970, W. B. Saunders Co.

Smith, David W., and Marshall, Richard E.: Introduction to clinical pediatrics, Philadelphia, 1972, W. B. Saunders Co.

Thorpe, Helene S., and Werner, Emmy E.: Developmental screening of preschool children: a critical review of inventories used in health and educational programs, Pediatrics **53:**362-370, 1974.

Traisman, Alfred S., Traisman, Howard S., and Getti, Richard: The well baby care of 530 infants: a study of immunization, feeding, behavioral, and sleep habits, J. Pediatrics **68:**608-614, 1966.

Tulkin, Steven R., and Cohler, Bertram J.: Child-rearing attitudes and mother-child interaction in the first year of life, Merrill-Palmer Q. Behav. Dev. **19:**95-106, April, 1973.

Washington Guide to Promoting Development in the Young Child, In Barnard, Kathryn E., and Erickson, Marcene L.: Teaching the child with developmental problems: a family care approach, ed. 2, St. Louis, 1976, The C. V. Mosby Co.

White, Burton L.: Human infants: experience and psychological development, Englewood Cliffs, New Jersey, 1971, Prentice-Hall, Inc.

Wigglesworth, R.: At risk registers, Dev. Med. Child Neurol. **10:**678-681, 1968.

Wolfensberger, Wolf, and Kurtz, Richard A.: Measurements of parents' perceptions of their children's development, Genet. Psychol. Monogr. **83:** 3-91, 1972.

Wolff, Peter H.: State and behavior in the neonate. In Smart, Mollie S., and Smart, Russel C., editor: Infants: development and relationships, New York, 1973, The Macmillan Co.

2

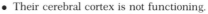

MODELS FOR ASSESSMENT OF THE NEWBORN AND THEIR CAREGIVERS

In the recent past child care professionals tended to rely on a generalized pediatric pathological model for assessment purposes, waiting for gross clinical manifestations to appear before making a diagnosis, collecting further data, and initiating an intervention plan. Furthermore, they did not share assessment data appropriately with their professional colleagues; they tended to communicate more about the sick newborn than about the well newborn.

It has been frustrating for all health care professionals working in the newborn setting to provide care that is ideal, and they have probably all experienced doing less than they would have liked to do. Nevertheless, they were content to view all infants, particularly newborns, as being alike; therefore planning care on an individualized basis was difficult, if not impossible. Professionals tended to go along with numerous myths about newborns such as the following:

- They are dominated totally by reflexes.
- They are all alike in looks and behavior.
- They all have the same needs.
- They experience no pain.
- They have no emotions, just reflexes.
- They are incapable of learning.

- Their cerebral cortex is not functioning.
- Their brain is completely controlled by subcortical operations.
- They do not discriminate visually.
- They cannot see (bright lights do not make a difference).
- They cannot hear.
- They do not distinguish between sounds.
- They do not respond to sounds or voices.
- They do not recognize who is taking care of them.
- They do not distinguish between males and females.
- They are not aware of their surroundings.
- They just lie and kick their feet—their responses have no meaning.
- They really do not have distinct personalities until they are older.
- They do not have behavior *yet*.
- They are either awake or asleep—no in-betweens.
- They should be kept in a quiet environment.
- They really do not smile; it is gas.
- They are not doers; people do things for them.
- They are not capable of loving.
- They do not experience anger.
- They are very fragile.
- They have no way of telling you what is wrong.
- Crying means the same for all infants.
- When they cry, they are hungry.
- The first cry is a cry of terror.

- They need to be consoled right away by others.
- A mother knows her infant because she can feed him.
- All they do is eat and sleep.
- It is the mother's fault if the infant is not happy.
- It is silly to talk to newborns; you are crazy if you do.

In short, health care professionals fell into the habit of looking only for the negative characteristics of newborns.

There was a tendency to rely heavily on subjective impressions and labeling of newborns and their parents. Professionals called newborns drowsy, "hyper," tense, irritable, sluggish, passive, cute, stubborn, or temperamental; they called their parents inadequate, nonaccepting, sensitive, overprotective, rejecting, uncooperative, hostile, immature, or good. What do such terms mean? How can one plan intervention for a passive infant? Labels not only interfere with individualized care of the newborn but also tend to negate the newborn's positive features and to set up self-fulfilling prophecies. In addition to labeling, professionals relied on using checklists to assess newborns, being satisfied to check either normal or abnormal for eyes, head, trunk, and other body parts. They also tended to focus on the newborn's gastrointestinal tract by recording whether he sucked well or poorly, how much formula he drank, how many stools he had, and how many times he urinated. Child care professionals were inclined to gather data on a one-shot basis before the infant was discharged home; worse yet, they planned care based on this fragmentary and incomplete information—a dangerous and hazardous practice, to say the least. There simply is no question that health professionals need impressive, documented, developmental assessment data about a newborn before planning a program of care.

During the assessment process, professionals focused on the newborn alone, forgetting about the parents' needs. Parents may experience severe anxieties about their newborn and may fear that they are *already* inadequate in their parenting roles. They may set unrealistic goals for the newborn or for themselves, making their new roles as parents *unnecessarily* difficult. Unfortunately, child care professionals did not effectively communicate with parents concerning data about the newborn's developmental and behavioral status. They tended to make global statements instead of defining and describing specific newborn behaviors and traits.

It is my opinion that child care professionals made the process of assessment extremely difficult for themselves. They may have been confused about their roles; they may have lacked support for what they were attempting to do. I think they have suffered needlessly and have been basically uncomfortable with the assessment process. It has been stressful for child care professionals, but it need not remain that way. There *are* alternatives. For example, professionals need not continue to record developmental or behavioral data inadequately or to ignore the use of standardized assessment tools. They can relegate subjective, ineffective practices to the past and begin to contribute vital, systematic, and objective information about newborns.

METHODS OF ASSESSMENT

Positive changes are now occurring in newborn assessment—I am observing that professionals are becoming more accountable and more competent and comfortable with assessment practices.

Nurses and physicians are relying more on the developmental model than on the pathological model. This developmental model focuses on even the smallest changes an infant can make. It allows health professionals to be more optimistic and to tune in to what an infant *can do*, not what *he cannot do*. Professionals look for the strengths of the newborn instead of his deficits. By using the developmental model, they are better able to individualize the infant, to decrease the use of labels, and to eliminate stereotyping.

They are also facilitating early intervention by acting on an increased index of suspicion. If a minor anomaly is detected, the newborn is automatically observed carefully for other minor variations. Marden, Smith, and McDonald,[1] in a study of 4,412 newborns, found that 13.4% had one minor anomaly on surface inspection. They suggested that two or more minor variations might indicate the presence of a major defect and would therefore necessitate continued observation and surveillance. This study emphasizes the need for ongoing and repeated observations of an infant over a period of time, and it points out that one minor variation is never diagnostic in itself. Marden, Smith, and McDonald's study[1] also revealed that 71% of minor anomalies are found in the facial area, including the eyes, ears, mouth, and hands. This finding has major implications, meaning that careful appraisal in the area of the face and hands for minor variations is necessary.

A study done by McIntosh and co-workers[2] on 5,964 newborns revealed that only 43.2% of minor anomalies were found on surface inspection alone at birth, also suggesting the need for continued surveillance. Anderson[3] reported that only 50% of the significant abnormalities found in a population of 6,668 during surface examinations were noted in the first 2 months of life, whereas a total of 80% of physical abnormalities were detected by the time newborns were 6 months old. Waldrop and Halverson[4] point to the need to look at clusters of minor malformation patterns that might signal a correlation with later behavior and developmental problems. These researchers found that young boys who had significant minor variations later showed hyperactive behaviors; their study was done when the children were 2½ years of age and then again at 7½ years of age. All of these studies suggest the need for ongoing surveillance from birth through the first year of life.

Child care professionals are currently practicing more objective methods of assessment, not just parts of an assessment procedure. For example, they do not simply perform a surface appraisal or see how the neonate startles; instead, they observe how the neonate is doing in his neurological responses, his interactions with his caregivers, his gross and fine motor coordination, and his sleeping feeding patterns. More attention is being paid to the "state" of the infant, his ability to orient to his environment, and his ability to habituate to stimuli that are surrounding him.

Professionals have finally realized that parents are naturally concerned about the physiological functioning of the gastrointestinal tract and that nurses on newborn units perpetuate this orientation. Nurses and physicians should, of course, respond appropriately to questions about digestion, breathing, and bowel movements, but they should also help to *redirect* parents' attention to other attributes and behaviors of the infant, such as his ability to settle down, his ability to process information, and his ability to hear, see, and interact with his caregivers.

Child care professionals are also becoming more sensitive to the need to support the parents during the early infant-parent acquaintance process. They are in a favorable position to help facilitate and reinforce the process whereby the parent and infant get to know and become attached to each other. It is imperative that professionals observe the quality and progress of these interactions. Do the parents observe their infant, talk to him, comment about his behavior? Are they interpreting their infant's behavior in an appropriate way?

Professionals are finally incorporating active parental participation in the assessment process, giving parents more opportunities to define their concerns, to state what solutions *they* think will work, to describe what *they* have tried, and to say what *they* want to do next. Parents are creative and resourceful; by including them, the professional encourages them to feel more responsible for the care their child receives. Intervention is no longer a matter of giving the infant to the professional to "fix-up" and give back to the parents. The aim is to help parents be problem solvers rather than future help seekers. Child care professionals are attempting to tap the parents' resourcefulness. Parents do want answers, but in my opinion, instant advice or reassurance can lead to instant failure in interacting with the parents. Instead, professionals need to be oriented toward thinking of better ways to collect data for appropriate problem solving *with* parents and their newborn.

There is evidence that professionals are working harder to share observational data with parents. By doing so they can reduce the mystique associated with the assessment process. Parents of newborns are basically asking, "Is my infant OK?" and "Am I OK as a person and as a parent?" The inclination has been to answer that everything is fine. Now child care professionals are more sensitive to parents' needs to have their questions answered in specific, concrete, comprehensive ways. Parents are entitled to have their questions answered and to feel assured that their infant's appearance is "normal" or average. They usually require extra support if irregular features or markings of a transient nature are present. The best way to answer parents' questions is to do a thorough surface assessment in their presence to demonstrate how the infant moves and what postures are appropriate and to give detailed information about surface features of the newborn. For example, the nurse or physician can point out the shape of the head, the measurements of the fontanels, the appropriate placement of the features of the face, the way the eyes line up on a transverse plane, the central location of the nose, the distance between the eyes, the shape and placement of the ears, the spacing of the nipples, the contour of the chest and abdomen, and the movements of the legs as they kick alternately rather than moving together like the hands. Parents find this basic information fascinating and reassuring, and it allows them the opportunity to ask questions. The added bonus is that the nurse or physician saves time because two essentials are achieved —assessment and teaching of parents. The result is that the professional kills two birds with one stone, in a manner of speaking.

If parents are included early in the newborn assessment process, as they should be, they come to accept being included in future assessments that are done on their children. It provides an excellent opportunity for encouraging the acquaintance process and for observing interactions between parents and infant. Parents seem to become more accountable for their own health and participate more readily in planning their children's health care if they are actively involved in the assessment and planning process.

Previously, nurses assessed the infant but somehow weakened their own impact and function by letting the physician assume the role of discussing the assessment results with the parents. Thus nurses gradually discounted themselves and disowned a highly important contribution that they could have been making all the way along.

There is no question that nurses have an important role to play in the parents' early learning process, and nurses' efforts do not necessarily duplicate those of the physician. Nurses and other child care professionals now have norms available to determine if an infant exhibits any minor variations. They can measure surface features and count behaviors. If they cannot describe their observations in words, they can make drawings. They now rely on a number of standardized tools that help them do a better, more comprehensive job of newborn assessment than ever before.

Neonatal Behavioral Assessment Scale

One of the most useful tools now available is the Neonatal Behavioral Assessment Scale, developed by T. Berry Brazelton (Chapter 3).[5] This scale has, practically overnight, changed professional perception of newborns' capabilities. For example, instead of relying on the old-established beliefs that the newborn cannot see,

hear, or interact in his environment, it is known with certainty that newborns have the following characteristics:

- They have unique, distinct, and individual personalities.
- They are aware of and respond to their environment.
- They respond to both animate and inanimate objects and stimuli.
- Their reflexes are protective and indicate status of central nervous system.
- They are not as fragile as formerly believed.
- They have several levels of consciousness. (We used to think that a mother knew her infant if she could feed him. We now know that she needs to be able to identify different "states" of her infant before discharge.)
- They have different levels of awake and asleep states.
- They emit distinct behavioral signs about their levels of alertness or drowsiness.
- They see, hear, and attend to stimuli in their environment.
- They "hook" on to objects and break their attention.
- They shut down and out on noxious sounds and other stimuli they dislike.
- They establish a memory trace in their brain to respond appropriately to stimuli.
- They can maintain attention for brief periods.
- They have alerting behaviors and periods when the brain is processing information.
- They coordinate certain motor movements.
- They initiate and terminate activity.
- They have purposeful movements.
- They adapt to new environments.
- They sense their own needs and try to communicate them as best they can.
- They quiet themselves in stressful situations and environments.
- They have different degrees of cuddling.

Most importantly health professionals have learned that all newborns are not like little cutouts!

The Neonatal Behavioral Assessment Scale is a valuable resource and guideline for teaching parents more effective and appropriate ways to interact with, and make adjustments to, their infants. For example, parents should realize that newborns are capable of becoming alert at different times and of turning toward a voice as early as 3 days. The nurse can help orient parents to the times when the infant may be processing information, and they can determine together the best times to interact with the infant and to present animate or inanimate stimuli. The assessment scale can also be used to help parents observe the ways the infant begins to orient to his environment and interact within it, the ways he shows beginning signs of attachment behavior, and the cues he gives that influence the early mother-infant acquaintance process.

If parents perceive their infant as not being cuddly, the child care professional can help them explore their own definition of cuddliness, their views and reactions, their expectations, and what the infant's behavior means to them. Together with the child care professional they can make systematic observations to discover that the newborn's individual way of interacting explains his behavior and to relieve their possible fears that his lack of cuddliness is their fault and that he is rejecting them.

Similarly, the assessment scale can help parents understand the impact of their voices on the infant, the value of touch, how to best position him, when to feed him, and how to console in graduated degrees to obtain the most favorable responses from him. Such learning can help parents perceive themselves early in the game as the most significant resource persons who can alter certain behaviors of the infant and help him master his early environment and experience more positive input from it.

I must point out that the emphasis of the Neonatal Behavioral Assessment Scale is on the infant and his neurological status, motor behaviors, states, and interactions with the environment. However, the opportunities it provides for teaching, counseling, reassuring, and supporting parents during the early acquaintance process are equally exciting. This is a personal bias, but I am convinced that the data obtained from the assessment scale must be shared with parents. It is not enough to record in the chart that the infant performed adequately or inadequately on the scale. Parents are intrigued by the many behaviors of which their infants are capable as early as the first few days of life, and they find it valuable to learn as quickly as possible about their infant's strengths and weaknesses. I have found from my own personal experience that parents observe the same behavior as I do when I use the scale in their presence. They describe accurately what their infant is doing, and they like to have their thinking validated. During the examination I ask parents if they saw what I did, if they agreed with my observation, and if they saw something I did not. These simple questions encourage parents to observe their infants'

early behaviors, and commenting on the observational skills of parents enhances their feelings of adequacy.

The Neonatal Behavioral Assessment Scale[5] enables child care professionals to help parents react in positive ways to their infants initially, thus contributing to the goal of healthy parent-infant interactions. I believe that the results of assessment can give parents confidence about what to expect from their infants and how to provide the most suitable responses. Also, the assessment scale can help child care professionals be more sensitive to an individual infant and his parents. By using the scale, professionals no longer play a passive role; instead, they are responsible and accountable, applying relevant knowledge in a vitally important setting, the newborn nursery. Although using the scale may add more responsibility to the assessment process, it simultaneously "takes health professionals off the hook." They no longer need to guess or to advise about care based on their intuition. Instead, they can make appropriate decisions based on systematic observations.

The availability of the Neonatal Behavioral Assessment Scale has worldwide implications for assessing infants.[6] By using it effectively, professionals can give parents and children a head start in optimal interaction with each other and can present to parents those items in which the infant lags in a way that creates a realistic challenge for improvement.

Neonatal Perception Inventory

Another exciting tool is the Neonatal Perception Inventory, referred to as the NPI (Chapter 4), which was developed by Dr. Elsie Broussard, a physician from the University of Pittsburgh.[7] The NPI is used to assess maternal perception of infants; its aim is to promote the mental health of the newborn child and to serve as an aid to appropriate early caregiving.

Once the NPI has shown that a mother does not rate her infant as better than average, prompt intervention should occur.[7] Ongoing intervention that focuses on the mother's needs and helps her interact with her infant may reduce stress and disturbances in the parent-infant relationship, whereas failure to intervene may result in irreversible damage to the child. Parents usually know when problems exist between them and their infants, but they need professional confirmation and permission to get help so that the problems can be resolved. The child care professional should turn the mother's attention to the infant's unique strengths in an empathetic and supportive way, while helping the mother sort out her concerns about herself and the infant. It is crucial that the mother begin to experience a positive orientation and to express positive feelings about the infant's unique features and behaviors. The professional should reinforce and accentuate these features of the infant that the mother points out. A mother who does not view her infant as better than average may be vulnerable herself so that the professional might need to reassure her that her infant really does like her, as is evident from the many positive ways he responds to her. The mother may need to hear many favorable comments about her infant before she attains a positive perspective. She may also need reassurance from one or several persons on a *continuing basis* that the behaviors she considers most negative are temporary and will be repeated only until the infant has adapted in a better way to his new environment.

Because the NPI is a significant instrument of prediction and prevention, child care professionals face the exciting possibility of being able to diagnose potential problems and work to prevent them, thus assuring more infants of their right to healthy development.[8]

DEVELOPMENTAL APPROACH

Assessment of the newborn is viewed as a crucial beginning step in early case finding and preventive care. The purpose of an objective and systematic newborn assessment is to get an in-depth, individualized picture of a newborn in his first minutes, hours, and days of life before discharge home. One meticulous thorough surface appraisal does not necessarily duplicate the efforts of another's examination but assists in supplementing data at different times for planning the care the infant needs. The quality and quantity of observations that are made in this early newborn period will influence the nursing care the newborn receives, the medical attention he will get, and the approaches his mother* selects in caring for him and may influence in a major way the adjustment the newborn makes in the early phase of his life.

Newborn assessment has been traditionally performed in the delivery room, newborn nur-

sery, and again in the home and/or well-child clinic. The major objective of the assessment is to obtain baseline information regarding surface features, appearance, movement patterns, and general health status for comparison with results of future examinations. Since the focus of health care, particularly nursing, is gradually shifting to promotion of health rather than merely care in illness, the importance of a systematic health appraisal program consisting of ongoing assessment at predetermined intervals cannot be overemphasized.

With this change in philosophy, traditional methods and models of assessment are being replaced with more effective methods characterized by greater accuracy and objectivity for obtaining comprehensive information on an individualized basis. To achieve this goal, nurses and physicians are increasingly using a developmental approach to assessment rather than adhering to the traditional disease-oriented model. As a result, more systematic assessment approaches are being integrated into more effective health care planning and delivery programs.

As part of this transition, health care professionals are beginning to describe their assessment findings with greater accuracy and detail. This change is significant in determining care priorities and planning and implementing more relevant health care practices.

Even though significant changes are being made in assessment philosophy, there is still a need for improving and refining skills in assessment practices so that they are more objective and systematic. A number of advances have been made in developing assessment tools utilizing more accurate methods for assessment such as the Gestational Age Scale and the Neonatal Behavioral Assessment Scale. However, it is evident that approaches have not been discovered that include uniform practices in which personnel consistently share their findings with each other. Child care professionals tend to do a more thorough job of sharing data regarding an infant who is sick or at risk; however, more progress can be made in sharing information regarding the level of wellness of a newborn. Collaboration and sharing of data are imperative for establishing an effective health promotion program.

One of the weakest areas in the present system is the lack of sufficient parental involvement, particularly of the mother. Many parents express the need to have more assistance in the early stages of their adjustment to their

---

*Generally, the term "mother" will be used throughout the text to delineate the infant's primary caregiver. However, this is not to say that the father is excluded in caregiving activities.

newborn. Parents need to know that child care professionals are willing to listen to them and respond appropriately. The parent-infant acquaintance process consists of gathering information, processing information, and responding to another person with certain perceptions and attitudes. The acquaintance process is greatly influenced by the parents' observations, reactions, attitudes, perceptions, and feelings about the infant's physical appearance. Parents are able to more readily identify physical characteristics before they are able to assimilate and respond to individual behavioral traits and temperamental characteristics of their infant. Parents are entitled to have their questions answered and to feel reassured that their infant's appearance is "normal" or average. They require support if irregular features or markings of a transient nature are present. It is a major responsibility to acquaint parents with physical features, offer reassurance and support, and encourage them to discuss the physical parameters that they can observe repeatedly. Including the parents in the physical assessment process and sharing their observations with other health care professionals will not only help parents to a natural start in the entire acquaintance process, but it will also facilitate compiling comprehensive baseline information for planning future care.

Assessment of the infant in the parents' presence is an excellent opportunity for initiating the acquaintance process and for observing parental reactions and interactions with the infant. This also provides the opportunity to discuss early perceptions and to begin anticipatory guidance in a mutual problem-solving framework based on the observations of both the parents and the examiner.

Since the length of time the mother and infant remain in the hospital after birth is so short and because so many changes are occurring rapidly, it is necessary to again emphasize the importance of infant assessment and evaluation on a regularly scheduled basis beginning in the hospital setting. Many studies suggest that not all minor physical anomalies or variations in surface structure are necessarily discovered during the newborn period. According to McIntosh and co-workers,[2] only 43.2% of the total number of congenital anomalies were discovered in a study of over 5,964 infants during the newborn period. Other studies emphasize the importance of observing for clusters, or groups, of signs and symptoms that suggest the presence of major variations. A critical time during which these observations can be made is while the newborn is in the newborn nursery. This allows for making comparisons in the infant's growth in terms of measurements (e.g., head circumference, height, and weight). There is a significant relationship between these early patterns and how the newborn later grows and develops. Since rates of growth or patterns of behavior vary from individual to individual and from one time period to another, regular scheduled assessments during the newborn period are essential. Signs of maturation, integration, and organization of the central nervous system can be observed, identified, and systematically recorded as baseline data. Baseline information gathered and documented during each assessment can be compared with previous and future assessments both in and out of the hospital, not only to determine the present status of health but also to provide the basis for identifying any particular deviations or variations that should be evaluated at future assessments.

Newborn assessment commences with observations of resting posture and movement patterns, upper and lower extremity movement patterns, and spontaneous movements. The appearance of the skin, its color, markings, and general condition should be noted and documented in detail. The appearance of the skull and face and respirations, reflexes, and postures in supine, prone, and upright positions are observed and documented. Measurements of height, weight, and head and chest circumferences are recorded and compared with standard table measurements.

For purposes of facilitating a systematic appraisal, the term "symmetry" can be used when describing equalness, evenness, or balance, and "asymmetry" can be used to refer to states of unequalness or difference. The terms "symmetry" and "asymmetry" can be overused and abused in the same way that the words "normal," "satisfactory," and "unsatisfactory" are abused and never should be considered an automatic substitute for specific words describing shape, size, form, or movement of any observed infant behavior.

A developmental approach to early assessment begins with attention to symmetry of motion and movement, as well as symmetry of relationships between features and surface features, and overall body alignment. The general assessment guidelines that are discussed in this chapter are presented to facilitate understanding and utilization of the developmental approach for neonatal assessment, the purpose of which is to establish accurate, objective, and comprehensive data to be used in identifying immediate priorities as well as providing a basis for well-child care. Following is a concise summary of assessment philosophy and key points that should assist the child care professional in developing comprehensive and objective assessment practices:

1. Assessment is a starting point and not an end in itself.

2. Regular and periodic assessment is crucial in monitoring and evaluating growth and adaptation, as well as in planning anticipatory and preventive care.

3. Single handicaps are less common than double or multiple handicaps, and all physical and congenital anomalies are not discovered during the newborn period.

4. The presence of clusters or patterns of minor physical anomalies may signal the presence of a major malformation.

5. The assessment process should include the use of screening tools that have predictive value for later behavioral adaptations.

6. Well-child assessment is recommended every 4 to 6 weeks during the first 6 months, every 2 months during the second half of the first year, every 3 months during the second year, and every 6 to 12 months thereafter to 6 years.

7. Valid data from prior assessment histories are invaluable in determining what is normal, abnormal, or unusual for a particular individual at any given time.

8. As children change in growth rates, behavior patterns, and adaptive capacities, simultaneous changes occur in parental responses to these differences.

9. Since parents' responses and needs change simultaneously with developmental changes in their children, parents should definitely be included in the assessment and planning process.

10. Effectively incorporating a family-centered approach not only requires developmental assessment of the child but also assessment of the child's environment to determine its capacity for sustaining growth and development.

11. Developmental assessment should include testing and screening of physical and inner competencies as they develop.

12. The assessment process does not end with knowing where a child is developmentally. Signs and clues indicating new capacities, advanced behaviors, and readiness for new tasks should be capitalized on in facilitating growth, development, and adaptation.

13. Health care professionals should develop expertise in areas of counseling and interaction with families to more effectively meet families' changing needs.

14. Health care professionals must collaborate and share observations and accurate data with each other and with parents to more effectively respond to needs of the well child and his family.

15. One tool alone is not sufficient for accurately evaluating a child's developmental status. Each tool, although standardized, is designed for different purposes and uses at different age periods.

16. The degree of successful care planning is directly proportional to the amount of objective and valid data that are collected. Confusion and error in data collection result in error and confusion in care planning and giving.

17. No single person, approach, assessment tool, or partial evaluation is sufficient to establish valid indicators for progress that has been made, is being made, or will be made. Holistic care includes physical, developmental, behavioral, environmental, and family assessment on a continuous *scheduled* basis.

18. Parents become more accountable for their own health and participate more readily in planning their child's health care if they actively participate in the assessment and planning process.

GENERAL GUIDELINES FOR ASSESSMENT OF SURFACE FEATURES AND MOVEMENT PATTERNS

It is imperative that assessment practices be modified to include consistent and objective techniques. To facilitate this objective, it is important to incorporate the following in the assessment process:

1. Examine alignment of parts and relationships between parts and measure the distances between them (either height or width).

2. Count movements that are observed.

3. Document height or width with numerical figures.

4. Record impressions of "smaller than" or "larger than," with actual measurements, using either millimeters, centimeters, or inches.

5. Recognize that it is important to compare any findings with the mother's or father's observations.

6. Use imaginary lines for measuring distances from a central reference point; for example, if examining a surface structure to the right, automatically compare measurements with the same surface structure on the left.

7. Establish a midline or reference point and make comparisons by looking from left to right, front to back, side to side, and top to bottom, and examine how each part looks on one side in comparison with the other side. How do the parts line up or match up, or how are they similar or different from the other side in shape, size, color, or configuration?

8. Consider the alternative of actually drawing a picture of what was seen, the exact location, and position of the surface of the body when an unusual feature or difference is noted (Fig. 2-1). This is especially recommended when a minor or major variation is recognized in the cranial, facial, ocular, or oral regions or if marks are present on the surface of the hands or feet. Changes in surface features particularly

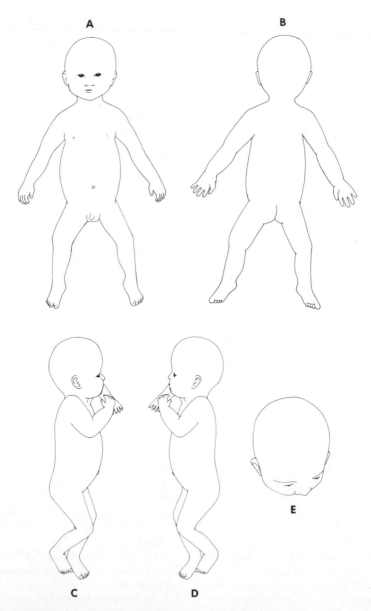

Fig. 2-1. Views for drawing pictures to indicate location of unusual surface features, variations, or markings. **A,** Front view; **B,** back view; **C,** right side view; **D,** left side view; and **E,** top view of head.

warrant scrutiny and continued observations over a period of time.

Drawing a part can be of particular value when there is doubt or uncertainty about an irregular shape; unusual appearance; lack of consistency in formation, contour, or configuration; or major differences. Drawings can also be of assistance when describing the locations of irregular or unusual skin markings or elevations or eruptions.

Too often, false impressions and reassurances are conveyed by subjective descriptions. More accurate descriptions can be used and dangerous practices can be avoided by counting, measuring, and actually drawing rather than using descriptive phrases that are vague and incomplete such as "a large amount," "a fair portion," or "the lower part is involved."

The skin is a typical example of a part of surface features with many variations that requires objective descriptions of color, texture, temperature, or turgor. Color can vary in intensity of predominant hues; it can range from light to dark, shiny or dull, or pale to light brown and can change in tone and intensity of color. Colors can vary in different locations of the body. The degree, location, color, and changes of pigmentation need accurate description. Degrees of cyanosis and where located, as well as the time they appeared, also need accurate description. Presence, amount, location, color, and degrees of flatness to degrees of elevation of eruptions should be accounted for. Consistency, uniformity of degrees of thickness to thinness, and amounts and location of peeling and scaling, should be observed and documented. The degree of smoothness or roughness, ability to spring back, amount of swelling, and numbers of changes in color state can be easily and thoroughly described.

It is not expected that each side of the body or part that is being examined will match up exactly in shape, size, or color; subtle differences are anticipated.

Monitoring of a neonate commences with observations of postural attitudes and the condition of the skin.

Posture and movement

In general, observe spontaneous motor activity for symmetry of movements, intensity of movements, and amount of movement. Observe if posture is symmetrical, if limbs are semiflexed, and if there is slight abduction of the hips when the infant is in a supine position with the head in the midline. Note degrees of coordination, smoothness, and rhythm of movements as compared to jerky, rapid, or tremulous, irregular movements. Observe movements of upper extremities for any tendency to move spontaneously together and of lower extremities for alternate movement and in separate, pedaling-like fashion. Note the presence of regular or irregular patterns in movement and their occurrence on both sides of the midline and whether the eyes, mouth, neck, chest, abdomen, legs, arms, hands, or feet are involved.

Measure the maximal range or the degree of an angle that both arms can extend upward, laterally, or medially. Observe neck movement by its ability to turn from the midline to the side and back again. Observe the movement of the legs extending and flexing separately and together from the front, back, and lateral positions. Observe for degrees of flexion and extension at the base of the neck, at the shoulders, and at the elbows and wrists, and note if fists are clenched or if they open and close spontaneously. As patterns of flexion are observed, determine the opposite or patterns of extension in movement that can be observed in the neck, shoulders, arms, back, hips, legs, and feet.

If the neonate is held in ventral suspension, note the infant's ability to elevate his head. Observe head movements in the supine position, and observe efforts in righting the head to the right and left, as well as anteroposterior movements that are made, and the length of time the head is held steadily before bouncing or falling forward. Observe both flexion and extension patterns of the neck and head and upper and lower extremities when the neonate is in the supine position, ventral suspension, or prone position, or held vertically. Note head movements when the infant is pulled to a sitting position and time how long he steadies his head before it bounces forward.

Observe head movements when changing the infant, dressing him, and holding him for feeding and when he is sleeping. Describe head movements when the infant is held in the curve of the arm or up against the chest. Spontaneous motor activity can be observed for speed, strength involved, and amount of movement in a selected time period.

The neonate should be assessed in terms of his response to and resistance to passive movements, the power of active movements, and the range of movements of the joints. One moves both the upper and lower limbs rhythmically and simultaneously through their full range of movements. Avoid jerky or too rapid movements. Resistance against passive movements and the neonate's own active power, strength, resistance, and range of movements of the joints are observed and recorded for the neck, trunk, shoulders, elbows, wrists, hips, knees, and ankles.

Make further in-depth observations when only extension is noticed, flexion is the primary postural attitude, the neonate stays in one movement pattern, he is unable to move from a midline position, he is inclined to stay in or on one side, or movement is noticed only in the upper extremities or only on the right or left side. Be alert for excessive irregular movements, overshooting, constant motion, continuous tremors, and jerkiness of the majority of movements made; and watch for one side, part, or extremity moving higher or lower or deviating significantly from the other side.

Be alert for and make continued observations of movement patterns of neonates with multiple minor malformations, positive central nervous system difficulties, major malformations, temperatures, illnesses, exaggerated movement patterns, inability to move out of flexion or extension, lack of movement patterns, hypotonicity, or definite asymmetrical responses of primitive reflexes. Make observations and document slowness or sluggish reactions of extremities to recoil.

Make in-depth continued observations on neonates whose mothers describe concern about their movement patterns, whether the mother has observed differences in movement during feeding, changing, undressing, or holding her infant. Describe and record accurately what she has reported. Mothers should receive support for their observational abilities and assurance and appropriate attention for their concerns.

Validate observations more than once with timing of movements in minutes and seconds, and record.

Skin

The appearance of the skin can give many valuable clues as to the status of health and well-being. The texture, turgor, and color can serve as reliable indices to the infant's physiological stability or lack of it and nutritional status. More importantly it can aid in detecting any minor or major variations of surface features and can help identify immediate or later care needs. The appearance of the skin also serves as a basis for modifying the external environment such as temperature change, position

change, caloric needs, fluids, medications, and other significant aspects of parental, nursing, or medical interventions. Many a parent's first questions are generated by the appearance of the infant's skin and are concerned with color, changes in color, markings, or lesions that may be present.

Explanations to parents are generally required in giving reassurance about common variations, which may be transitory and are nonpathological. Most parents benefit from knowing that variations will disappear within the first few months if not days or weeks. Explaining the common variations such as a mottled or marbled appearance of the skin and some blueness to the palms of hands and soles of feet should be done in a manner that is simple yet clear and helpful in reducing parental anxieties.

The skin should be observed for color, eruptions, cyanosis, erythema, icterus, petechiae, cysts, markings, and scars. An accurate, objective, detailed description of the appearance of the skin is more significant in its implications than a subjective interpretation of the observation; for example, pallor is not necessarily diagnostic of anemia. The infant may be observed to have a uniform pink color to his entire body, but circumoral pallor or circumoral cyanosis might be present. An infant requiring oxygen does not necessarily have to be blue all over.

At birth the skin of a so-called normal infant is purplish red in color, brightening to red with expansion and improved oxygenation of the circulatory and vascular system. The skin gradually assumes a pink color. Depending on race, a newborn's skin can range from light pink to the darkest shade of brown. Mottling occurs in newborns, particularly with temperature changes. Skin color varies from pink to red and changes according to activity levels, temperature of the environment, and the infant's condition.

In general, observation of the skin color should include the degree of color changes and uniformity of color. It is important to observe whether the color is different than it was at an earlier time and whether it is the same all over the body surface, from top to bottom, and from front to back. If cyanosis is present, it is significant to determine the degree of blueness, whether deep or light, and where it is located. It should be determined if cyanosis is present in the extremities only, palms of hands only, soles of feet only, or all three areas. If pallor is noticed, it should be evaluated with regard to where it is noted and whether present over the entire body surface or in parts such as face, hands, or feet. (The newborn is often ruddy and mottled during the first few days.)

Attention should be given to the number of times the newborn has a change in color, the frequency of color state changes, and when they occur, whether when he is crying, being undressed, or fed or during bathing or sleeping. If a color state is noticed, it is informative to know the length of time it took for the color of the skin to return to its earlier observed color, when the color state began to change, the environmental conditions that may have influenced it, whether aversive stimulation occurred (undressing, examined for reflexes, pulled to sit), or whether color state change was spontaneous in nature.

Brazelton[5] suggests the following rating scale to determine the number and frequency of color changes in the newborn:

1. Pale, cyanotic, and does not change during exam.
2. Good color which changes only minimally during exam.
3. Healthy skin color; no changes except change to slight blue around mouth or extremities when uncovered, or to red when crying; recovery of original color is rapid.
4. Mild cyanosis around mouth or extremities when undressed; slight change in chest or abdomen, but rapid recovery.
5. Healthy color but changes color all over when uncovered or crying; face, lips, extremities may pale or redden, mottling may appear on face, chest, limbs; original color returns quickly.
6. Change in color during exam, but color returns with soothing or covering.
7. Healthy color at outset, changes color to very red or blue when uncovered or crying; recovers slowly if covered or soothed.
8. Good color which rapidly changes with uncovering; recovery is slow but does finally recover when dressed.
9. Marked, rapid changes to very red or blue; no recovery to good color during rest of exam.*

Frequency of color state changes should be noted during the first weeks of life. Of equal importance are observations and descriptions of the presence of skin eruptions. It is helpful to

pinpoint exactly where skin eruptions are discovered, their color, whether elevated, regularity or irregularity of patterns, and whether eruptions change color (i.e., become darker or lighter with overall body color change).

Skin color can be described according to variations that are seen. It can vary from pallor to uniform pink to variable pink or reddish hues and may be pink over ears, lips, palms, or soles while reddish hues may be present over the face or trunk. If jaundice is present, the amount and degree of pigmentation and time of onset of appearance should be noted, as well as specific areas it covers (e.g., over forehead, cheeks, chin, abdomen, sclera, and membranes). Jaundice appearing 48 to 72 hours after birth is common and is most readily observed on the face and brow and, in lesser amounts, on the hands and feet.

Opacity of the skin can vary from numerous veins over the abdominal area being clearly visible to only a few veins or vessels being obvious to a few large vessels being noticeable. The turgor of the skin can be assessed by grasping 2.54 to 5.1 cm (1 to 2 inches) of it over the abdominal wall and releasing it. This helps estimate the skin's ability to spring back to its original contour. Generally, the texture of the skin is smooth, soft, flexible, and firm. It can vary from smoothness to roughness and may be scaly or dry and may even have more severe degrees of deep cracking. Markings or spots of the skin should be described for size, coloration, exact location, shape, and when noticed and/or disappeared. Descriptions of eruptions of the skin should include when noticed, when disappeared, exact location, amount of spreading, color, size of each, shape, degree of flatness, degrees of elevation, or degrees of coolness to warmness. Note if skin elevations contain fluid. Edema of the skin surface should be described according to location, degrees of pitting, nonpitting, and amount of puffiness or swelling noticed. If impressions of a finger mark were to remain, notations should include how long, the location, how much was involved, when it was first noticed, and any changes in degrees. Evidence of hydration should be described according to estimated degrees and exact location where the surface of the skin is dry, scaling, and/or peeling.

Hair present on the body surface should be described according to length, thickness, color, and patterns on different parts of the body.

---

*From Brazelton, T. Berry: The Neonatal Behavioral Assessment Scale, London, 1973, William Heinemann Ltd., and Philadelphia, 1973, J. B. Lippincott Co., p. 60.

Nails should be described according to flatness, completeness of formation, and convexity of shape on the outer surface.

Lymph nodes

At birth the size of both individual and groups of lymph nodes ranges from minute unobservable proportions to sizes covering an area 1 × 1 cm. The largest single formation is generally the superficial inguinal lymph nodes. Another sizable group of nodes is found in the axilla. Nodes that are barely observable are located in the head and neck, upper limbs, thorax, abdomen, pelvis, and lower limbs. The natural color of the nodes is usually pink.[9] Palpate and observe the presence, number, and ease of moving palpable nodes; note the temperature (cool to warm), and observe size (small to large) and exact measurements on both the right and left sides of the head, neck, axillas, arms, and inguinal areas.

Skin temperature

The temperature of the full-term infant at birth is either the same or a degree above that of its mother, or about 98.8° F (37.1° C). An automatic drop of 3° F in the temperature of the infant occurs in spite of any efforts to keep it maintained. About an hour after birth, the rectal temperature is usually about 95.8° F (35.4° C). According to Crelin,[9] during the first 2 hours after birth there may be a drop of as much as 5° F without any substantial changes in the environmental temperature. Temperatures of 92° F to 94° F are common in the newborn. They rise as the newborn is warmed up.

Be alert to rapid and frequent color changes or to the absence of color changes during the neonatal period. Observe for any sudden changes to white, blue, or beefy red tones. Make further in-depth serial observations when extremes are seen; major differences occur; the skin feels excessively dry, moist, warm, or cool; color changes are abrupt or sudden or cyanosis persists; extremes are noticed in lightness or darkness; skin is extremely loose, tight, or swollen over an area; elevations in the skin are felt or drainage is present; or major differences are seen or felt in one part and not in its opposite part, whether to the right or left or below or above it. Continue to make observations of skin if the parents report concern, if differences are noted from one period to another, or if differences are noted by others.

Serial observations are necessary if persistent cyanosis is evident, if equal cyanosis in the hands persists beyond 4 hours after birth, if persistent pallor is evident, and if cyanosis lessens or increases when the infant cries. Blueness of the tongue, oral mucosa, and nail beds require further attention. A beefy red color over the entire skin surface, excessive edema, or edema localized in hands and feet warrants further observations. Pitting edema requires continued observations. Poor turgor and excessive wrinkling and jaundice appearing at birth or within 12 hours merit extensive observations. Jaundice lasting 10 days requires further observation. Skin with dry, coarse, rough, scaling, or cracking characteristics warrants further observations. Vernix caseosa that has a yellow shade merits continued observation.

The presence of small, light brown patches of skin requires ongoing observations. A temperature differential between abdominal skin and extremities signals the need for further measurements and observations.

Height, weight, and body proportions

The average full-term newborn infant weighs 3.4 kg (7½ pounds). The length from the top of the head to the sole of the foot is about 50 cm (20 inches). The relative size relationships between the head, trunk, and limbs are approximately the same. The greatest proportion of subcutaneous adipose tissue develops during the last weeks of pregnancy. This tissue formation accounts for the full-term newborn appearing more hardy than an infant of lesser gestational age.[9]

Linear growth is the best single indicator of chronic aberrations affecting skeletal growth. More than 200 different disorders may initially be suspected by virtue of linear growth deficiency.[10] It is important to recognize that linear measurement basically evaluates bone growth. It reflects changes in the height of the skull, vertebral bodies, femora, and tibia and thus represents a more refined measurement than one which simply reflects overall mass such as weight. The mean birth length is 50 cm (20 inches). Rates of change can be predicted with serial height measurements as follows[11]:

1. By 1 year of age—50% increase to 75 cm (30 inches)
2. By 4 years of age—100% increase to 100 cm (40 inches)
3. By 13 years of age—200% increase to 150 cm (60 inches)

It is essential that length is measured three

times with the infant lying in a recumbent position with the crown of his head flat against a surface and the knees flat and soles of feet pressed against a flat surface. Only this method will ensure optimal, accurate records of this increasingly recognized crucial measurement.

Head

The distance from the top of the skull to the upper margin of the orbit is 5 cm, and the measurement from the superior margin of the orbit to the lower surface of the mandible is about 4 cm.[9]

Observations are made of the general configuration of the head from all angles. The head is viewed from the top, side, front, and back. Contours, shape, and configuration are described (Fig. 2-2). Measurements are obtained and recorded and compared with standardized norms.

An examination is carried out and observations for degrees of roundness, flatness, regularity to shape, smoothness, and roughness,

and a tendency for the configuration to be the same or different are noted for the left and right sides, front and back, and top and base of head. The distance of the separations between the skull sutures is measured and recorded. Overriding of sutures is described according to location. Degrees of moulding are noted, with the location described and recorded. Changes in moulding are noted from one day to the next (Fig. 2-3). Degrees of flatness or roundness and bulging of the occiput are described. The head is observed for signs of control in sitting and other upright positions, and the examiner notes whether movement from forward to back position occurs, whether there is righting of head movements, the ease of movement, whether movements are smooth or jerky, whether tremors are seen, and most particularly what occurs when the neonate is held vertically and pulled to sit and when his face is placed in midline in the prone position. Note efforts of the newborn to right his head to one side or another and the distance the head can be raised off the surface of a bassinet.

The scalp is examined for abrasions, elevations, eruptions, markings, depressions, holes, ridges, and masses, and their shape, size, location, color, and the temperature of elevations from cool to warm is noted. One side is examined for the degree to which it matches or compares with another, even though differences are expected. Observations are made from the front, midline, right to left, side to side, and anterior to posterior. The shape of the head may be described using geometrical terms such as "ovoid" or "circular," or other terms.

Measurement of head circumference. According to Smith,[10] "Head circumference is the best presently utilized indicator of brain size. The brain is in a rapid growth phase throughout early infancy and this is a period when it is most important to monitor its progress in growth."

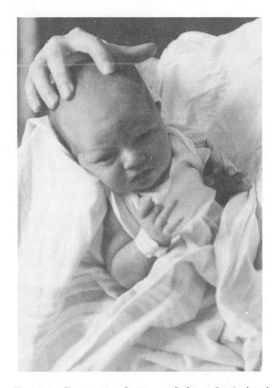

Fig. 2-2. Examining features of the infant's head (palpating the infant's anterior fontanel). (From Chinn, Peggy L.: Child health maintenance: concepts in family-centered care, ed. 2, St. Louis, 1979, The C. V. Mosby Co.)

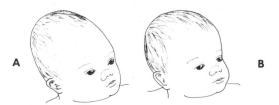

Fig. 2-3. A, Front and top view of moulding of infant's head. **B,** Front and top view of infant's head after moulding.

Both interexaminer and intraexaminer variations may be influenced by the technique of measurement used, as well as material of the tape used. Different measurements may result if objective techniques are not routinely carried out. It is important that the tape be passed from the most prominent part of the occiput around the area above the eyebrows (supraorbital ridges) (Fig. 2-4). It is essential that this measurement be done at least three times for purposes of objectivity and interreliability with one's own measurements beginning with first to last. The largest figure obtained is recorded on a standardized head chart for either females or males. The infant whose head circumference falls below two standard deviations (the third percentile below the mean) merits serial, ongoing, repeated measurements because of the implications of a small brain mass. Head circumference graphs are shown in Fig. 2-5.

Fontanel measurements. The width of the fingers can be measured in centimeters to obtain an accurate measurement. These early measurements of the fontanels can serve as indicators of the closure of the fontanels over a period of time and are recorded as they reduce in size and close. The size of the fontanels may reflect evidence of altered intracranial pressure.

The technique most helpful in identifying the status of the cranial bones, sutures, and fontanels separating them is palpation. The anterior fontanel, which is a diamond-shaped structure lying between the two sections of the frontal and parietal bones, is palpated for bulging, depression, or minor pulsations. The anteroposterior and transverse dimensions are measured from anteroposterior margins and transverse margins. The anterior fontanel rarely reaches a diameter of more than 5 to 6 cm.[9] Popich and Smith[12] report that the anterior fontanel is usually variable in size and shape. They found that the mean anterior fontanel size of newborns is 2.1 cm, with two standard deviations above and below the mean being at 0.6 and 3.6 cm, respectively. The mean posterior fontanel measurements obtained by Popich and Smith rarely exceeded 0.5 cm in size.

Although the anterior fontanel may increase in size during the initial postnatal months, alarm is not necessary because it will plateau and decrease slowly until closure is evident between 14 and 18 months. Each time the occipital frontal circumference (OFC) is obtained, fontanel measurements can be obtained

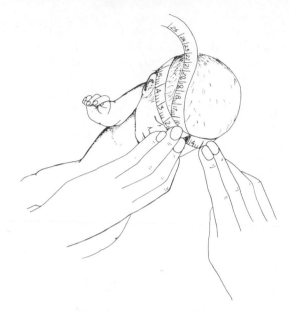

Fig. 2-4. Proper techniques are essential for accurate head measurements.

during the first 18 months as evidence of the progressive, expected reduction in size. Popich and Smith[12] report that the pressure of an unusually large fontanel without increased intracranial pressure can serve as a valuable clue in the identification of a number of serious skeletal disorders, chromosomal abnormalities, and other syndromes. The single finding of an enlarged fontanel cannot be viewed alone as a sign of pathology. The range of variability both in size and shape of fontanels is considerable, and extra precaution is needed in interpreting information that could prove to be misleading and unnecessarily alarming.

Continued surveillance should be performed on infants who have difficulties in head balance in the seated position, who maintain the head in a fixed position, or who extend and maintain static head position with arching of the back. Observations should be made on a serial basis in case of the following: the infant's head falls downward in an inverted U shape when in ventral suspension, there is no neck righting when the infant is brought or pulled to a sitting position, primarily flexion is noted, extension is the predominant posture, or spontaneous movements are not observed.

More detailed observations are imperative if premature, irregular closure of fontanels is

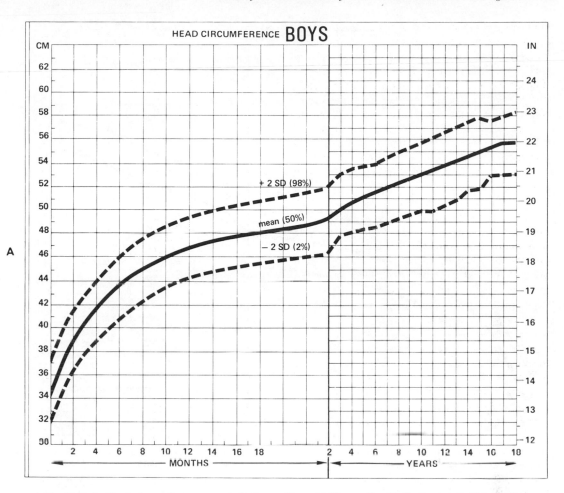

Fig. 2-5. A, Head circumference graph for boys. (From Nellhaus, Gerald: Pediatrics **41**:106, 1968.)
Continued.

noted, there is wide open spacing of fontanels, a fontanel measurement of 6 cm is obtained, or irregular pulsations, tightness, bulging, or depression of any fontanel is noticed.

A cranium that is large or small or two standard deviations above or below the norm for a normal head circumference merits further serial observations and measurements.

A head circumference that changes from one growth rate channel to another within short periods of time deserves continued observation and measurements.

A flat or prominent occiput, skull with delayed closure of fontanels, or a wide spread to sagittal or coronal or lamboidal sutures deserves continued observations and measurements. Unusually large fontanels merit serial measurements along with the head circumference.

Frontal bossing or a prominent or receding central forehead calls for further observations.

Continued surveillance and observations are indicated for an infant with sluggish responses in eating or one who exhibits a high-pitched cry, little or no cry, a coarse or low cry, or a growling cry. Asymmetrical responses to the Moro reflex or sluggishness and hyperirritability require in-depth, repeated observations.

Hair

The hair is inspected for length of hairs, thinness to thickness of each strand, and regularity or irregularity of hair patterns. Notations are made as to the formation of patterns of hair, how much is present from the top of the head to the midnape of the neck, whether it is present in equal amounts; where it begins from the fore-

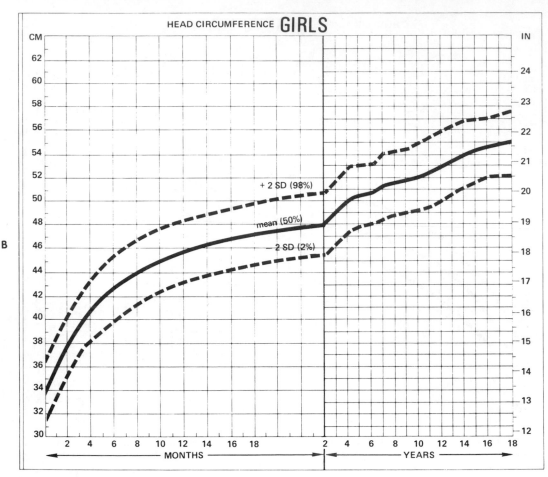

Fig. 2-5, cont'd. B, Head circumference graph for girls.

head and across the occiput and down to the neck, the texture and separability of strands, and the evenness of distribution from side to side. The hair is visualized for hair whirl patterns, where they are located, how many, and whether patchiness is seen. Observe if the hair strands are thick, thin, straight, fine, even, coarse, or curly. The color is noted and observed for light brown, red, or black pigmentations. The hair is also observed for one color or combination of colors together.

Additional observations are carried out when variations in surface structure such as the following appear: excessive length of hair; excessively low posterior hairline; hair covering forehead to face; nonseparable strands of hair in a white newborn; irregular patches of hair; red rusty color of hair; a white forelock; coarse, dry, or brittle hair; flatness on one side or another; or an excessively low hairline.

Face

Like the head, the face is examined for symmetry of parts, shape, regularity of features, evenness, and sameness or differences in features. Judgments about distance of spaces between parts are significant.

The face is examined for relationships of parts as they are compared to the whole general appearance. Observations are made according to how different features are distributed or placed, the distance between parts, and the degree of similarity of or difference between one part with another. Heights and widths can be used to quantify distances. Observations are made from the midline, from right to left, from side to side, and from anterior to posterior. The top of the forehead to the bottom of the chin is inspected and described and can be measured. Establishment of details requires palpation and measurements. The width of the newborn face is approximately 8 cm.[9] The main contours of the face are governed by bony landmarks or prominences. A study by Marden and associates[1] indicated 71% of minor anomalies to be located on the face, ears, and hands; thus the need for close scrutiny of the face is recognized.

The eyes generally line up on the same horizontal plane, the ears are evenly lined up with the outer orbit of the eyes, and the nose and mouth are aligned centrally on the face. Although subtle differences are noted on the right and left sides of the face, any unusual differences merit further examination. Repeated notations by description and drawings are useful if they clarify, identify, or add information. The eyebrows are examined for equal distance from the top of the eyebrow to the top of the eyelid on each side. The formation, arch, and width of the eyebrow across the top of the eye and the distance from the brow to the eyelid can be measured. The amount of hair present, length of eyebrow strands, and color are noted.

Eyes

The muscles of facial expression are relatively well developed at the time of birth. The orbicularis oculi muscles can contract firmly to protect the eyes. The eyeball is proportionately large at birth. The anteroposterior diameter of the newborn eyeball is about 16.4 mm, the horizontal diameter 16 mm, and the vertical diameter 15.4 mm.[9] Even though the newborn eyeball is relatively smaller than that of the adult, its shape and relative size are found to be similar. At birth the orbit at its margin measures 1.9 cm in height and measures 2.3 cm in width, and its greatest depth is about 3 cm.[9]

The eyes are observed for their appearance when lined up on a horizontal plane and the relationship that can be seen when shape, configuration, contour, size, and colors of each eye are compared. The placement and alignment of the eyes and how proportionate they appear when contrasted with other features of the face are also noted. They are compared for shape (e.g., rounded, oval, or spherical), size (if one is larger or smaller), or difference in color.

The luster, clarity, shininess, and exterior appearance of both eyes are noted. The color of the sclera is judged on each side. The size of the right pupil in comparison with the left in response to light and darkness is observed and recorded. The degree of opacity of the lens under natural light is estimated. The presence

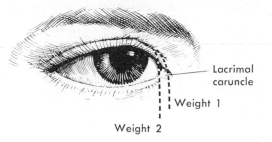

Fig. 2-6. Varying degrees of epicanthic folds. A weight of 2 demonstrates a greater degree of epicanthic fold than does a weight of *1*. (From Waldrop, Mary Ford, and Halverson, Charles, F.: In Hellmuth, Jerome, editor: Exceptional children: studies in abnormalities, vol. 2, New York, 1971, Brunner/Mazel, Inc.)

of the red reflex with ophthalmoscopic examination is noted.

The distance between the palpebral fissures can be measured. The degree of slant of the palpebral fissures is judged by drawing an imaginary line across the outer orbit of the eyes and aligning each eye on this transverse plane. The right eye is examined for its position on the horizontal plane and the degree of slant in an upward or downward direction. This is repeated and compared with the left eye.

Eyelids. These are examined for amount of movability, placement over eyes, evenness in size, and whether the upper is larger than the lower.

Eyelashes. The length of the eyelashes is compared, distribution of hairs on each eyelash is compared, and length of the upper eyelash is compared to length of the lower. Observations are made for short, thick, curved hairs arranged in a double or triple row. The lashes above are generally more numerous than lower ones and curve upward; the lower lashes curve downward.

Pupils. Pupils are noted for position in the middle of the orbit; whether they move to extreme right or left; whether movement of the eye is vertical, rotary, or lateral; and if movements are continuous or change with position or handling. Shape and size of each are compared. Reactions to light are observed. Prechtl and Beintema[13] suggest placing a hand over one pupil to observe for reaction to shading. A bright light elicits a blink of the eye. The outer two thirds of the irises are observed for color, markings, or spots.

Epicanthic folds. The degree, amount, place-

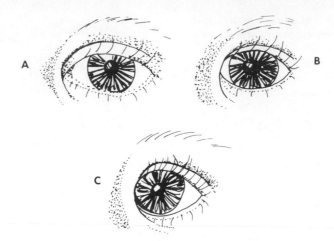

Fig. 2-7. A, Normal eye without epicanthic fold. **B,** Partial epicanthic fold of eye. **C,** Epicanthic fold completely covers lacrimal caruncle. (Modified from Smith, David W.: Recognizable patterns of human malformation, vol. 7, Philadelphia, 1970, W. B. Saunders Co.)

ment, and thickness of the epicanthic folds are described after measurement (Fig. 2-6).

There is increasing evidence, according to Smith,[10] "that epicanthic folds represent a redundancy of skin tissue which tends to be less apparent as the child gets older."

Epicanthic folds must be carefully judged as to the degree of partial or complete covering of the point of juncture at the nose. Degrees of thickness must be estimated to determine minor or greater significance. Folds can exist and vary in size and subsequently be clarified as minor variations (Fig. 2-7).

Measurement of inner and outer orbital distances. A false impression of ocular hypertelorism can be avoided by measuring the distance between the inner canthi of both eyes. Laestadius and co-workers[14] report the mean distance between the inner canthi for a full-term newborn to be 2 cm. Graphs giving inner and outer orbital distances are shown in Fig. 2-8. A measurement of 3 cm was judged to represent true ocular hypertelorism in newborns in a study reported by Marden and associates.[1]

Ocular region. The ocular region warrants further inspection, observations, and measurements if one or more of the following are evident: a wide distance between the eyes in relationship to the breadth of the face, short palpebral fissures, a lateral displacement of inner canthi, inner epicanthal folds covering the lacrimal duct, slanted palpebral fissures,

shallow orbital ridges, prominent eyes, eyebrows extending to the midline, or ptosis of the eyelid (Fig. 2-9).

General observations. Continued observation of the eye is necessary when strabismus, nystagmus, or colobomas of the iris are evident, cloudiness is present, opacities of the cornea are visualized, cataracts are present in one or both eyes, differences in retinal pigmentation are observed, and a constant "setting sun" sign is present.

The need for close surveillance and monitoring for other minor surface variations is imperative if eyes are judged to be closely or widely spaced, epicanthic folds entirely cover lacrimal ducts or eyes slant upward or downward when compared against a horizontal line on a non-oriental infant, one eye is larger or smaller, one pupil is smaller than the other, or eyebrows meet in the center or overlap.

If a white reflex is seen or the red reflex is absent, cloudiness of the cornea is observed, or opacities are visualized, further data are obtained.

Observations are made for the presence of other minor variations around the eyes and ears.

If eyelashes are not evenly distributed or are missing or if eyebrows are thick, joined, or placed in unusual formations above the eyes, further careful observations are necessary. When a low nasal bridge exists, measurements of the distance between the eyes must be obtained.

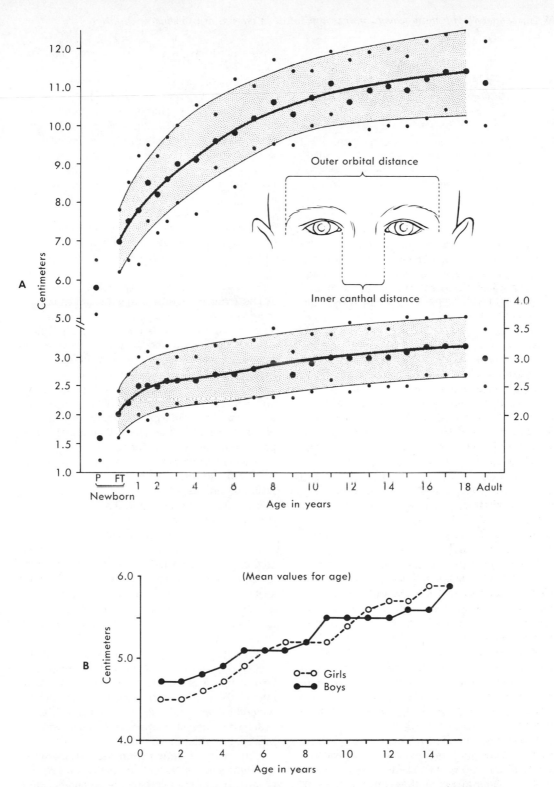

Fig. 2-8. A, Graph of inner canthal and outer orbital distances. The large points represent the mean value for each age group, and the smaller points represent two standard deviations from the mean. The heavy line approximates thc fiftieth percentile, and the shaded area roughly encompasses the range from the third to the ninety-seventh percentile. *P,* premature; *FT,* full term. Note that 70% of the adult inner canthal distance is achieved by 2 years of age. **B,** Graph of interpupillary distance measurements (mean values for age) from 5,570 normal white children. (From Laestadius, Nancy D., Aase, Jon M., and Smith, David W.: J. Pediatr. **74:**465-471, 1969.)

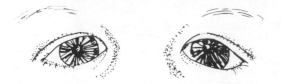

Fig. 2-9. Downward slant to palpebral fissures and wide space between eyes. (Modified from Smith, David W.: Recognizable patterns of human malformation, vol. 7, Philadelphia, 1970, W. B. Saunders Co.)

Nose

Observations are made of the bridge of the nose, which is located below the frontonasal suture. The degree of convexity from side to side and the concavoconvex angles and contours seen from looking above and downward are noted.

The nasal cavities are noted to be two irregular spaces situated on either side of the midline of the face. The nose is separated by a thin vertical septum, which can be visualized as long and straight. According to Crelin,[9] the height and width of each choana, or posterior naris, are about equal in measurement (5 to 7 mm). The nasal cavities of the newborn infant are described as low, broad, and relatively long. The height of each cavity measures 18 to 19 mm. The anterior nasal aperture is large, broad, and round, with a distinct anterior nasal spine. Its height is 1.4 cm, and its broadest width is 1.1 cm.

The nose is examined and notations are made regarding central placement on the face. An imaginary line drawn vertically through the nose is a help in observing details of position on the face, size, shape, length, and general appearance of one side of the nose as compared to the other side. The nose should be observed to be at the middle and upper part of the face. The external appearance of the nose can be described in degrees of concavoconvexity from above downward and convexity from side to side.

The openings, or nares, can be observed for their general shape and size.

Observe and note respiratory activity, rates, and color changes when examining for patency of the nasopharynx. If choanal atresia exists, it will be evident if one of the nares is closed off. Note color changes in the lips, extremities, or nail beds, and observe for change in respiratory efforts. Repeat examination on the other side of the nostril. Notations are made if nares are higher or lower on one side than another or if flaring of either nostril is observed or both are expanded.

Continued surveillance is imperative in the following situations: respiratory distress is evident when one of the nares is momentarily blocked, a low nasal bridge is seen, the left side of the nasal septum is strikingly different from the right side, a small nose or prominent nose is viewed from either side or the anterior surface, the bridge of the nose is estimated to be low, alar hypoplasia exists, or a prominent nose or one that is beaklike in appearance is seen. One should remember that one unusual feature by itself is not diagnostic; it simply leads to further observations of facial features.

Ears

The external acoustic meatus is proportionately long at birth. It is about 16.8 mm in size. The external meatus is usually straight, and it courses downward and forward. The newborn middle ear or tympanic cavity is similar in size to that of the adult. It is an elongated cavity that is narrow at the midpoint. The anteroposterior and vertical diameters at birth are equal and are 1 cm. The transverse diameter is usually 6 mm at the roof of the cavity, 2 mm at its midpoint, and 4 mm on the floor.[9]

Observations of both ears include inspection, palpation, and measurements of size, shape, position, degree of slant, height, width, and placement on the cranium. The configuration, contour, and degrees of completeness of the helix of both ears as well as the general appearance of the auricles are noted. The ear or pinna of the ear is inspected for shape and whether its larger end is directed upward. The lateral surface is inspected for the degree to which it is concave. The numerous eminences and depressions that can be visualized and palpated are examined.

The extension of the wall above the eardrum, the epitympanic recess, is well developed at birth as is the mastoid strium. The bony openings of the medial wall or oval window are reported by Crelin[9] to be 2.5 mm long and 1.5 mm wide. The fenestra tympanum or round window has a 2 mm diameter.

A line can be drawn from the outer orbit of the right eye and extended across the greatest prominence of the occiput. This imaginary line serves as a reference point to determine if ears are set and aligned in a proportionate relationship with the eyes, nose, and cranium. If the ears cross this line or line up evenly, no further observations are necessary. If the tip of the

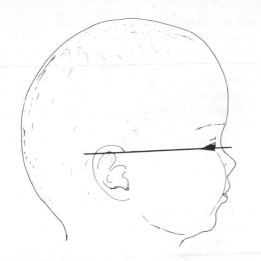

Fig. 2-10. Determining if ears are set and aligned in proportionate relationship with the eyes.

pinna does not cross this line, this finding would indicate low placement (Fig. 2-10).

Estimation of the degree of the slant of the ear is made by drawing an imaginary line from the outer orbit of the eye and intersecting this same line with one line drawn vertically on the cranium. Estimate the degree to which the ears are aligned vertically or slanted in relationship to the perpendicular. Ten degrees or more from this perpendicular angle is evidence of a slanted ear.

The firmness of the ear is judged in varying degrees from the ability to fold it easily with no recoil, to some recoil when folded, and to instant recoil. Firmness is also estimated by noting the firmness of the edge of the pinna and whether this firmness is even. Note whether the pinna is soft in some places and not in others.

Notations should also be made describing the amount of flatness or incurving on the edge of the pinna or incurving of parts, and one should judge whether incurving is partial or extends to the whole or upper pinna. Attention is also directed to the degree of fullness or completeness of the ear lobe, and observations are made for adherent ear lobes (Fig. 2-11). The skin surface

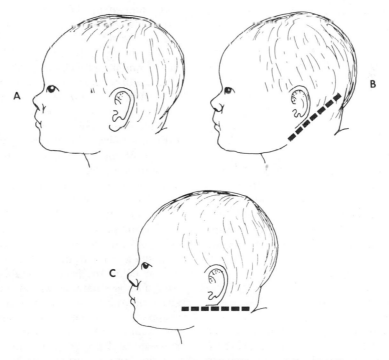

Fig. 2-11. A, "Normal" set of ears, alignment, and lack of adherent earlobes. **B,** Adherent earlobe with an upward and backward slant toward the cranium. **C,** Adherent lobe extends forward from the back of the head and neck. (Modified from Waldrop, Mary Ford, and Halverson, Charles F.: In Hellmuth, Jerome, editor: Exceptional infant: studies in abnormalities, vol. 2, New York, 1971, Brunner/Mazel, Inc.)

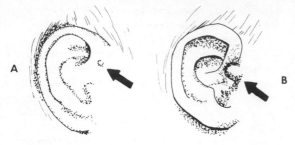

Fig. 2-12. A, Presence of cutaneous pit on surface of ear. **B,** Cutaneous tag present on surface of ear. (Modified from Smith, David W.: Recognizable patterns of human malformation, vol. 7, Philadelphia, 1970, W. B. Saunders Co.)

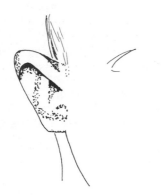

Fig. 2-13. Prominent ear. (Modified from Smith, David W.: Recognizable patterns of human malformation, vol. 7, Philadelphia, 1970, W. B. Saunders Co.)

surrounding the ears is noted for small openings, extra tags, or sinuses of any size (Fig. 2-12). Extensive observations are made if ears are noted to be low set or slanted, auricles are incomplete or malformed, one ear is larger than the other, a lobulus is missing or is hypoplastic, or if extra skin tags are located, sinuses are found, or the exterior structure of the ear is judged to be unusual in size or shape (Fig. 2-13).

Mouth and oral cavity

The muscles of the lips, jaws, tongue, palate, and pharynx are well developed in the newborn infant for suckling and swallowing. The exterior appearance of the mouth is observed for shape, movements, and size. The alignment of the right corner of the upper lip is compared with the left corner of the upper lip, and this is repeated for the lower lip. The color of the lips during sleep, undressing, alertness, and feeding is noted, and the ability to close the lips on and around a nipple is observed. Observations of size are noted, and the shape of the mouth is described. If there are tags, grooves, fissures, or ridges present or if there is drooping or unevenness to the external surface of the mouth, the lips are also inspected for edema.

Tongue

A light and tongue blade are helpful in observing the tongue. Its size, shape, and movement anteriorly and posteriorly or from side to side are observed. The degree of any coating is noted. The degree of roughness or smoothness to the surface of the tongue is estimated.

The tongue of the newborn is relatively short and broad. Crelin[9] reports that with the mouth closed, the tongue is about 4 cm long, 2.5 cm wide, and 1 cm thick. The hard palate is noted to be short, wide, and only slightly arched at birth, whereas it is deeply arched both anteroposteriorly and transversely in the adult. The hard palate is usually 2.3 cm long, and its width is 2.2 cm. The hard palate is visually inspected and explored by the examiner's forefinger for the shape of the palate and its evenness or sloping on one side as compared to the other (Fig. 2-14). The uvula is observed for its placement in the midline of the soft palate and its ability to move upward. The length is noted. Degrees of evenness, completeness, and absence of ridges and bumps are noted, and intactness in all directions is documented.

Further observations are made and documented if one or more of the following are present: the mother or the nursing or medical staff note difficulty or slow rates of sucking on nipple; one side of the mouth droops lower than the other; clefts are discovered in the lips or hard or soft palate; gagging reflex is not elicited; color is cyanotic or pale or color of the lips changes to an extreme dark or light bright red or blue color; the palate is high, flat, and steepled and is characterized by abrupt angles, shape of arch is marked by abrupt angles, and shape of arch is marked by abrupt flat and narrow ceiling; tongue is beef red or blue; bumps are seen and palpated on tongue; tongue has tremors; tongue thrusts forward; movement is irregular in any direction, or there are asymmetrical movements of the tongue; mouth is dry; or gums are not smooth.

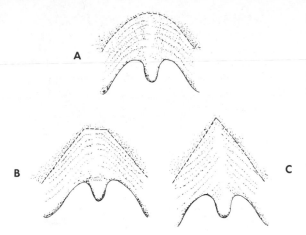

Fig. 2-14. A, Dome-shaped palate. **B,** Narrow flat part across the top of palate. **C,** High-steepled palate. (Modified from Waldrop, Mary Ford, and Halverson, Charles F.: In Hellmuth, Jerome, editor: Exceptional infant: studies in abnormalities, New York, 1971, Brunner/Mazel, Inc.)

Continued inspection about the mouth is essential in cases of the following: clefts are present in the hard or soft palate, ridges are felt along gum lines, teeth are present, there is an inability to close the lips and seal around a nipple, the tongue is short or thick and protruding, and uncoordinated movements of mouth and tongue are noted.

Cheeks

The cheeks on the face are palpated for equal degrees of fullness of the tissue, and the shape of each side is noted. Further observations are of value if the left side is uneven or not as full as the right side, edema is present over the cheeks, or shape is conspicuously different.

Chin

Observe the profile of the face for the shape and degree of recession of the chin in relationship to the other parts of the face. Note observations of a chin that recedes to a questionable degree.

Continued surveillance should be planned if one or more of the following occur: cleft palate, bifid uvula without cleft in lip, macroglossia, or hypertrophied alveolar ridges are seen; lips are bright red, pale, or blue or extremes in color changes are noticed; a cleft lip with or without a cleft palate is noted; an abnormally short or long philtrum is seen; lips are full and prominent; there are lower lip pits; the corners of the mouth remain downturned; or the mouth

is exceptionally small or large in comparison to the remainder of the face.

Continued observations are made if the face appears flat, round, broad, triangular, or coarse; if the face looks masklike; or if maxilla and mandible malar hypoplasia, micrognathia, and prognathism are evident.

Neck

Since the neck of the newborn is not as easily visualized lying down, it is better to lift the infant, with one hand supporting the back and shoulders. This position allows the head to gently fall back into extension and makes the shoulders and thorax more prominent.

The neck is inspected visually and palpated for size, suppleness, degrees of freedom of movement, and ability to flex and extend. Movements to the left or right from the midline position are observed. Responsivity to passive movement is noted as well as spontaneous movements that are seen.

The trachea is examined. According to Crelin,[9] the average length of the trachea in the full-term newborn is about 4 cm. The trachea is broader above than below, and its width from one side to the other side is a little larger (5 mm) than from front to back (3.6 mm).

Notations are made of the location of the trachea.

The muscles on the right and left sides of the neck are visualized and palpated for masses or lumps on either side as the sternocleidomastoid muscle is examined by turning the head left and right. Exact location, size, and shape of any lumps are described and written down. Note whether masses are located on the upper or lower third of the neck.

Pulsation on both sides of the neck is counted, described, and recorded. Evidence of creases, extra folds, or webbing is noted on the posterior surface.

Note presence and degree of distention in neck veins.

Clavicles

The clavicles are inspected for width, smoothness of prominences, and equalness of thickness of skin covering each bone. Depressions, separations, ridges, or degrees of unevenness of placement are noted.

Movement of both shoulders is observed. The clavicles are observed for alignment on a horizontal line from either the front, side, or back.

Continued observations of the clavicles are

made if webbing of the neck is seen, masses are palpated, clavicles are found to be hypoplastic, the trachea is deviated to the left or right, or vertebral defects are noted. If veins are distended, continued observations are made for cardiac problems.

Observations are made if neck veins are distended, masses are felt in the neck, and resistance to passive movement to the right or left is felt.

Thorax

Crelin[9] describes the thorax of the newborn as looking like a truncated cone with a wide base that is slightly flattened anteroposteriorly. The posterior wall of the thorax is reported to be as long in proportion to the trunk as it is in the adult. The horizontal circumference of the thorax at the level of the mammary glands, with respiration totally functional, is 34 to 35 cm. Before the first inspiration of air, this measurement is about 30 cm and, after the first breath, 31.2 cm. The thorax appears almost circular because of the relatively greater anteroposterior diameter. Crelin describes the sternum as a flexible strip of cartilage 5 cm long.

According to Crelin, after respiration begins, the apices of the lungs are positioned 5 to 8 mm above the level of the superior margin of the sternum, and the inferior margins are at the level of the eleventh rib posteriorly. The respiratory rate of a full-term infant is 40 to 44 breaths per minute.

An imaginary line can be placed down the middle of the thorax in determining symmetry of movement, shape, and distance between nipples.

Observations are made on the evenness of respiratory activity between the thoracic cavity and diaphragm (Fig. 2-15). Respiratory rates are counted and recorded.

Measurement of the chest circumference is obtained by placing a tape measure at the lower end of the scapula and directly over the nipple line anteriorly. Three measurements are taken, and the average is recorded.

The chest is noted for the degree of expansion on both sides and if costal respiration is evident (Fig. 2-16). The degree of the circular shape of chest is noted and described. Note the color, formation, and degrees of swelling about nipples. Note whether breast tissue is firm, flat, and made up of round masses of tissue about 1 cm in diameter and 7 mm thick.[9] Observe for a depres-

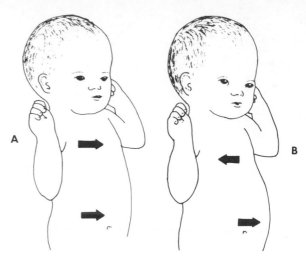

Fig. 2-15. A, Normal breathing pattern with protrusion of the abdominal wall and a rise in the chest wall. Movements are synchronized. **B,** Asymmetrical seesaw movements in which the chest falls while the abdomen rises.

sion in the center of the areola, which contains the nipple.

The distance between the nipples may be considered to be widely set when intermamillary index is above 28, according to Mehes and Kitzveger.[15] The intermamillary index is calculated by the following formula:

Intermamillary index =

$$\frac{\text{Intermamillary distance (cm} \times 100)}{\text{Circumference of chest (cm)}}$$

Indentations, depressions, and shortness or longness of the sternal area deserve further observations.

If the nipple is a dark color, further observations are warranted. Observations, counting of respiratory rates, and notation of seesawlike movements between the thoracic cavity and diaphragm warrant continued follow-up and repeated observations. Retractions of the sternum, ribs showing, and a respiratory grunt indicate need for emergency care.

Heart

According to Crelin,[9] the cardiac output of blood in a newborn is usually 550 ml per minute, and blood pressure is about 80/46. The pulse is normally irregular. Near term the fetal pulse rate is 150 beats per minute. At birth it is about 180 beats per minute; about 10 minutes

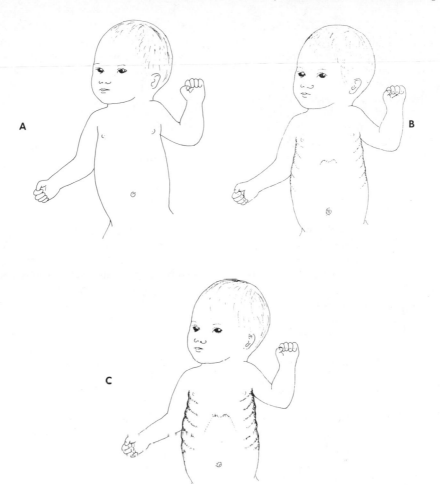

Fig. 2-16. Observations of retractions. **A,** No retractions are visible. **B,** Retractions are visible. **C,** Retractions are marked. (Modified from Silverman, W. A., and Anderson, D. H.: Pediatrics **17**:1, 1956.)

after birth the pulse rate drops to between 120 and 140 beats per minute. From 6 months to 1 year of age the pulse rate is between 113 and 127 beats per minute.

Abdomen

Muscle tone, contour, tissue turgor, flatness, distention, condition of umbilicus, presence of two arteries and one vein, masses, vessels seen, bulges, color, presence of hair, presence of umbilical hernia, and respiratory activity are noted.

Genitals

Male genitals. Observe whether the penis appears slender in the newborn. Note whether the glans is tapered at the tip. Crelin[9] reports that the length is approximately 2.5 cm, and width is usually 1 cm. The entire length of the urethra is approximately 6.2 cm. The width at the base of the scrotum is about 2 cm, and length is approximately 3 cm. The testes at birth average about 10 mm in length and 5 mm in width. Note if the left testis has migrated into the scrotum.

Generalized masses in the scrotal sac are carefully described. Each side of the scrotum is observed for size, shape, length, elevation, and presence of ridges, and the condition of the spermatic cord is described.

The male genitals can vary with at least one testis down in the scrotum, one testis felt high in the scrotum, or neither testis palpated in the scrotum.

Observations and palpations for presence of the testes in both scrotal sacs are done after placing the index finger and thumb together in the position of an inverted V above the center of the inguinal ligament. The procedure of blocking the inguinal canals on both sides is noted, and the location and shape of the testis on each side are described.

Further observations are made if the meatus is located to the side, dorsally, or ventrally. If the direction of the urinary stream is not centered directly out, further observations are carried out.

Female genitals. Observe if the labia majora cover the labia minora. Crelin[9] has reported that the labia minora are about 2.5 mm thick; their length is about 2 cm, and the widest part of the flap measures 1.2 cm. Observe if the orifice of the vagina has a circumference of about 0.5 cm.

In addition to observing for size and shape, the appearance of the external structures of the female genitals is observed for skin discoloration, the presence and amount of edema, and the presence of masses. Note the color of edges of the labia minora and if they are of a darker pigmentation than the labia majora. Note if the labia minora protrude from the labia majora and the degrees of protrusion. Observe and record the placement and shape of urethral meatus and the presence of a vagina.

Observe for the degree of separation between the labia majora, whether labia majora are completely or partially covering minora, and the degree to which the labia minora are visible.

The amount, color, and changes in vaginal discharges are judged, described, and recorded.

Femoral pulses

The femoral pulses are best counted by applying gentle pressure over the femoral area on each side. An absent femoral pulse indicates coarctation of the aorta.

Vertebral column

The average length of the free vertebral column is 19 or 20 cm.[9] Note the presence or lack of fixed curves. It is not until after birth that the thoracic area forms a fixed curve. When the infant begins to lift his head, a flexible cervical curve can be observed. At approximately the end of the first year, a flexible lumbar curve is noticed.

Vertebral posture is observed from the front, sides, and back in flexed position. If curves are exaggerated forward or backward, observe and feel for presence of spinous processes.

Back

The spinal column is observed, palpated, and described according to shape, placement, alignment, outline, and whether unusual prominences or depressions or masses are noted.

Coccyx

This area is examined and palpated, and observations are made of shape, presence of tufts of hair, dimples, cysts, and sinuses or fistulas.

Extremities

Lower extremities. Note the position of the lower limbs. Observe if limbs are flexed and abducted at hip joints, knees are flexed, and feet are inverted. Observe for spontaneous movement patterns and response to passive movements. Observe for appearance of bowed legs created by the position of the limb joints and shape of soft tissues. The distance between the hip joint and the heel of an extended limb is about 16.5 cm (6½ inches). The distance between the knee and ankle measures about 7.5 cm (3 inches).[9]

The length of the feet from the heel to the tip of the big toe averages about 6.5 cm (2½ inches). The greatest width is reported to be 2.5 cm (1 inch). The sole is markedly tapered at the heel.[9] Depths of creases are measured for soles of feet. Creases can be drawn to depict location and depth on foot.

Upper extremities. Observe for evidence that the upper limbs are longer in comparison to the trunk and lower extremities. The upper extremities measure approximately the same length as the lower ones. A measurement of 16.5 cm (6½ inches) is average, according to Crelin.[9]

Observe if the fingers have a slender appearance. The middle finger measures about 2.2 cm in length and is 6 mm wide at its base.

Creases in palms of hands are described as to amount, width across palm, location, and similarity or difference of right hand with left hand.

The topography of a crease should be described according to the extent it covers the surface of the palm, whether it is horizontal or vertical, the angle at which it is joined, and whether it completely covers, bridges, or partially covers a surface of the palm across or up and down (Fig. 2-17).

Fingers and toes. The length, distance between, curvature, number of joints on a digit,

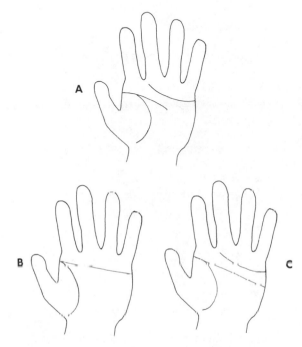

Fig. 2-17. A, Normal crease of palm traversed by two horizontal and one vertical crease. **B,** A single palmar crease traverses the palm from the radial to the ulnar margin. **C,** The Sydney line is characterized by a proximal transverse crease that extends beyond the ulnar margin of the palm. (Modified from Johnson, Charles F., and Optiz, Erica: Unusual palm creases and unusual children, Clin. Pediatr. **12:**102, 1973.)

evidence of overlapping or fusion, and height of fusion are noted.

Appearance of the fingers is described, that is, whether they are long, narrow, short, stubby, clubbed, fused, or spiderlike (long and thin). Also note if the fifth finger is incurved or there is overlapping of second and third fingers.

If clubfoot is evident or if there is joint hypermobility or joint dislocation at the shoulder, hip, or elbow, continued observations are made.

Nails and creases. The surface of nails is examined for color, shape, thickness, length, and size. Observe for partial or complete covering of nail bed.

Continued observations are made on nails that are not completely developed or when a single crease is noted on the upper palm or distal palmar axial triradius.

General observations. Continued observations are made if limbs are short, hands are small, feet are small, fifth finger hypoplasia exists, there is thumb hypoplasia, polydactyly exists, broad thumb or toes are evident, or syndactyly exists or if there are wide variations in creases of hands.

Hips

Observe the degree of equalness in movement with the infant in the supine position with both thighs rotated. Note the number of gluteal creases or folds on each side. Observe the legs when brought together at the midline and the hips and both legs when extended. Observe the length of both legs when both soles are lined up.

Note the maximal degree of range of abduction when the hip is flexed and abducted on the right or left (Fig. 2-18). Characteristic movement of lower extremities should be described. Observe and note the amount of resistance when the knees are flexed and the hips are abducted up and out, when resistance is met, and at what angle it occurs. Note if a thud, snap, or click is heard on flexion and abduction as the femur slips out of the acetabulum. Observe unequal gluteal folds. Observe for an increase or decrease in range of motion at different time periods. Note crawling movements forward when neonate is placed in supine position.

Continue to make appropriate observations if unevenness of folds and differences are noted; if a click, snap, or thud is heard; or if one leg is noticed to be longer than the other.

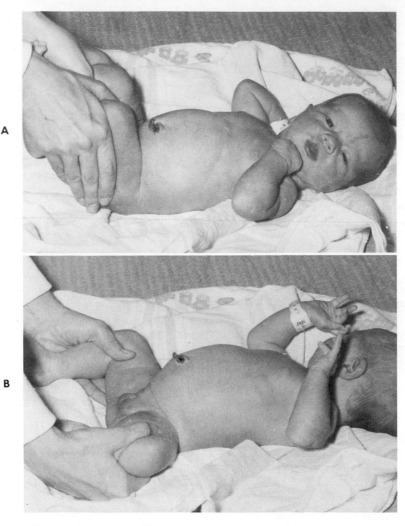

Fig. 2-18. Observation of the motion of the hip joints is conducted by full abduction with palpation. **A,** The examiner's index finger is placed along the thigh with the finger palpating hip motion as, **B,** the hips are brought to a full 90-degree angle. (From Chinn, Peggy L.: Child health maintenance: concepts in family-centered care, ed. 2, St. Louis, 1979, The C. V. Mosby Co.)

Skin and hair. Continued observations are made if a deep sacral dimple is discovered, pilonidal cyst is observed, unusually sparse hair is evident, hirsutism is noticed, or there are abnormalities to hair form, color, or patterns.

Cry

The cry of a neonate is monitored for intensity of pitch, when it begins and ends, characteristic patterns when tone or pitch changes, and whether these changes go to a higher, lower, or medium level of pitch. Differences in the cry of the neonate when excited, distressed,

moved about, hungry, completely undressed, or brought to a sitting position are described. Validate parents' impression of differences in a newborn's cry before discharge home.

Muscle tone

Limp, flaccid, or hypertonic tone of the newborn deserves accurate observations.

Rectum

Patency of anus; position, shape, and presence of skin tags; fissures; tears; and color that is present should be described.

Table 2-1. List of anomalies and scoring weights*

Anomaly	Weight	Anomaly	Weight
Head		Ears—cont'd	
Fine electric hair:		Adherent ear lobes:	
Very fine hair that will not comb down	2	Lower edge of ears extend:	
Fine hair that is soon awry after combing	1	Upward and back toward crown of head	2
Two or more hair whorls		Straight back toward rear of neck	1
Head circumference outside normal range:		Malformed ears	1
>1.5σ	2	Asymmetrical ears	1
>1.0σ ≦1.5σ	1	Soft and pliable ears	0
Eyes		Mouth	
Epicanthus:		High-steepled palate:	
Where upper and lower lids join the nose, point of union is:		Roof of mouth:	
Deeply covered	2	Definitely steepled	2
Partly covered	1	Flat and narrow at the top	1
Hypertelorism:		Furrowed tongue (one with deep ridges)	1
Approximate distance between tear ducts:		Tongue with smooth-rough spots	0
>1.5σ	2	Hands	
>1.0σ ≦1.5σ	1	Curved fifth finger:	
Ears		Markedly curved inward toward other fingers	2
Low seated ears:		Slightly curved inward toward other fingers	1
Point where ear joins the head not in line with corner of eye and nose bridge:		Single transverse palmar crease	1
Lower by >0.5 cm	2	Feet	
Lower by ≦0.5 cm	1	Third toe longer than second.	
		Definitely longer than second toe	2
		Appears equal in length to second toe	1
		Partial syndactylia of two middle toes	1
		Big gap between first and second toes	1

*From Waldrop, Mary Ford, and Halverson, Charles F.: Minor physical abnormalities and hyperactive behavior in young children. In Hellmuth, Jerome, editor: Exceptional infant: studies in abnormalities, vol. 2, New York, 1971, Brunner/Mazel, Inc., p. 359.

Anomalies

Waldrop and Halverson[4] compiled a selected list of eighteen congenital anomalies and assigned corresponding weights to them (Table 2-1).

INCLUDING PARENTS IN ASSESSMENT PROCESS

Information regarding the systematic data obtained from the assessment of the infant's surface features from the top of his head to his feet and from front to back should be shared and validated with the parents. Their observations should be noted. They should be included in further assessments and instructed in observational techniques, how to record, and exactly what to note. Their notations, observations, and recordings should be discussed in following and subsequent planning of the child's care.

In addition to surface appraisal, the parents should be included in observations regarding the neonate's responses to his early environment.

Information about the status of the neonate's early reflexes; his ability to cuddle, hold up his head, and respond to auditory and visual stimulation; his capacity to shut out disturbing stimuli such as noise and light; and the graduated measures necessary for consoling the infant such as talking to him, holding, rocking, placing one's hand over his chest and hands, or using a pacifier as a means to settle him down from crying should be explored with the mother.

The parents' impression of the infant's movement, alertness, and response to eye contact should be validated, and their impression of his needs for stimulation and what they have done or thought of doing to meet them could be discussed.

It is imperative that stereotyped methods of observation be replaced with comprehensive individual profiles. Use of objective and systematic assessment approaches will influence present and future care practices and outcomes.

Table 2-2. Observational guide to assess the newborn

Surface features	Surface inspection	Description of observations
General appearance	Postural attitudes, muscle tone, activity levels, and state of comfort responsiveness	Partial flexion; consistent and firm muscle tone, active; slightly irritable when picked up; cries when bathed and undressed
Skin	Degree and uniformity of color; degrees of cyanosis or pallor (generalized or peripheral); eruptions; hydration; hemorrhagic manifestations; rash, inflammation; pigmentation, nevi, subcutaneous nodules, desquamation; presence, absence, and degree of jaundice; striae, wrinkling, vernix caseosa; texture; turgor; elasticity; lanugo (quantity and distribution); sensitivity; temperature; parchment; opacity; edema	Uniformly pink and smooth over face, trunk, and extremities; dry and cracked around ankles; petechiae over cheeks of face; small area of erythema toxicum on outer aspects of buttocks; light purplish blue spots on right buttocks, 3.5 ×4.5 cm area; uniformly jaundiced; tissue turgor on abdomen and calf, with skin consistently springing back; small amount of lanugo on upper back, right side; skin mottled when undressed; small amount of desquamation on arms; no obvious edema of hands and feet; veins and tributaries seen
Head	Size, shape, circumference, control and movement, sutures, forceps' marks, moulding	
Skull	Contours, symmetry, moulding, resistance of skull bones to gentle pressure	Round and symmetrical on all planes, 34.5 cm (OFC)
Scalp	Presence, quantity, texture, distribution of hair, and location of hairline	Fine, soft, separate, silky hair, evenly distributed; covers scalp but is receding over both temporal bones
Fontanels	Cephalhematoma, subcutaneous nodules around occiput; tension, size (centimeters), pulsations; closure and number	Sagittal and coronal sutures palpable Anterior fontanel Anterior posterior plane, 2 cm Transverse plane, 1.5 cm Posterior fontanel, 0.5 cm
Face	Shape and symmetry of parts, distance between mouth and nose, depth of nasolabial fold, distribution of hair; size of mandible, fullness of cheeks, facial movements when resting and crying to evaluate integrity of innervation of the facial musculature	Symmetrical, hair receding on temporal bones, eyebrows and eyelashes present, facial movements even when resting or crying
Eyes	Placement, symmetry, distance between inner canthus, lacrimation, clarity and luster of corneas, pupillary reaction, opacity of lenses, placement of eyebrows and eyelids, distribution of eyelashes, color of iris, muscular control, position of pupils in relationship to palpebral fissures	Both eyes bright and clear; even placement; left eye 2 cm wide, right eye 2 cm wide, and distance between inner canthi 2 cm; eyelashes tend to clump together; scant amount of drainage from both eyes; slate blue; slight nystagmus present; both pupils constrict to light and dilate equally in darkened room
Nose	Exterior appearance, shape, patency, discharge, placement in relationship to eyes and mouth, symmetry, septum	Nose in midline, nares patent, breathes easily, even placement in relation to eyes and mouth, septum intact, no discharge, button shape, mucous membranes moist and pink
Ears	Placement, form, position and size of pinna, symmetry, firmness	Firm, well-defined curving of upper pinna of both ears; cartilage firm; recoil rapid for both ears
Mouth	Size, shape, placement, symmetry, color of mucosa, anterior mouth cavity, pharynx, lip margins	Lips pink, hard palate dome shaped, and lip margins well defined; sucks with force when stimulated
Tongue	Size, mobility, color, coating, grooves	Tongue proportionate size, pink and uncoated, freely movable and moves in anteroposterior direction
Chin	Size and distance from lips	Chin recedes in comparison to other bones of face

Table 2-2. Observational guide to assess the newborn—cont'd

Surface features	Surface inspection	Description of observations
Neck	Size, position, movement, contour, flexion	Short, straight, head moves easily from side to side from midline
Thorax	Shape, symmetry, retractions and pulsations, size, position and distance between nipples, length of sternum, palpation of breast tissue, respiratory activity (depth and rate), chest circumference	Right thorax more elevated than left; sternum 8 cm in length; distance between nipples 8 cm; breast tissue palpable, 0.5 cm in width; chest circumference 32.5 cm; respiratory rate 38 per minute; trachea in midline; diaphragmatic breathing patterns
Abdomen and navel	Size and contour, respiratory movements, musculature, tension, pulsations, presence of the umbilical vein, two umbilical arteries, surface of umbilicus	Size proportionate, rounded, soft abdominal breathing irregular, cord dry and healed
Genitals	Male: circumcision, meatal opening, foreskin, surface and size of scrotum, position of testes in scrotum	
	Female: size of labia majora and labia minora, secretions, edema of genitals	Some edema over labia majora, labia majora large but labia minora visible anteriorly, whitish secretions
Rectum	Patency	Patent
Hips	Posture, motion, movement, flexion, symmetry	Full abduction and flexion of hips; gluteal folds even; when flexed, some resistance to movement but can be taken through full range of motion
Extremities	Range of motion, movement, length, symmetry, posture, tremors, number of digits, flexion, creases of hands, quality of nails, resistance to passive movement	Nail beds pink; size and shape even; ten fingers, ten toes; tremors apparent when agitated; nails on fingers and toes well defined; M creases present on both hands; upper extremities move together; lower extremities move alternately
Back and spine	Posture, symmetry, mobility, alignment	Straight, easily flexed, symmetrical
Cry	Tone, pitch, frequency, duration, intensity, alternate periods of excitability and quietness, lacrimation	Moderate tone and pitch, cries when disturbed, quiets when left alone, lacrimation not present when crying, shortest crying periods 3 to 5 minutes, longest crying periods 5 to 7 minutes before outside consoling measures are necessary
Height		49.6 cm
Weight		3,400 kg
Heart rate		120 beats per minute
Temperature		98.6° F
Respiratory rate		38 breaths per minute
Head circumference		34.5 cm
Chest circumference		32.5 cm

INTERPRETING DATA TO PARENTS

One paramount concern of parents is whether the newborn is healthy and normal. Although a difference from the norm may be noted, this does not mean the infant is abnormal, nor is "different" to be equated with "bad." Parents deserve to have their concerns and questions answered as completely and specifically as the assessment allows.

Having collected early, ongoing, and regular information, nurses, physicians, and other health care professionals are in a better posi-tion to answer questions regarding parental observations, to validate mothers' and fathers' early observations, and to offer appropriate feedback and individualized anticipatory guidance.

A RECORDING FORM FOR NEWBORN ASSESSMENT

The observational guide shown in Table 2-2 offers a method of observing, recording, and describing assessment of the newborn in a systematic, objective way. Note that entries in the third column are examples of descriptions of a newborn after assessment.

CLINICAL ASSESSMENT FOR GESTATIONAL AGE

Objective methods for determining gestational age are available to gauge care responses according to age and care needs. Specific problems can be anticipated and complications avoided or eliminated if the infant is routinely observed for signs of immaturity or levels of increased maturity. Well-defined external signs help determine the care planning that is vital to the newborn's individual needs.

A scale for clinical assessment for gestational age was developed by Dubowitz and associates[16] to aid in objectively identifying signs of both immaturity and maturity for the newly born. Used in a systematic way, it promotes accuracy in defining short-term care as well as long-term goals for the newborn.

The objective of the clinical assessment is to determine that the newborn's gestational age is accurate. The observation, rating, and scoring time is approximately 10 minutes once skills in using it are mastered.

A major reason for using this objective and reliable assessment scale is to assist medical and nursing health care professionals to identify gestational age and corresponding problems that can be anticipated for certain ages or maturity levels. The tool can be used to anticipate problems that can occur, whether it be for a small-for-date infant or for an infant who is born prematurely. It is highly useful in differentiating the infant who is plump, weighs 9 pounds, but is not 40 weeks and term. Some infants of diabetic mothers merit ratings by the Clinical Assessment Scale because their plump appearance can be misleading and can result in errors in care planning that are inappropriate for their actual gestational age.

It is useful in discriminating the infant who is malnourished and meets weight criteria for a premature baby but who may not necessarily be premature. Similarly, the Clinical Assessment Scale can be of value in assessing age, needs, and appropriate care for an infant who appears younger but is actually dehydrated.

If nursing or medical health care personnel are curious or are trying to estimate whether a full-term infant has a lesser gestational status, the clinical assessment scale can be used to determine and answer questions in a reliable, objective manner.

The Clinical Assessment Scale, which is in increasing use, is particularly valuable in helping nursing personnel be more secure in their estimates of an infant's condition. It helps in making serial objective comparisons from one week to the next and is a tremendous advantage in planning appropriate ways of interacting with the infant, providing adequate amounts of appropriate stimulation to the infant (including touching, holding, or moving the infant around), and planning optimal feeding schedules. Its value in explaining unique features of the infant clearly and simply to parents is being increasingly recognized. If an infant has been born prematurely, the results from the clinical assessment can be encouraging and of valuable assistance to parents, who also find it intriguing to see their infants assessed. The Clinical Assessment Scale, when used weekly in the presence of parents, can serve as a reassuring foundation that change, even though slow in nature, is actually occurring in their infant. Parents customarily need concrete evidence that change is occurring. Parents are encouraged to note signs of strength, improvement, and increments in progress.

Dubowitz and co-workers[16] chose two categories that would be helpful in estimating gestational age: neurological signs and external characteristics. These two categories were chosen because they were easily identified, and observations could easily be carried out in a prescribed manner. In addition, the investigators selected criteria for these categories that could easily be observed, rated, and scored.

There is evidence that external characteristics of the infant are a better indicator of maturation levels than neurological reflexes, but both together provide a reliable, comprehensive profile of an infant's gestational age.

The external criteria include items such as whether the infant is edematous, the texture of the skin, the presence or absence of plantar creases, the amount and presence of lanugo, whether ears stay in place or snap back when bent, and others. The appearance of the external genitals is also observed and scored. The scoring system for external criteria is shown in Table 2-3.

The neurological criteria of the assessment scale are included in a list of postures and reflexes that are to be observed in each infant (Fig. 2-19). The majority are obvious and simple to score. These include observations of the in-

Table 2-3. Scoring system for external criteria*

External sign	Score†				
	0	1	2	3	4
Edema	Obvious edema of hands and feet; pitting over tibia	No obvious edema of hands and feet; pitting over tibia	No edema		
Skin texture	Very thin, gelatinous	Thin and smooth	Smooth; medium thickness; rash or superficial peeling	Slight thickening; superficial cracking and peeling especially of hands and feet	Thick and parchment-like; superficial or deep cracking
Skin color	Dark red	Uniformly pink	Pale pink; variable over body	Pale; only pink over ears, lips, palms, or soles	
Skin opacity (trunk)	Numerous veins and venules clearly seen, especially over abdomen	Veins and tributaries seen	Few large vessels clearly seen over abdomen	A few large vessels seen indistinctly over abdomen	No blood vessels seen
Lanugo (over back)	No lanugo	Abundant; long and thick over whole back	Hair thinning especially over lower back	Small amount of lanugo and bald areas	At least ½ of back devoid of lanugo
Plantar creases	No skin creases	Faint red marks over anterior ½ of sole	Definite red marks over > anterior ½; indentations over < anterior ⅓	Indentations over anterior ⅓	Definite deep indentations over > anterior ⅓
Nipple formation	Nipple barely visible; no areola	Nipple well defined; areola smooth and flat; diameter <0.75 cm	Areola stippled; edge not raised; diameter <0.75 cm	Areola stippled; edge raised; diameter >0.75 cm	
Breast size	No breast tissue palpable	Breast tissue on one or both sides; <0.5 cm diameter	Breast tissue both sides; one or both 0.5-1.0 cm	Breast tissue both sides; one or both >1 cm	
Ear form	Pinna flat and shapeless; little or no incurving of edge	Incurving of part of edge of pinna	Partial incurving whole of upper pinna	Well-defined incurving whole of upper pinna	
Ear firmness	Pinna soft, easily folded; no recoil	Pinna soft, easily folded; slow recoil	Cartilage to edge of pinna, but soft in places; ready recoil	Pinna firm, cartilage to edge; instant recoil	
Genitals					
Male	Neither testis in scrotum	At least one testis high in scrotum	At least one testis right down		
Female (with hips ½ abducted)	Labia majora widely separated; labia minora protruding	Labia majora almost cover labia minora	Labia majora completely cover labia minora		

*From Dubowitz, Lilly, Dubowitz, Victor, and Goldberg, Cissie: Clinical assessment of gestational age in the newborn infant, J. Pediatr. **77:**1-10, 1970; modified from Farr and associates: Dev. Med. Child Neurol. **8:**507, 1966.
†If score differs on two sides, take the mean.

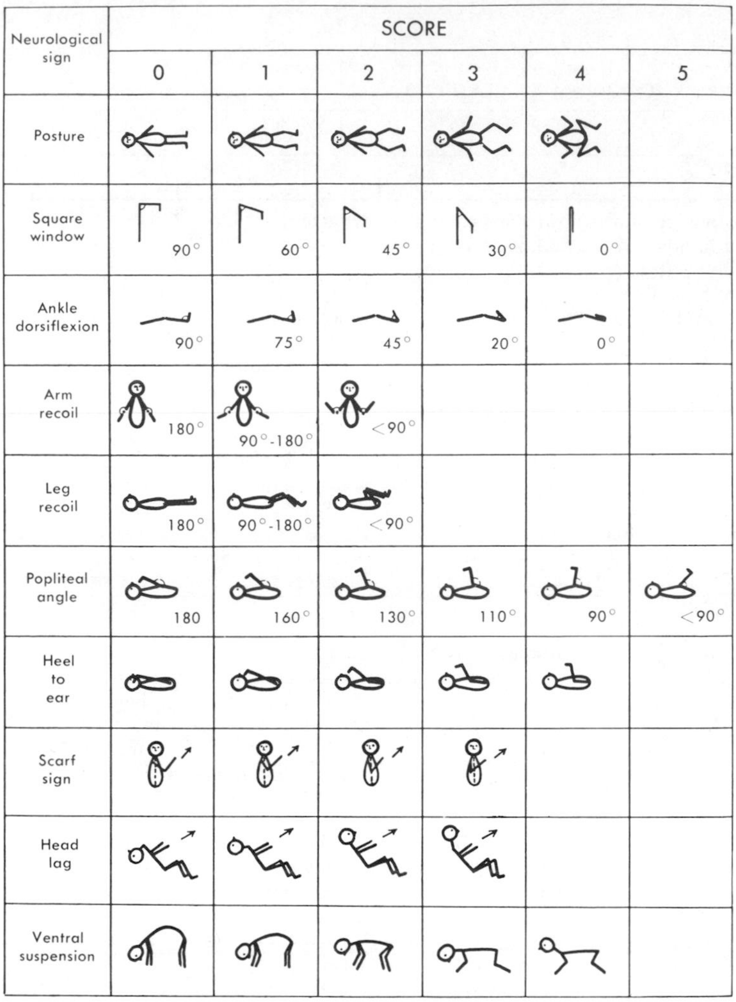

Fig. 2-19. Scoring system for neurological signs of the infant. (From Dubowitz, Lilly, Dubowitz, Victor, and Goldberg, Cissie: J. Pediatr. **77:**1-10, 1970.)

fant's posture, the degree of dorsiflexion of the feet, how fast the arm or leg recoils from a standardized position, the distance the heel can be moved to the ear, how far one arm can be crossed to the opposite shoulder, the degree of head lag when sitting, and the position of the head in ventral suspension. Techniques for scoring the neurological signs shown in Fig. 2-19 are as follows:

Posture. Observed with infant quiet and in supine position. *Score 0:* arms and legs extended; *1:* beginning of flexion of hips and knees, arms extended; *2:* stronger flexion of legs, arms extended; *3:* arms slightly flexed, legs flexed and abducted; *4:* full flexion of arms and legs.

Square window. The hand is flexed on the forearm

between the thumb and index finger of the examiner. Enough pressure is applied to get as full a flexion as possible, and the angle between the hypothenar eminence and the ventral aspect of the forearm is measured and graded according to diagram. (Care is taken not to rotate the infant's wrist while doing this maneuver.)

Ankle dorsiflexion. The foot is dorsiflexed onto the anterior aspect of the leg, with the examiner's thumb on the sole of the foot and other fingers behind the leg. Enough pressure is applied to get as full flexion as possible, and the angle between the dorsum of the foot and the anterior aspect of the leg is measured.

Arm recoil. With the infant in the supine position the forearms are first flexed for 5 seconds, then fully extended by pulling on the hands, and then released. The sign is fully positive if the arms return briskly to full flexion (*Score 2*). If the arms return to incomplete flexion or the response is sluggish it is graded as *Score 1*. If they remain extended or are only followed by random movements the score is 0.

Leg recoil. With the infant supine, the hips and knees are fully flexed for 5 seconds, then extended by traction on the feet, and released. A maximal response is one of full flexion of the hips and knees (*Score 2*). A partial flexion scores *1*, and minimal or no movement scores *0*.

Popliteal angle. With the infant supine and his pelvis flat on the examining couch, the thigh is held in the knee-chest position by the examiner's left index finger and thumb supporting the knee. The leg is then extended by gentle pressure from the examiner's right index finger behind the ankle and the popliteal angle is measured.

Heel to ear maneuver. With the baby supine, draw the baby's foot as near to the head as it will go without forcing it. Observe the distance between the foot and the head as well as the degree of extension at the knee. Grade according to diagram. Note that the knee is left free and may draw down alongside the abdomen.

Scarf sign. With the baby supine, take the infant's hand and try to put it around the neck and as far posteriorly as possible around the opposite shoulder. Assist this maneuver by lifting the elbow across the body. See how far the elbow will go across and grade according to illustrations. *Score 0*: elbow reaches opposite axillary line; *1*: elbow between midline and opposite axillary line; *2*: elbow reaches midline; *3*: elbow will not reach midline.

Head lag. With the baby lying supine, grasp the hands (or the arms if a very small infant) and pull him slowly towards the sitting position. Observe the position of the head in relation to the trunk and grade accordingly. In a small infant the head may initially be supported by one hand. *Score 0*: complete lag; *1*: partial head control; *2*: able to maintain head in line with body; *3*: brings head anterior to body.

Ventral suspension. The infant is suspended in the prone position, with examiner's hand under the infant's chest (one hand in a small infant, two in a large infant). Observe the degree of extension of the back and the amount of flexion of the arms and legs. Also note the relation of the head to the trunk. Grade according to diagrams.

If score differs on the two sides, take the mean.[*]

When scores are obtained for each category (neurological criteria and external criteria), the infant's estimated age in weeks should be recorded on a graph for accuracy of gestational maturity. Fig. 2-20 shows how to obtain gestational age from the total score.

---

[*]From Dubowitz, Lilly, Dubowitz, Victor, and Goldberg, Cissie: Clinical assessment of gestational age in the newborn infant, J. Pediatr. **77:**5, 1970.

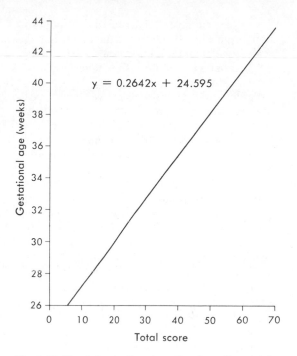

$$y = 0.2642x + 24.595$$

Fig. 2-20. Graph for reading gestational age from total score obtained on the gestational age scale. Formula for obtaining gestational age score is shown above, with x as the total score and y as the gestational age score. (From Dubowitz, Lilly, Dubowitz, Victor, and Goldberg, Cissie. J. Pediatr. **77:**1 10, 1070.)

The total score obtained by one person and compared with another after acquaintance with use of the scale rarely varies more than two points.

It is recommended that initial attempts in observation and scoring be done with another individual to increase objectivity of measurement techniques and to increase reliability and reduce subjectivity of the observer rating the infant.

The Clinical Assessment Scale is most effectively used and its results most accurate and reliable when it is used within the first 5 days of a neonate's life.

It is recommended that health care professionals using the Clinical Assessment Scale refrain from reading charts on the infant or talking first to parents about the expected date of confinement (EDC). The practice of getting information about the infant before he is assessed may influence and actually diminish the maximum objectivity that can be attained in rating an infant.

It is also suggested that guesses about gestational age not be attempted before using the scale. In addition, it is important that the mother not be queried as to her estimate of how many weeks old the infant is.

Parents are generally receptive, have a positive orientation to the results of scores being shared, and are relieved to know that their infant can be rated according to objective means. They feel more secure in knowing that such refined tools for measuring infants' ages are available. Observation during the use of the tool can add valuably to parents' perceptions, attitudes, and appreciation of the assets that their infants have from one time period to the next. Proper use of the tool fosters a more positive orientation for nursing and medical professionals, as well as for parents. Those in the field of health care are equally delighted to see observable, progressive, and incremental changes occur, however slight.

The clinical assessment of gestational age scale is recommended to be routinely used with other assessment tools. A younger infant may be showing different neurological signs, less response to the environment, more difficulty in feeding, irregularity in sleep patterns, unusual postural attitudes, and color and state changes, which are initially viewed as pathological in nature. The systematic use of the Clinical Assessment Scale is designed to correct these errors in judgment and make it easier for health care professionals to accurately identify, plan, and implement care according to what is directly observed, not what is assumed to be present.

SUMMARY

Child care professionals now see assessment as a multifaceted, multidimensional process that is a starting point and not an end in itself. It is heartening to note that professionals are incorporating more parental participation in the assessment process. They are not content to give lip service about including parents but are actually asking for parental input, either verbally or in record keeping. Professionals are attempting to give parents appropriate support for their child-rearing concerns, goals, and values and are acknowledging parents' competencies, strengths, and abilities in the numerous decision-making processes that they encounter on a moment-to-moment, day-by-day basis.

Child care professionals are also paying more attention to developing their skills in presenting assessment information to parents or other caregivers. For instance, they attempt to be supportive when interpreting assessment findings. They try to share results with both parents present and to point out an infant's strengths and assets before talking about deficits or weaknesses.

More than anything else professionals have replaced myths about early infant development with objective, systematic observations that can be used to initiate innovative services in preventive health care.

In summary, the major trends in newborn assessment are as follows:

1. Use of the developmental model
2. Greater objectivity
3. Use of a variety of standardized, predictive tools, incorporating interrater reliability
4. Not focusing on the child alone
5. Giving parents more credit
6. Use of the mutual participation model in place of conveying a mystique about observations
7. Viewing assessment as a multifaceted process—no single assessment is sufficient
8. Viewing assessment as a starting point
9. Including fathers in assessment and care practices of infants.

REFERENCES

1. Marden, Phillip M., Smith, David W., and McDonald, Michael J.: Congenital anomalies in the newborn infant, including minor variations, J. Pediatr. **64:**357-371, 1964.
2. McIntosh, R. K., Merritt, K., Richards, M. R., Samuels, M. H., and Bellows, M. S.: The incidence of congenital malformations: a study of 5,964 pregnancies, Pediatrics **14:**505-522, 1954.
3. Anderson, Frederick P.: Evaluation of the routine physical examination of infants in the first year of life, Pediatrics **45:**950-960, 1960.
4. Waldrop, Mary Ford, and Halverson, Charles F.: Minor physical anomalies and hyperactive behavior in young children. In Hellmuth, Jerome, editor: Exceptional infant: studies in abnormalities, vol. 2, New York, 1971, Brunner/Mazel, Inc.
5. Brazelton, T. Berry: The Neonatal Behavioral Assessment Scale, London, 1973, William Heinemann Ltd., and Philadelphia, 1973, J. B. Lippincott Co.
6. Tronick, Edward, and Brazelton, T. Berry: Clinical uses of the Brazelton Neonatal Assessment Scale. In Friedlander, E. Z., editor: Exceptional infant: assessment and intervention, vol. 3, New York, 1975, Brunner/Mazel, Inc.
7. Broussard, Elsie R., and Hartner, Miriam Sergay

Sturgeon: Further considerations regarding maternal perception of the first born. In Hellmuth, Jerome, editor: Exceptional infant: studies in abnormalities, vol. 2, New York, 1971, Brunner/Mazel, Inc.

8. Broussard, Elsie R., and Sturgeon, Miriam Sergay: Maternal perception of the neonate as related to development, Child Psychiatry Hum. Dev. **1:**16-25, Fall, 1970.

9. Crelin, Edmund S.: Functional anatomy of the newborn, New Haven, Conn., 1973, Yale University Press.

10. Smith, David W.: Personal communication, Jan., 1975.

11. McClean, H. E.: Physical growth and its evaluation: a manual for nurses, Vancouver, British Columbia, 1971, City of Vancouver Health Department.

12. Popich, Gregory A., and Smith, David W.: Fontanels: range of normal size, J. Pediatr. **80:**749-752, 1972.

13. Prechtl, Heinz, and Beintema, David: The neurological examination of the full-term newborn infant, London, 1964, The Spastics Society International Medical Publications in association with William Heinemann Ltd.

14. Laestadius, Nancy, Aase, Jon, and Smith, David: Normal inner canthal and outer orbital dimensions, J. Pediatr. **74:**465-468, 1969.

15. Mehes, Karoly, and Kitzveger, Erzsebet: Inner canthal and intermamillary indices in the newborn infant, J. Pediatr. **85:**90-91, 1974.

16. Dubowitz, Lilly, Dubowitz, Victor, and Goldberg, Cissie: Clinical assessment of gestational age in the newborn infant, J. Pediatr. **77:**1-10, 1970.

3

THE NEONATAL
BEHAVIORAL
ASSESSMENT
SCALE

One of the most exciting and revolutionary developments to emerge from the infant and early childhood assessment field is the work of Dr. T. Berry Brazelton. The Neonatal Behavioral Assessment Scale, developed by Brazelton[1] and associates over the past twenty years, is the first major tool of its kind to focus on the newborn. Data collected from this assessment scale show beyond a doubt that a 1-day-old infant is not the passive recipient of environmental stimuli as has commonly been accepted. As a result of Brazelton's work, many traditional beliefs about the nature of the newborn are being relegated to the realm of myth.

In the early 1950s Brazelton, a pediatrician and expert in normal child development, began his search for a tool to assess newborn behavior. He was initially looking for a means of determining how the environment shaped the child, as well as a means of documenting observable individual differences in neonates. After years of observing the neonate both in his studies and private practice, Brazelton became convinced that the neonate shapes his environment much more than the environment shapes him and that the implications of such a finding would have tremendous impact both on the quality of care the infant initially receives and on

the early interactions between the infant and his early care providers and the infant and his parents. Furthermore, Brazelton believed that the predictive aspects of the parent-infant interaction would have major diagnostic and management possibilities for child health and development professionals in ensuring that the parent-infant relationship start out on the right foot and continue in a healthy, prosperous fashion.

In 1955 Brazelton and associates began to develop a neonatal behavior scale to assess reflex responses within a behavioral context, particularly in their relationship to predicting cognitive and emotional patterns in the infant. This early attempt at assessing and predicting infant behavior, along with the work of many other early pioneers in the field such as Dr. Bettye Caldwell, established a certain credibility to the concept that the infant has the ability to shape his environment. Over the next decade, the initial neonatal assessment scale was used in longitudinal studies of the normal development of infants and was redesigned and retested on numerous occasions with a variety of infant populations around the world. In every case its use was improved and its predictive value, even in transcultural situations, maintained and strengthened. The tool was particularly scrutinized for reliability.

In studies of Mayan infants in southern Mexico in 1965 the scale was found to be more sensitive than classic neurological evaluations. During these studies Brazelton and associates found the scale of value in reflecting the subtle behavioral changes in infants as the effect of delivery medication began to wear off.

In 1966 the scale was used to assess the behaviors of Greek infants in an ongoing study in Athens.

In following years the scale was used by paraprofessional observers in a Chicago study, and as a result the techniques for application of the assessment tool were refined. It has also been used to assess high-risk infants such as those who are premature and those of lower socioeconomic backgrounds.

Although the concept and objectives of the assessment tool have been accepted as valid from the start, the tool has undergone many revisions primarily in an attempt to make it applicable to almost any culture and usable for a variety of professional observers, with a scale that can be applied to observations in an easy, accurate, and consistently reliable fashion. Throughout the vigorous testing period, the tool has emerged as the best means yet of assessing the subtler behavioral responses of the neonate as he adjusts to and shapes his environment, gains mastery over himself, and enters the critically important formative period of cognitive and emotional development in infancy. Its implications for improving early health and developmental care and the all-important interface of the parent-child interaction are just beginning to be felt.

The Neonatal Behavioral Assessment Scale measures a total of twenty-seven behavioral responses of the infant. The behavioral items include the infant's inherent neurological capacities, as well as his responses to certain sets of stimuli. In each case, the items on the test are repeated several times so that the infant is rated on his best and not his average performance. This is done to provide a prediction of what the infant is capable of doing given optimal circumstances. The twenty-seven scale items are organized according to the following six categories:

1. *Habituation*. Scale items are included that assess how soon the infant diminishes responses to stimuli of light, sound, and a pinprick to the heel.

2. *Orientation*. Both auditory and visual items are presented to determine how much and when the infant attends to, focuses on, and gives feedback in response to animate or inanimate stimuli.

3. *Motor maturity*. Several scale items assess the degree and organization of the infant's motor coordination and control of motor activities throughout the examination.

4. *Variation*. Selected scale items assess the infant's rate and amount of change during periods of alertness and his states, color, activity, and peaks of excitement throughout the examination.

5. *Self-quieting abilities*. Scale items are included to assess how much, how soon, and how effectively the infant uses his own resources to quiet and console himself when upset or distressed. This category also includes the graduated efforts of the caregiver to intervene and quiet the infant.

6. *Social behaviors*. Scale items to assess the infant's smiling and amount of cuddling behaviors are included. These are important to assess because both are social cues that the parents assess while they hold or interact with their infant.

As mentioned previously, perhaps the most interesting and exciting result of data thus far collected in studies utilizing the Brazelton scale is the demystification of the life period of infancy. In the face of overwhelming objective evidence, many traditional concepts about infants now seem little more than well-intentioned fairytales, used always to keep a child at his dependent, submissive, pliable, and grateful best.

What are some of these so-called established truths? An infant is totally dependent on and reactive to his environment. An infant cannot see, hear, or recognize individuals or objects for several months. An infant does not know how to protect himself or how to adapt to circumstances in his environment. An infant does not know his needs, and even if he does, he cannot communicate them. And finally, that gem of all generalizations—all infants are alike!

As a result of the work of Brazelton and others, it is now known that infants can see, hear, and attend to both animate and inanimate objects. They can shut out noxious sounds and other stimuli they do not like; they can maintain attention for relatively long periods of time; they can coordinate certain motor movements; they can initiate activity and readily adapt to most situations; they sense their needs and try their best to communicate them; and they can quiet and console themselves in a stressful environment. Child care professionals now know beyond a doubt that an infant has some influence over his environment, particularly on how he and his parents respond to each other.

The Brazelton Neonatal Behavioral Assessment Scale is in increasing demand as an instrument to observe and assess the more subtle adjustments that the newborn makes in response to his extrauterine environment. This chapter will discuss the use of the Brazelton scale, its reliability, its value as a predictive tool particularly for high-risk infants, and its implications for improving the quality of early care the infant receives as well as his environment in a way that is most beneficial for both the infant and his parents.

PURPOSE OF THE NEONATAL BEHAVIORAL ASSESSMENT SCALE

The assessment scale was developed for the purpose of observing, making judgments, and scoring selected reflexes, motor responses, and interactive behavioral responses of newborn infants. The main emphasis of the scale is on the observation and rating of an infant's interactive behavior. How does the infant's environment affect him? How in turn does the infant respond to that environment? By increasing certain behaviors? By decreasing others? Or by not responding at all? To answer these questions Brazelton developed an assessment scale that offers a systematic approach to assessment and a reliable way of rating infant behaviors. In addition, it helps structure ways to observe the infant's subtle responses that he emits within his environment, the success he has, the unique features he has which affect how others respond to him, the progress he has made in the early maternal-infant acquaintance process, and most importantly, the signs he shows of how he attempts to control his own environment.

WHAT CAN BE LEARNED BY USING THE NEONATAL BEHAVIORAL ASSESSMENT SCALE?

By using the assessment scale it is possible to observe how an infant attends to environmental stimuli, how he shuts out environmental stimuli, and how the infant responds to stimuli, particularly if it is repeated. As a memory trace of a stimulus is established, the infant in all probability differentiates the need not to continue to respond to an irritating stimulus, and his responses diminish. The scale is designed with items that require the repeated presentation of stimuli to an infant as many as ten times. Most newborns habituate to repeated stimuli, particularly disturbing or aversive ones. Infants tend to "shut down" on certain stimuli in the scale, such as a bright light, the sound of a rattle presented repeatedly, or the sound of a bell ringing at each ear. If an infant becomes more alert or agitated to disturbing stimuli, it might suggest the need for further observations. In addition, this infant may present particular difficulties to parents or caregivers. In such cases in which the infant cannot habituate to irrelevant, noxious stimuli, changes in the environment such as dimming lights, lessening sounds, or lowering voices when interacting with the infant should be considered.

By using the scale, an examiner learns without a doubt that neonates are variable from moment to moment, they change from one time to another, and they are sometimes unpredictable, but their behavior does not necessarily have to be interpreted and stereotyped as a buzzing mass of confusion. Use of the scale has shown that there is a regular hierarchy of states that each newborn will go through in a variable, individual way. All the behavioral items are administered according to the infant's "state," or level of consciousness, which is a major departure from other infant assessment scales.

Brazelton shows with the scale that the newborn's capability to control responses to external stimuli within his own environment is varied and complex. Thus the scale offers a relatively new way for professionals and parents to perceive the newborn. Newborn behaviors traditionally have been underestimated, and infants have not been acknowledged for the unique capacities they present as early as 3 days of age.

By using the scale, it can be seen how the newborn can use a stimulus such as a bell, pinprick, rattle, or light to bring himself down (that is, reduce his own responses to these stimuli) and maintain himself in a controlled way without having to depend on others to interfere, rescue, or interrupt aversive stimuli for him. Other knowledge obtained from Brazelton's findings is that infants smile early and mothers can pick up on these smiles and respond to them spontaneously. Infants' smiles foster the beginnings of positive social experiences within the first few days.

With the assessment scale, infants can be observed to maintain mechanisms of consolability either by themselves or by another person. An infant can be observed to bring his hand to his mouth and manifest other sets of organized behaviors, which can be interpreted as attempts to console himself. Brazelton suggests graduated measures for consoling a truly fussy infant such as presenting the face alone; adding the voice; placing a hand on the abdomen; holding both of the baby's hands to shut off more response; putting clothes or blankets on to minimize motor behaviors of hands and feet; picking up, rocking, and talking to see if the infant quiets down and stops crying; and using a pacifier after the previous measures have been implemented.

Brazelton emphasizes that state changes and color state changes are sensitive indicators to autonomic stress, and thus they are counted and recorded for each infant during the examination period.

The Neonatal Behavioral Assessment Scale is equally valuable in helping professionals

NEONATAL BEHAVIORAL ASSESSMENT SCALE SCORING SHEET*

Scale (note state)	1	2	3	4	5	6	7	8	9
Response decrement to light (2, 3)									
Response decrement to rattle (2, 3)									
Response decrement to bell (2, 3)									
Response decrement to pinprick (1, 2, 3)									
Orientation—inanimate visual (4 only)									
Orientation—inanimate auditory (4, 5)									
Orientation—animate visual (4 only)									
Orientation—animate auditory (4, 5)									
Orientation—animate visual and auditory (4 only)									
Alertness (4 only)									
General tonus (4, 5)									
Motor maturity (4, 5)									
Pull-to-sit (3, 5)									
Cuddliness (4, 5)									
Defensive movements (4)									
Consolability (6 to 5, 4, 3, 2)									
Peak of excitement (6)									
Rapidity of buildup (from 1, 2 to 6)									
Irritability (3, 4, 5)									
Activity (alert states)									
Tremulousness (all states)									
Startles (3, 4, 5, 6)									
Lability of skin color (from 1 to 6)									
Lability of states (all states)									
Self-quieting activity (6, 5 to 4, 3, 2, 1)									
Hand-mouth facility (all states)									
Smiles (all states)									

*Modified from Brazelton, T. Berry: Neonatal Behavioral Assessment Scale, London, 1973, William Heinemann Ltd., and Philadelphia, 1973, J. B. Lippincott Co.

and parents observe and acknowledge the beginnings of infants' mastery of internal controls and how infants use external stimuli to keep themselves under control. It is notable how hard infants actually work and how resourceful they are from the beginning in using practically everything from their outside environment to help them master and cope with incoming stimuli.

By using the scale, one can observe how the infant is set up with many powerful mechanisms to shut out kinesthetic, visual, auditory, and other disturbing stimuli. The infant can also be observed for the ways he alerts, orients, and attends to cues in his environment.

OVERVIEW OF THE NEONATAL BEHAVIORAL ASSESSMENT SCALE

The Neonatal Behavioral Assessment Scale involves a procedure of examination and testing that results in ratings on twenty-seven items. Each of these twenty-seven items is rated on a nine-point scale corresponding to the nine choices given with each item. The scale also includes ratings on twenty elicited reflexes and movements on a three-point scale.

The scale contains a scoring sheet for the twenty-seven test items, shown on p. 61, on which one indicates the sleep or awake state in which a response is elicited. The numbers in parentheses represent the optimal states for eliciting a reponse. Briefly the states and corresponding numbers are as follows: 1, deep sleep; 2, light sleep; 3, drowsiness or semi-dozing; 4, alertness; 5, high activity level; and 6, intense crying (see p. 66 for further explanation of states).

It is essential that each examiner have a wealth of experience in assessing normal infants against which to establish norms for scoring an infant. For most of the items, the rating scales are arranged so that the midpoint is the mean whereas the two ends of the scale represent deviations from the mean. The mean score is based on the expected behavior of an infant, that is, an "average" 7-pound or more, full-term (40 weeks' gestation), normal, white infant whose mother did not have more than 100 mg of barbiturates for pain or 50 mg of other sedative drugs as premedication in the 4 hours prior to delivery and whose Apgar ratings were no lower than 7-8-8 at 1, 5, and 15 minutes after delivery. To meet assessment criteria, infants should not require special care after delivery and should have had a normal intrauterine

existence. Hydration, nutrition, color, and physiological responses should be given careful consideration. The infant's behavior on the third day is acceptable as the mean.[1]

Twenty elicited reflexes and movements are observed and rated as part of the assessment scale.[*] Scores for reflexes are obtained from a three-point scale corresponding to ratings of hypoactive, normal, and hyperactive.

The twenty elicited reflexes and their scoring criteria are as follows[†]:

X = omitted
O = not able to elicit reflex
L = 1 = low
M = 2 = medium
H = 3 = high
A = asymmetrical response

	X	O	L	M	H	A
Plantar grasp			1	2	3	
Hand grasp			1	2	3	
Ankle clonus			1	2	3	
Babinski			1	2	3	
Standing			1	2	3	
Automatic walking			1	2	3	
Placing			1	2	3	
Incurvation			1	2	3	
Crawling			1	2	3	
Glabella			1	2	3	
Tonic deviation of head and eyes			1	2	3	
Nystagmus			1	2	3	
Tonic neck reflex			1	2	3	
Moro			1	2	3	
Rooting (intensity)			1	2	3	
Sucking (intensity)			1	2	3	
Passive movement						
Arms R			1	2	3	
L			1	2	3	
Legs R			1	2	3	
L			1	2	3	

GENERAL PROCEDURE AND ORDER OF TESTING

To ensure optimal assessment outcomes for each infant, it is recommended that the examination begin when the infant is asleep at a time

---

[*] See Prechtl and Beintema[2] for reference to the reflex to be examined, the infant's state, position of the infant, activity of the examiner, expected response of the infant, recording of observed behaviors, and clinical importance.

[†] From Brazelton, T. Berry: The Neonatal Behavioral Assessment Scale, London, 1973, William Heinemann Ltd., and Philadelphia, 1973, J. B. Lippincott Co., p. 11.

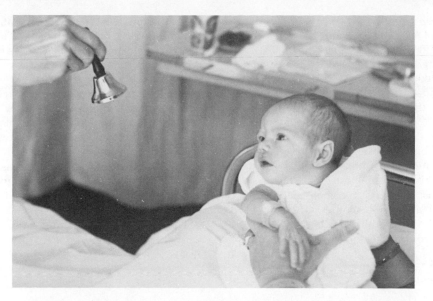

Fig. 3-1. The infant is alerting, and his head and eyes turn to the bell.

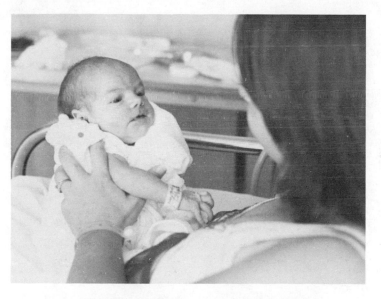

Fig. 3-2. Orientation and head turning to voice and face.

midway between two feedings. Ideally a given order of stimulus presentations is followed, according to the protocol outlined by Brazelton.[1] Brazelton encourages examiners to get into flexible working interaction with the infant to optimize the infant's best performance throughout the entire testing session.

Brazelton also urges that health care professionals who are examining the infant take every opportunity to see how the infant reacts to stress. For example, does he spit up? Does he move his arm and hands up and down? Does he bring his hand to his mouth or suck, hiccough, make mouthing movements, or cry?

The examiner begins by assessing the initial state of the infant for 2 minutes. The state of the infant is then recorded on the scoring sheet.

The initial presentation of a flashlight to the eyes, a rattle to the ears, and a bell to the ears is done while the infant is in a state of 1, 2, or 3.

After these stimuli are presented, the infant is uncovered and his relevant reactions are observed and recorded. While the infant is still quiet, a light pinprick is applied to his foot four times. Ankle clonus, foot grasp, and the Babinski response are then determined before undressing the infant. As the infant is being undressed, he is observed for relevant reactions such as state changes, lability of skin color, and speed of buildup. His general tone is also assessed while being undressed. Passive movements of the infant are rated while he is awake but not disturbed. It is recommended that he be tested for auditory responses to the rattle and bell while in the awake state to determine responses to inanimate, visual, and auditory stimuli (Fig. 3-1). While he is still in the awake state, the infant is then pulled to sit. The next items to assess include the infant's standing, walking, and placing reflexes. After elicitation of these, incurvation, body tone across the examiner's hand, and prone responses of the infant are then assessed. Next the infant is picked up, held, and spun around slowly for vestibular responses and nystagmus. The infant should then be held while assessing his responses to the orientation animate behavioral items. He should systematically be tested for his responses to animate stimulus, visual stimulus, auditory stimulus, and then visual and auditory stimuli in combination (Fig. 3-2).

The most disturbing maneuvers are used last with the infant. The infant is assessed as he reacts to a cloth on the face, in addition to an

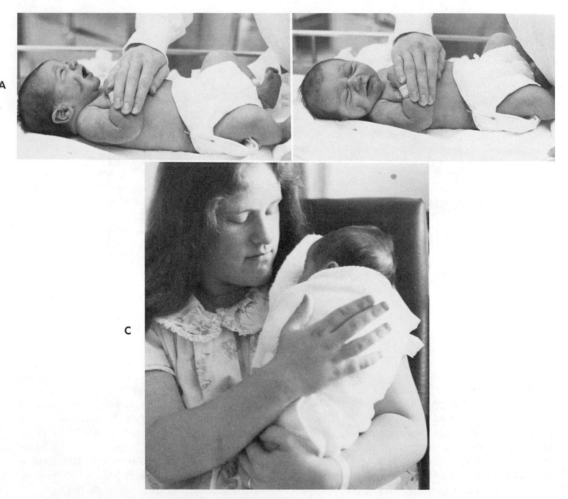

Fig. 3-3. A, Assessing consolability with intervention. The infant is assessed in an upset state. **B,** The infant is responding and crying less when the examiner's hand is placed on arms and abdomen. **C,** The infant is consolable after being picked up, held, and patted.

assessment of the infant's reaction to the elicitation of the tonic neck reflex and the Moro
reflex. The infant's reactions to aversive stimuli
offer an excellent time to observe his graded
attempts to quiet himself.

Whenever the infant becomes upset, the
examiner should wait 15 seconds before intervening with comforting measures. This allows
the infant an opportunity to quiet himself. If no
self-quieting behavior occurs, the examiner
should comfort the infant, using graded measures to quiet him (Fig. 3-3), such as the
examiner placing his face in front of the infant; using both his face and voice; placing his
hand on the infant's abdomen; restraining one
of the infant's arms; restraining both arms;
holding the infant; holding and rocking the infant; and holding, rocking, and talking to the
infant. These are graded estimates of the infant's need for external consoling.

The infant's responses such as hand-to-mouth
movements, tremulousness, amount of startle,
vigor, and amount of activity are observed
throughout the entire examination. In addition,
the number of discrete state changes that occur
are documented.

Conditions for assessment

It is recommended that the infant be observed
and assessed in a quiet, somewhat darkened
room. If these conditions cannot be met, the
disturbing aspects of a noisy, brightly lighted
room or interruptions should be documented as
part of the stimuli to which the infant might be
reacting.[1]

The entire examination usually takes about
20 to 30 minutes. Except for the first four items,
which can be scored immediately by the examiner, most of the items are scored at the conclusion of the testing. Scoring may take from 10
to 15 minutes. Some of the twenty-seven items
are scored during a specific interaction with the
infant, such as his head turning to a voice, but
others are scored according to total continuous
observations that are made throughout the
entire assessment examination. For example,
state changes, color changes, periods of alertness, and peaks of excitement are observed
throughout the examination and are scored at
the conclusion of the examination.

Consideration of sleep and awake states

Because the infant's state of consciousness
is the single most important variable in the behavioral examination, it is carried out within
the framework of the state the infant is in and

the level of arousal that is present or absent.
By consideration of a framework of the infant's
state, another major difference from other assessment tools is clearly appreciated. How the
infant reacts to any of the twenty-seven behavioral items will depend on his corresponding
state at the time he is presented with a stimulus.
An infant is either in a sleep state or an awake
state, according to Prechtl and Beintema.[2] An
infant can meet the criteria for being asleep by
either being in a deep sleep state or a light sleep
state. An infant can meet the criteria for being
in an awake state by either being drowsy, alert,
having his eyes open, or crying. It is important
to take into consideration a range of environmental variables, events, conditions, or changes
that may affect the infant's state. The time that
has lapsed since the infant's last feeding, the
presence of stressful stimuli, the infant's body
position, temperature, lightness, darkness, and
noise levels are examples of environmental
variables that can affect changes in the infant's
state.

Examiner training

All persons who are using the scale should be
trained in the proper administration of test
items, order of examination procedures, optimal
conditions of treating, and method of scoring.
Examiners using the scale should also be
familiar with special considerations that are
included during an assessment of an infant.
Before an examiner can be assured of independent reliable ratings, it is essential that practice
with testing of at least 10 infants be completed.
By practicing with 10 infants an examiner can
be trained to achieve higher interscorer reliability.*

SELECTED ITEMS FROM BRAZELTON NEONATAL BEHAVIORAL ASSESSMENT SCALE

Nine selected items are presented from the
Neonatal Behavioral Assessment Scale. In addition, the neurological component of the examination is considered. The purpose is to acquaint
the reader with behavioral items contained in
the scale, to illustrate the behavioral responses

---

*A list of trained examiners who can provide training
can be obtained by writing directly to the principal
investigator, Brazelton. In addition, four training films
are available for use with the published manual.
These can be obtained by writing to the Educational
Development Corporation, 8 Mifflin Place, Cambridge,
Mass. 02138.

that are scored, and to introduce the method of scoring. These scale items represent only a part of the neonatal assessment scale and are not intended to be a substitute for the Neonatal Behavioral Assessment Scale manual.

Sleep and awake states

Newborns can be observed in different sleep states, which range from deep to lighter sleep states, and different awake states, which range from semidozing to intense crying. According to Brazelton,[1] who refers to Prechtl and Beintema's[2] definitions, there are certain criteria for behavior that if present indicate whether a newborn is in a deep, medium, or light sleep state or which awake state he is in. The criteria for sleep states and awake states are listed as follows:

Sleep states

1. Deep sleep with regular breathing, eyes closed, no spontaneous activity except startles or jerky movements at quite regular intervals; external stimuli produce startles with some delay; suppression of startles is rapid, and state changes are less likely than from other states. No eye movements. . . .

2. Light sleep with eyes closed; rapid eye movements can be observed under closed lids; low activity level, with random movements and startles or startle equivalents; movements are likely to be smoother and more monitored than in state 1; responds to internal and external stimuli with startle equivalents, often with a resulting change of state. Respirations are irregular, sucking movements occur off and on. . . .

Awake states

3. Drowsy or semi-dozing; eyes may be open or closed, eyelids fluttering; activity level variable, with interspersed, mild startles from time to time; reactive to sensory stimuli, but response often delayed; state change after stimulation frequently noted. Movements are usually smooth. . . .

4. Alert, with bright look; seems to focus attention on source of stimulation, such as an object to be sucked or a visual or auditory stimulus; impinging stimuli may break through, but with some delay in response. Motor activity is at a minimum. . . .

5. Eyes open; considerable motor activity, with thrusting movements of the extremities, and even a few spontaneous startles; reactive to external stimulation with increase in startles or motor activity, but discrete reactions difficult to distinguish because of general high activity level.

6. Crying; characterized by intense crying which is difficult to break through with stimulation.*

---

*From Brazelton, T. Berry: The Neonatal Behavioral Assessment Scale, London, 1973, William Heinemann Ltd.; Philadelphia, 1973, J. B. Lippincott Co., pp. 7-8.

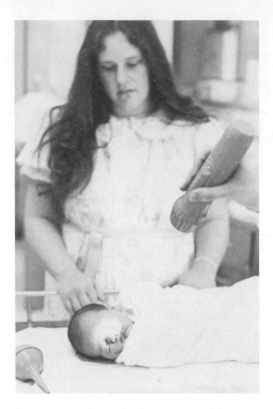

Fig. 3-4. Assessment of infant's response decrement to light with parent observing. Blink reaction of both eyelids is seen.

Response decrement to light (states 1, 2, or 3)

The response decrement to light is an observational item that is important in learning the infant's capacity to shut out disturbing stimuli (Fig. 3-4).

A flashlight is shown briefly to both eyes, in a downward swipe of the flashlight if the baby is on his side or across both eyes with a horizontal movement of the flashlight. The passing of two trials without any observable response is considered criterion for "shutdown." Up to ten stimuli are allowed.

Scoring

1 No diminution in high responses over ten stimuli.

2 Startles delayed; rest of responses still present (*i.e.* body movement, eye blinks, and respiratory changes continue over 10 trials).

3 No startles; other responses, including body movement, still present after 10 trials.

4 No startles; body movement delayed; respiratory changes and blinks continue unchanged over 10 trials.

5 Shutdown of body movements; some diminution

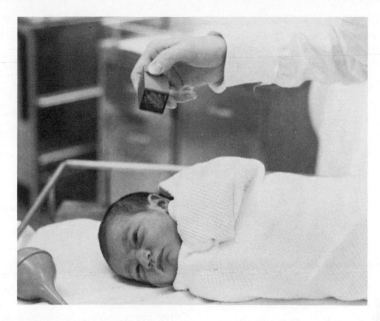

Fig. 3-5. Assessment of infant's response decrement to rattle. The infant is observed as she tries to shut out a disturbing auditory stimulus.

in blinks and respiratory changes after 9-10 stimuli.
6 Shutdown of body movements; some diminution in blinks and respiratory changes after 7-8 stimuli.
7 Shutdown of body movements; some diminution in blinks and respiratory changes after 5-6 stimuli.
8 Shutdown of body movements; some diminution in blinks and respiratory changes after 3-4 stimuli.
9 Shutdown of body movements; some diminution in blinks and respiratory changes after 1-2 stimuli.*

Response decrement to rattle
(states 1, 2, and 3)

The rattle should be presented in a brief and discrete manner (Fig. 3-5). Each sound should be presented 5 seconds after the end of the response to the previous sounds of the rattle. The test should continue until the infant does not make any observable response to two consecutive stimuli.

Scoring
1 No diminution in high responses over 10 stimuli.
2 Startles delayed; rest of responses still present (*i.e.* body movements, eye blinks and respiratory changes continue over 10 trials).

3 Startles no longer present but rest are still present, including body movement in 10 trials.
4 No startles, body movement delayed, respiratory and blinks same in 10 trials.
5 Shutdown of body movements; some diminution in blinks and respiratory changes in 9-10 stimuli.
6 .... in 7-8 stimuli.
7 .... in 5-6 stimuli.
8 .... in 3-4 stimuli.
9 .... in 1-2 stimuli.*

Response decrement to bell
(states 1, 2, and 3)

The bell should be similar to the one used in a standard Gesell test. The sound of the bell should be presented 5 seconds after the end of the response to the previous sound of the bell. The test, like that with the rattle, should continue until the infant has ceased to make any responses to two consecutive stimuli. Only ten stimuli are allowed.

Scoring
1 No diminution in high responses over 10 stimuli.
2 Startles delayed; rest of responses still present (*i.e.* body movements, eye blinks and respiratory changes continue over 10 trials).
3 Startles no longer present but rest are still present, including body movement in 10 trials.

---
*Ibid., p. 13.

---
*Ibid., p. 16.

4 No startles, body movement delayed, respiratory and blinks same in 10 trials.
5 Shutdown of body movements; some diminution in blinks and respiratory changes in 9-10 stimuli.
6 .... in 7-8 stimuli.
7 .... in 5-6 stimuli.
8 .... in 3-4 stimuli.
9 .... in 1-2 stimuli.*

Orientation response—inanimate visual (state 4 only)

Since most neonates will demonstrate some ability to fix on a visual object, a contrasting bright or shiny object (e.g., a bell, red ball, white mask) can be used to assess the newborn's ability to follow it horizontally or vertically (Fig. 3-6). This test is significantly state related and may be repeated under optimal conditions such as a quiet semidark room. Vertical following of the ball is anticipated. When the infant will not attend or follow a red ball in his bassinet, he may be held on the examiner's lap slightly propped up. By holding the infant up on the examiner's shoulder, another examiner can validate the infant's ability to focus, still, follow, follow horizontally, and follow vertically and can note whether head movements are smooth.

*Ibid., p. 16.

Scoring
1 Does not focus on or follow stimulus.
2 Stills with stimulus and brightens.
3 Stills, focuses on stimulus when presented, little spontaneous interest, no following.
4 Stills, focuses on stimulus, follows for 30° arc, jerky movements.
5 Focuses and follows with eyes horizontally for at least a 30° arc. Smooth movement, loses stimulus but finds it again.
6 Follows for 30° arcs with eyes and head. Eye movements are smooth.
7 Follows with eyes and head at least 60° horizontally, maybe briefly vertically, partly continuous movement, loses stimulus occasionally, head turns to follow.
8 Follows with eyes and head 60° horizontally and 30° vertically.
9 Focuses on stimulus and follows with smooth, continuous head movement horizontally, vertically, and in a circle. Follows for 120° arc.*

Orientation response—animate auditory (states 4 and 5)

A useful scale item that helps assess orientation to the environment is that which tests the infant's ability to respond to clues given by others.

*Ibid., p. 19.

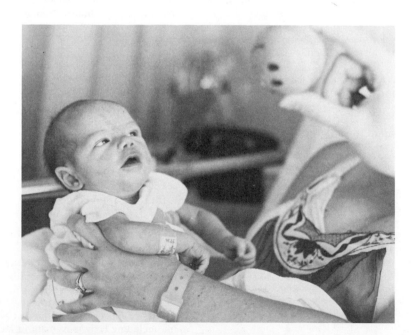

Fig. 3-6. The infant is observed while she follows the ball intently in an alert state. The assessment is being done in front of the infant's mother.

The examiner removes his face from the infant's line of sight and talks to him from one side (6 to 12 inches from the infant's ear). Continuous soft and high-pitched speech is recommended as the best stimulus (Fig. 3-7). Also the examiner should use the infant's name. The examiner should be certain the infant's head is in the midline when he begins to elicit the infant's responses to voice.

Scoring
1 No reaction.
2 Respiratory change or blink only.
3 General quieting as well as blink and respiratory changes.
4 Stills, brightens, no attempt to locate source.
5 Shifting of eyes to sound, as well as stills and brightens.
6 Alerting and shifting of eyes and head turn to source.

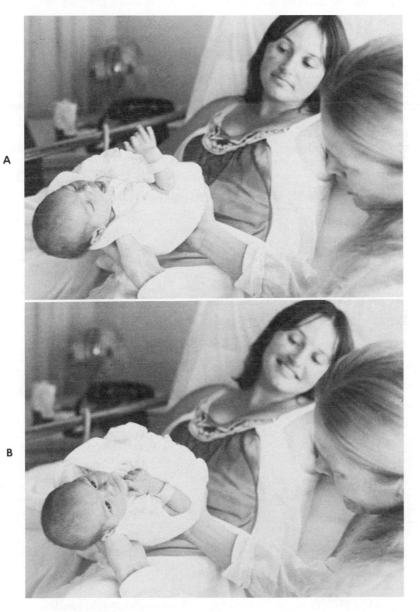

Fig. 3-7. A, The infant is observed as the examiner removes her face from infant's line of sight. **B,** Continuous soft and high-pitched speech is used to elicit prolonged alerting and eye and head turning of the infant to the auditory stimulus. The parent is present during the assessment.

7 Alerting, head turns to stimulus, and search with eyes.
8 Alerting prolonged, head and eyes turn to stimulus repeatedly.
9 Turning and alerting to stimulus presented on both sides on every presentation of stimulus.*

Parents can learn that the newborn is capable of alerting at different times and turns toward a voice as early as 3 days of age. Infants may vary in the degree or intensity of their behaviors in response to a sound, depending on the state they are in.

Alertness (state 4 only)

This scale item assesses the frequency of the best periods of alertness as shown by the baby's responses to the examiner (Fig. 3-8). Any period of alertness is considered part of the infant's capacity for responsiveness. "Alerting" is defined as "brightening and widening of eyes," in contrast to "orientation," which is used to define the response of turning toward the direction of the stimulus.[1]

*Ibid., p. 23.

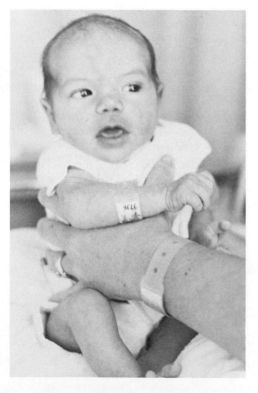

Fig. 3-8. Alertness of the infant. Note the brightening and widening of the eyes.

Scoring
1 Inattentive—rarely or never responsive to direct stimulation.
2 When alert, responsivity brief and generally quite delayed—alerting and orientation very brief and general. Not specific to stimuli.
3 When alert, responsivity brief and somewhat delayed—quality of alertness variable.
4 When alert, responsivity somewhat brief but not generally delayed though variable.
5 When alert, responsivity of moderate duration and response generally not delayed and less variable.
6 When alert, responsivity moderately sustained and not delayed. May use stimulation to come to alert state.
7 When alert, episodes are of generally sustained duration, etc.
8 Always has sustained periods of alertness in best periods. Alerting and orientation frequent and reliable. Stimulation brings infant to alert state and quiets infant.
9 Always alert in best periods. Stimulation always elicits alerting, orientating. Infant reliably uses stimulation to quiet self or maintain quiet state.*

Cuddliness (states 4 and 5)

This is an assessment of the infant's response to being held (Fig. 3-9). The item is used to score the summary of responses to being held in a cuddled position against the examiner's chest and up on his shoulder. The responses can be observed and interpreted to be negative, positive, or none at all.

Scoring
1 Actually resists being held, continuously pushing away, thrashing or stiffening.
2 Resists being held most but not all of the time.
3 Doesn't resist but doesn't participate either, lies passively in arms and against shoulder (like a sack of meal).
4 Eventually moulds into arms, but after a lot of nestling and cuddling by examiner.
5 Usually moulds and relaxes when first held, i.e., nestles head in crook of neck and of elbow of examiner. Turns toward body when held horizontally, on shoulder he seems to lean forward.
6 Always moulds initially with above activity.
7 Always moulds initially with nestling, and turning toward body, and leaning forward.
8 In addition to moulding and relaxing, he nestles and turns head, leans forward on shoulder, fits feet into cavity of other arm, all of body participates.
9 All of the above, and baby grasps hold of the examiner to cling to him.*

*Ibid., p. 25.

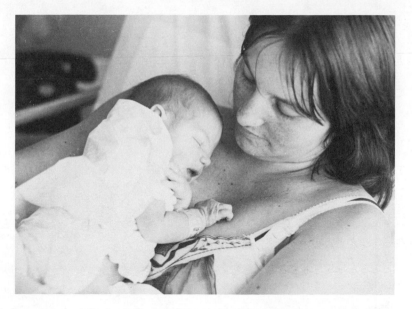

Fig. 3-9. Assessing the infant's response to being held. The mother is attempting to determine the degree of cuddliness of her infant.

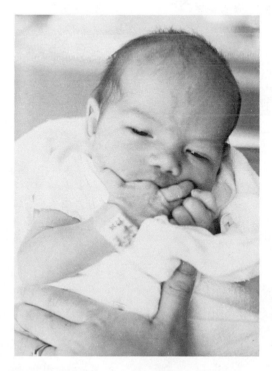

Fig. 3-10. The infant's self-quieting activities are assessed. The infant has brought her fist to her mouth, and fingers are inserted. The infant is sucking vigorously and for prolonged periods.

Self-quieting activity (states 6 and 5 to 4, 3, 2, 1)

This is a measure of the activity that the infant in a fussing state initiates himself and uses in an observable effort to quiet himself (Fig. 3-10). The number of observable activities that he uses is counted. The infant's success is measured by any observable state changes that persist for at least 5 seconds. Activities of the infant that can be counted are (1) hand-to-mouth efforts, (2) sucking on fist or tongue, and (3) the use of visual or auditory stimulus from the environment to quiet himself (more than a simple response is necessary to determine this).

Scoring
1 Cannot quiet self, makes no attempt, and intervention is always necessary.
2 A brief attempt to quiet self (less than 5 secs.) but with no success.
3 Several attempts to quiet self, but with no success.
4 One brief success in quieting self for period of 5 secs. or more.
5 Several brief successes in quieting self.

---

*Ibid., pp. 29-30.

Text continued on p. 77.

Table 3-1. Observing and recording selected newborn reflexes and examining their clinical importance*

Reflex	Infant's state	Position of infant	Activity of examiner	Expected response of infant	Recording observed behaviors	Clinical importance
Plantar grasp	Not important	Supine	Place thumbs against balls of infant's feet near toes	Flexion of all toes at same time	− Absent + Weak and unsustained ++ Good, sustained +++ Very strong	Absent in defects of lower spinal column; observe for asymmetries
Palmar grasp	Optimal in 3 and 4; avoid testing in 1, 2, and 5	Supine; maintain head in midline; arms semiflexed	Place fingers from ulnar side into hands and press palmar surface; do not touch dorsal surface of hands	Flexion of all fingers around examiner's fingers	− Absent + Short, weak flexion ++ Strong and sustained for 10 seconds +++ Sustained grasp with the tip of infant's fingers going white	Observe for difference of intensity between two hands; if no effect, attempt again; sucking movements enhance grasping reflex
Ankle clonus	Not important	Supine	Press both thumbs with rapid, abrupt movement against distal part of soles of feet	Quick dorsiflexion of foot	− Absent + Present	If present, record average number of beats for which it is sustained by eliciting response two or three times
Babinski reflex	Not important	Supine; legs semiflexed	Scratch sole of foot on lateral side starting from toes toward heel; do not rely on pressure alone; be certain scratch occurred	Dorsal flexion of big toe and fanning of smaller toes	− Absent + Weak dorsal flexion and some spreading ++ Good dorsal flexion with marked spreading of toes +++ Sustained dorsal flexion with sustained spreading of toes	Observe for asymmetries; absence suggests defects of lower spinal cord
Placing response	Optimal in 4; avoid testing in 1, 2, and 3	Hold infant with both hands under arms and around chest; support back of head with thumbs	Lift infant so that dorsal part of foot lightly touches protruding edge; avoid eliciting plantar response	Foot lifts up by simultaneous flexion of knees and hips and moves downward	Record left and right foot separately − Absent + Present	Not known at present

Response	Testing note	Position	Procedure	Expected response	Scoring	Comments
Spontaneous crawling and Bauer's response	Optimal in 4 and 5; avoid testing in 1, 2, or 3	Prone	Observe spontaneous activity of baby for 30 seconds; press hands gently on soles of feet determine if this stimulus increases crawling movements forward	Crawling movements forward	− Absent + Weak crawl + + Coordinated crawling movements + + + Locomotion for at least 30 cm occurring within 1 minute Record separately spontaneous and reinforced crawling movements	Crawling is absent in weak or depressed infants
Tonic neck reflex	Optimal in 2 or 3; avoid testing in 1 or 5	Supine suspension	Turn infant's face slowly to right side and hold it in extreme position with jaw over right shoulder; repeat, turning face toward left shoulder	Jaw (face), arm, and leg extend; occipital arm flexes at elbow; responses of lower limbs are more constant than those of upper limbs	Record separately for responses elicited in turning face to right and to left directions − Absent + Sustained response	May be present or absent in newborn; consistently obligate, well-marked tonic neck response may be clue of neurological dysfunction
Recoil of forearm at elbow	Optimal in 3 and 4; do not test during 1 and 2	Symmetrical supine; exclude asymmetrical positions	Examiner passively extends both forearms simultaneously at elbows and releases both at same time	Brisk flexion at both elbows	− Absent + Weak recoil (up to 45-degree angle) + + Marked, quick flexion in both arms (average) + + + Rapid and forceful flexion	Asymmetry should be recorded; asymmetry occurs in hemisyndromes or parents with one arm
Rooting response	Optimal in 3, 4, and 5; avoid testing during 1 and 2	Supine, with head symmetrical in midline and hands above chest	Stroke perioral skin at corners of mouth, upper lip, and lower lip in prescribed sequence; hold baby's hands against his chest with other hand	Directed head turning toward the stimulated side; mouth opens and jaw drops after stimulation of lower lip; baby attempts to suck stimulating finger in each instance	− Absent + Only a weak turn toward stimulated side and grasp with lips + + + Very vigorous turning and grasping	Absent in depressed infants

Continued.

*Modified from Prechtl, Heinz, and Beintema, David L.: The neurological examination of the full-term newborn infant, London, 1965, The Spastics International Medical Publications in association with William Heinemann Ltd., pp. 1-75.

Table 3-1. Observing and recording selected newborn reflexes and examining their clinical importance—cont'd

Reflex	Infant's state	Position of infant	Activity of examiner	Expected response of infant	Recording observed behaviors	Clinical importance
Sucking response	Optimal in 3 and 4; avoid testing in 1 and 2	Supine	Place index finger about 3 or 4 cm into mouth	Rhythmical sucking	Following components are recorded independently of each other: 1. Stripping action of tongue forcing upward and back 2. Rate 3. Amount of suction (negative pressure) 4. Grouping of sucks *First and third components:* − Absent + Low or barely discernible function + + Intermediate range of function; adequate and sufficient performance + + + Exaggerated performance *Second component (record number of sucks per 10 seconds):* − Absent + Up to 8 sucks per 10 seconds + + 9 to 12 sucks per 10 seconds	Sucking is poor (weak, slow, and with short periods) or even absent in apathetic infant; barbiturates seem to depress sucking, and infant may thus be affected if he is being breast-fed and mother is receiving any of these drugs

				+++ More than 12 sucks per 10 seconds *Fourth component:* − Absent + Groups in range of 1 to 6 sucks per group ++ Groups in range of 7 to 14 sucks per group +++ Groups in range of 15 to 30 sucks per group	
Moro response (head drop)	Optimal in 3 and 4; avoid testing in 1 and 2	Symmetrical with arms in front of or beside chest; head in midline	Body is supported by one hand, with other hand and arm supporting back and buttocks; head is held by other hand and then dropped a few centimeters with sudden, rapid, but not too forceful movement; head should be dropped back only at moment when neck muscles are relaxed and head is in midline position; test should be carried out at least 3 times to obtain	Complete Moro reflex consists of abduction of upper limb at shoulder, extension of forearm at elbow, and extension of fingers; subsequently arm at shoulder is abducted; sometimes these movements are preceded by quick flexion of forearm at elbow	Record separately for initial flexion at elbow, abduction at shoulder, extension at elbow, and adduction of upper limbs *Flexion at elbow:* − Absent + Weak, just discernible ++ Fully developed movement *Abduction at shoulder:* − Absent + Only anteflexion at shoulder ++ To about 45-degree angle from trunk +++ To 90-degree angle from trunk *Extension at elbow:* − Absent + To 90-degree angle ++ To about 135-degree angle	Look for asymmetry, which is present in Erb's paresis and clavicular fractures; absent or constantly weak Moro reflex indicates disturbances of central nervous system

Continued.

Table 3-1. Observing and recording selected newborn reflexes and examining their clinical importance—cont'd

Reflex	Infant's state	Position of infant	Activity of examiner	Expected response of infant	Recording observed behaviors	Clinical importance
Moro response (head drop)—cont'd					+++ Full extension of elbow to 180-degree angle *Abduction at shoulder:* − Absent + Half range of abduction ++ Full adduction through range of abduction +++ Across midline Threshold for Moro response should be marked as low (easily elicitable), medium, or high (after five or more trials, only with strong stimuli elicitable); if tremor is present during response, note frequency and amplitude	

6 An attempt to quiet self which results in a sustained successful quieting with the infant returning to state 4 or below.

7 One sustained and several brief successes in quieting self.

8 At least two sustained successes in quieting self.

9 Consistently quiets self for sustained periods.*

Neurological assessment

The neurological component of the examination presented in the Brazelton scale is modeled after the work of Prechtl and Beintema.[2] Guidelines for observing and recording selected newborn reflexes and examining their clinical significance are presented in Table 3-1.

NEED FOR REPEATED ASSESSMENTS

Repeated assessments are of considerably more value than just one assessment completed in the usual 20 or 30 minutes. Repeated assessments for up to 1 month can yield information about the various mechanisms an infant is developing to adapt to his own needs and to the conditions of his particular environment.

VALUE IN PREDICTING BEHAVIORAL OUTCOMES

More recently, the tool is recognized for its value in predicting behavioral outcomes. Findings from a study conducted by Tronick and Brazelton[3] suggest that the Neonatal Behavioral Assessment Scale is an excellent instrument for predicting developmental outcomes in the neonatal period. It is thus viewed as a sensitive instrument for discriminating between abnormal and suspect infants.

The Neonatal Behavioral Assessment Scale has greater value for predicting future behaviors of an infant if it is used in its entirety, than if just parts of the scale are employed, in which case the instrument has diminishing predictive value.

USE OF ASSESSMENT SCALE IN TEACHING PARENTS

The Brazelton assessment tool is considered to be a valuable resource and guideline for teaching mothers and fathers about their newborn's state changes, temperament, and individual behavioral patterns. An individualized approach of interacting with the infant, when to present stimuli, when to refrain from stimulation, when to pick up and console the infant while crying, and when not to pick up and console the infant are among the more practical applications that are inherent in using this assessment tool. Parents can learn effective and easier ways to interact with and to make adjustments to their infants. They can also learn how to consider alternative ways to best meet their newborn's needs.

Parental learning can be facilitated by the continuity of observations made by nursing and medical staff assigned to the same mother-infant pair during a consecutive stay in the maternity setting.

If individual behavioral assessments using the neonatal scale are not feasible, parents can learn about individual differences in infants in a group session. The major points of an infant assessment can be discussed, using one infant for demonstration purposes.

Mothers vary in their degrees of receptiveness to being taught about their infant's responses to different stimuli. Mothers are amenable and receptive to teaching according to their own needs. It is recognized that there are time periods in which each mother's ability, interest, and responsivity to learn are at higher peaks. This should be taken into consideration when encouraging the mother to verbalize, express, and communicate her perceptions, attitudes, and feelings about her infant's behavior and needs.

It is important that parents learn that the newborn is capable of alerting at different times and turns toward a voice as early as 3 days. Infants may vary in the degree or intensity of their behaviors in response to a sound, depending on the state they are in.

The alertness scale is impressive in that it can help orient the parents to the periods of time in which an infant may be processing information. The infant's alert periods may be the best times to interact with the infant, to present animate or inanimate stimuli, or to encourage more optimal parent-infant interactions.

Parents can be informed that the assessment scale helps structure ways of watching how the infant feeds back cues to his environment that will either encourage or discourage the parents or others to increase or to decrease their responsiveness toward the infant.

The assessment scale is also useful for parents to observe the variety of ways that the infant begins to orient to his environment and interact with it, how he shows beginning signs of attach-

---

*Ibid., p. 41.

ment behavior, and the cues he gives that influence the early mother-infant acquaintance process.

If a mother perceives her baby as not being cuddly, she may need to know that the infant's cuddliness is uniformly the same with other caregivers. The mother can make systematic observations about how she has identified her infant's cuddliness and be encouraged to discuss it in a way helpful to her.

An objective rating of a newborn's response to being held by the mother can be useful, particularly if the mother experiences disappointment with consistent noncuddling behaviors. The mother can be assisted in exploring her reaction and expectations and can be encouraged in learning that it is the newborn's individuality that causes its behavior and that the infant is not necessarily rejecting her.

Parents could profit from knowing specifically what external events trigger certain responses in their baby and also how external stimuli can be used to generate easier and more pleasant interactions between their infants and themselves. Parents can learn more effective uses of their voices, and the value of touch, position of the baby, and consoling in graduated degrees to obtain the most favorable responses from their infant. At the same time, they can learn to perceive themselves as significant resource persons who can alter certain behaviors and help the infant to gain mastery of and experience greater amounts of positive input from their early environment.

The emphasis of the assessment scale is on the infant and his neurological status, motor behaviors, states, and interactions with the environment. The implications, however, for teaching, counseling, reassuring, talking with, listening to, and providing appropriate responses to parents' questions during the early acquaintance process are equally as significant an aspect of the assessment tool. A mother who learns, for example, that her newborn typically does not cuddle with nursery personnel or others can learn to verbalize and express her disappointment with this single behavior alone instead of continuing to think her baby does not like her. The nurse or physician can facilitate a better understanding and promote healthier, more appropriate interactions between mother and infant, between father and infant, and among parents, infants, and professional care providers in a hospital setting or at home.

IMPLICATIONS FOR IMPROVING QUALITY OF CARE OF INFANTS

Parents can be helped to consider more effective measures to use in responding to or interacting with their infants. Results of the assessment can provide parents with confidence about what to expect from an infant, which in turn can help parents find the most suitable responses to their infant. The assessment scale helps make child care professionals more sensitive to an infant and his parents. By using the scale a child care professional is no longer a passive caregiver but a responsible one with relevant, applicable knowledge. Although the use of the scale may add more responsibility to caregiving, at the same time it takes the care provider "off the hook" because there is more certainty about what to expect from an infant.

Parents and the child care professional can explore together the best ways to respond to an infant's changes in sleep or awake states and his crying and ways to promote optimal parent-infant interactions.

This assessment tool is extremely appealing to personnel in newborn settings because of its usefulness in the early discovery, prevention, and management of concerns or problems that can occur between the mother and newborn as early as the first few days and up to the fourth week of life.

The nurse or physician can utilize findings about the infant's consolability, habituation to light and sound, attention to animate and inanimate stimuli, ability to cuddle, and responses to aversive stimuli in ways that enhance the infant's care. The data obtained can be helpful in providing an environment that meets the infant's special needs. In addition, these findings help the nurse or physician to communicate more effectively about each newborn with his parents.

The Brazelton tool can serve as an adjunct in effective modeling for parents, for teaching parents, for imparting information, and for helping parents perceive themselves as the most significant resources for the maximal well-being of their infant.

Parents require input about the infant's characteristics and a number of opportunities to discuss how they feel about how they are doing, whether they feel adequate in how they are responding in their various new roles, and what expectations they have for themselves. Mothers especially need specific, objective feedback about how they are responding to their infant in interactions such as feeding, holding, attempting to comfort, placing the infant to sleep, and giving his routine bath.

Parents also need to talk about how they view the infant's behaviors. What significance does it have for them? Many parents may respond with anger if they cannot meet an infant's needs or do not know what to do. This must be explored. Parents' frustrations and the ways they have elected to initiate changes in interactions with their infant are important topics for discussion. They may need assistance to rid themselves of the idea that it is their fault and that their infant is simply reacting to their poor parenting. They may need to gain perspective on their own resourcefulness for coping effectively with their infant's unique needs.

If a mother asks how to handle an infant who is not alert, is fussy, is not cuddly, "sleeps all the time," pushes her away, resists being held, or cries a lot, it is important that her concerns be acknowledged as valid. The steps involved in helping the mother to become more comfortable and able to generate more effective approaches with an infant begin with asking her to share her observations.

The mother can then be asked what she thinks is most important to change first, that is, what her first specific goal is. She can be reminded that she cannot change the entire infant, but alterations in her responses can occur, and the environment can be changed.

Sometimes the mother finds it valuable to keep records of her infant's behavior throughout the day so that she has concrete data for reference in regard to amount, frequency, and duration of sleep times; how often the infant is fed; and how many times the mother consoles and for what and what works best for her. Could she simply talk to the infant instead of picking him up, rocking, and feeding? To what extremes does the mother go in consoling? Has she observed that the infant has his own style and behaviors for self-quieting? Does she interact during the infant's alert periods?

Many parents find it helpful to be oriented to the positive features of their infants. They also need to be reinforced for their own effective parenting behaviors. It is important to state the infant's assets repeatedly and then ask the parents if they agree with these positive descriptions. The mother may need to explore what is easiest for her to do, whether it is consoling, feeding, quieting, or settling her infant down.

The mother should be questioned about what she considers positive about her infant's behaviors and activities that she has observed. A quiet infant may be positive and appealing to one mother, whereas an alert infant may not create the same feelings. What the mother considers positive or negative may vary with how the examiner imparts his perception of the infant. Following are some salient questions for consideration: What has the mother observed so far about her infant in its ability to shut out disturbing stimuli? When is the infant most likely to be awake? What position does the infant like to be held in? What position does the mother prefer for holding the infant? Has the mother noticed the baby smiling? Does the infant fall asleep before, during, or after feeding? Does the mother have to spend all her time trying to keep the infant awake? Does she talk to the infant? Does he turn toward her? Do his eyes fix on her eyes or her face? Does he cuddle next to her? How long does the infant seem to be alert to his surroundings? What does the mother like best about her ways of interacting with the infant? Can she tell when the infant's needs are different?

It is recommended that the Neonatal Behavioral Assessment Scale be used more than once before the mother and infant are discharged home.

It is especially useful for the examiner to take time out and share systematic observations that have been generated within the structured observation period while using the Brazelton tool. The examiner can effectively communicate and share with the mother and father the appealing, attractive traits they have observed about an infant.

Those using the tool are urged to share with parents just where the infant is in his development. Parents need to know both the strengths as well as the deficits of the infant so that parents do not end up believing that everyone else sees the assets or deficits but them. Those items that the infant is lagging in can be presented to the parents in a way that creates a realistic challenge for improvement for the infant.

The amount of state changes a baby consistently is observed to show may directly influence the attitudes, perceptions, and feelings that a caretaker might develop in response to these changes. The infant's state changes also evoke differences, adjustments, or adaptations on the part of the caregiver. If an infant consistently remains in lower states and the caregiver expects more alertness, special attention may be required to learn the best times and ways to present stimuli to which a certain infant will respond. The infant may need more stimulation according to his own temperament and receptivity to stimuli.

An infant who changes rapidly from one state to another may produce frustration for his caregivers. The parent, nurse, or physician may need observational data to substantiate frequent state changes. It is important that parents effectively communicate any frustrations they have in dealing with the infant, since these may affect the infant's response patterns. Parents may require special assurance that the infant's state is unique to the infant and is not necessarily the result of parental inadequacies. Parents' resourcefulness in responding more effectively to an infant's state changes can be acknowledged.

It is increasingly helpful for parents to learn to identify their infant's states to plan interactions, activities, and events in a way that is best suited to the unique needs of an infant.

A mother, for example, may find it disappointing and frustrating and may begin to believe she has failed in her early mothering capacities if she cannot successfully feed a newborn as she expected to during the infant's first 2 to 3 days of life. One variable that may be affecting the infant's capacity, ability, or efforts to maintain vigorous sucking on a nipple may be that he is in a sleep state of 1 or 2 and needs extra stimulation from the mother, or she needs to wait until he reaches an increased level of alertness to respond to her efforts at introducing formula or attempts to breast-feed. It is also important that feeding be delayed until an increased level of alertness has been reached so that the infant has more optimal chances of coordinated sucking movements of tongue with lip and mouth movements.

An infant who has a tendency to stay or return to a lowered sleep state may need extra stimulation at different periods throughout the day. Usually the mother is the best judge of his needs for extra stimulation, particularly if he falls off to sleep when she is attempting to get his attention, to get his eyes to focus on hers, or to get him to follow her eyes with eye tracking and stimultaneous head turning. Extra stimulation can be provided by the mother in ways that she judges best such as unwrapping him, touching his feet, or moving him into a different position. Some infants are drowsy by nature, and the

mother needs to express how she views this behavior, what it means to her, how frustrating it is, and what she has already thought of to obtain maximal responses while the infant is awake, how to keep him awake, what stimulation to provide him with to keep his attention focused, and how to reinforce an optimal learning state.

Parents of an infant who cannot shut out disturbing stimuli also require opportunities to discuss problem solving, their views of the infant's behavior, and their alternatives in caring for the infant. In addition, parents' choices in facilitating the infant's adjustments should be acknowledged.

Both parents and infants can benefit from discussions about infant crying. Data about crying can be shared with parents. It is helpful to discuss the significance of an individual newborn's cry pattern with parents in an effort to help them distinguish differences between pain, distress, hunger, fretfulness, and illness or danger. Sometimes parents need to know that their infant cries before he leaves the hospital environment. A mother might think that other infants cry in the nursery but not her infant. If an infant is reported to be "crying all the time," the mother may find it difficult to console the infant when he is crying. The mother may begin to feel frustrated that there is little she can do or, worse yet, believe that she is the cause of the crying. The mother might say the only time the baby is not crying is when he is asleep or feeding.

This mother can learn that she can use graduated approaches to help the infant console himself. First, she can talk to him gently. Next she can place her hands on his hands and across his chest or place both arms across his chest. If she finds that undressing produces crying, she can avoid complete undressing at times. If face and voice, hands on the abdomen, and swaddling with blankets are not effective after she has waited 15 to 20 seconds for the measures to work, she can pick up the baby, hold him, rock him gently, and, lastly, offer him a pacifier. Some infants have learned ways to console themselves and need not be picked up from the crib the minute they begin to fuss, fret, or cry. The mother can learn to allow the infant to cry before actual picking up occurs. The mother might discover that he consoles himself when held in a certain position

If continuous, high, shrieking, piercing crying continues and none of these measures seems to work, medical consultation should be considered. Sometimes mothers express the belief that the infant does not like them and is showing it by his continuous crying. Most mothers need reassurance that the crying is a facet of the baby's unique personality or, perhaps, illness.

IMPACT OF THE NEONATAL BEHAVIORAL ASSESSMENT SCALE ON THE FIELD OF CHILD DEVELOPMENT

The availability of the Brazelton Neonatal Behavioral Assessment Scale has created worldwide implications for testing infants. Its reliability is known, and its predictive ability for identifying infants at risk has been established. The scale has vast implications for use in transcultural settings. Its major implications seem to be those which focus on giving parents and children a head start interacting with each other in more optimal ways. Most parents want to provide the best care environment possible for their infant, as long as they know what to expect. The Neonatal Behavioral Assessment Scale assists parents in the early acquaintance process with their infants. The Brazelton tool enables child care professionals to promote the quality of early care for all infants. It assists in the detection of infants at risk in their early development and can be used to assess special groups at risk such as infants who are heavily medicated, infants of low birth weight, and premature infants.

As a result of this scale, many myths about early child development have been replaced by scientific observations that can be accurately applied to produce innovative services in preventive health care. The results of Brazelton's research have the potential to revitalize those efforts and early care practices that will truly promote and ensure optimal services, which henceforth have only been an ideal. The chances to implement measures that will promote the maximal well-being of the newborn as he adapts to the extrauterine environment are now available. Brazelton's work has just begun to have an impact around the world; new ideas on early prevention abound, and creativity in the care of the infant and parents is an increasingly central issue in newborn and maternity settings.

REFERENCES

1. Brazelton, T. Berry: The Neonatal Behavioral Assessment Scale, London, 1973, William Heinemann Ltd., and Philadelphia, 1973, J. B. Lippincott Co.
2. Prechtl, Heinz, and Beintema, David L.: The neurological examination of the full-term newborn infant, London, 1965, The Spastics International Medical Publications in association with William Heinemann Ltd.
3. Tronick, Edward, and Brazelton, T. Berry: Clinical uses of the Brazelton neonatal assessment. In Friedlander, E. Z., editor: Exceptional infant: assessment and intervention, vol. 3, New York, 1975, Brunner/Mazel, Inc.

4

ASSESSMENT OF MATERNAL PERCEPTIONS OF INFANTS

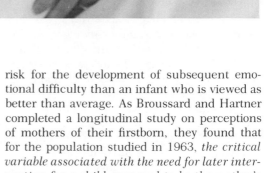

The Neonatal Perception Inventory (NPI) is a significant screening tool with numerous implications for the early interactional patterns occurring between mothers and their children. The NPI, developed by Dr. Elsie Broussard, is aimed at promoting the mental health of both the newborn and his mother and is designed as an early case finding tool that can detect potential disturbances in a child's developmental course, thus acting as a significant instrument of prevention.[1]

Broussard became convinced that detection of potential problems of infants before their development provides an opportunity for early preventive intervention, thus providing more children a better chance for healthy development during the most important and formative periods in their lives. It is for this reason that Broussard and Hartner[2] carried out a longitudinal study of mothers and infants to ensure a method of early screening, diagnosis, and intervention of children considered to be at risk in their development.

Broussard developed a conviction growing out of years of experience in observing mothers and children, a conviction that increasingly is supported by a steadily growing body of empirical evidence. This conviction is simply that an infant who is not perceived by his mother as being better than average is at much higher risk for the development of subsequent emotional difficulty than an infant who is viewed as better than average. As Broussard and Hartner completed a longitudinal study on perceptions of mothers of their firstborn, they found that for the population studied in 1963, *the critical variable associated with the need for later intervention for a child appeared to be the mother's perception of her infant at 1 month of age.*

While designing the NPI, Broussard gave consideration to a number of factors that affect the perception a mother has toward her infant. The mother's perception is based on such factors as how the mother feels about herself, which is influenced by the quality of the mothering that she herself received. Perception is also based on her total life experiences, as well as cultural values. It is Broussard's opinion that "for optimal mothering to occur it is essential that the mother be able to idealize her newborn infant to a certain extent."* Broussard pointed out that "In our culture, great emphasis is placed on 'being better than average'."† Hence

---

*From Broussard, Elsie R.: Personal communication, Feb., 1976.

†From Broussard, Elsie R., and Hartner, Miriam Sergay: Further considerations regarding maternal perception of the first born. In Hellmuth, Jerome, editor: Exceptional infant: studies in abnormalities, vol. 2, New York, 1971, Brunner/Mazel, Inc., p. 434.

"the choice of the average infant to serve as a comparison against her own infant was selected as a societal value which was thought to be universally used by parents. The concept of the average infant was also used as a method for tapping the mother's unconscious fantasies regarding her newborn."*

Broussard and Hartner have endeavored to make use of the findings from their study in their teaching, in the clinical supervision of psychiatrists and members of other caregiving disciplines, and in guiding child care professionals as they work with mothers, infants, and families.

Now it remains to discuss in more depth the NPI, its salient findings, and implications for child care professionals to intervene and provide services when mothers do not rate their infants as better than average.

THE MATERNAL-INFANT ACQUAINTANCE PROCESS

The NPI was developed by Broussard on the premise that for a short period of time after the birth of an infant, the development of optimal mother-infant interactions is vulnerable because of the lasting influence the mother's initial perception has on her subsequent parenting of her child. The tool was designed on the premise that as early as birth, an acquaintance process between a mother and her infant begins. This process of acquaintance forms the basis of subsequent interpersonal behaviors between mother and child. The ways that the mother interacts with her infant will be influenced by her perceptions of the infant's appearance and behaviors. The infant's behavior will then be influenced by the way the mother interacts and handles the infant.

From the mother's point of view, how she relates to her infant is based on a number and variety of perceptions of the infant. After delivery, each mother, particularly the first-time mother, is attempting to discover what her infant is really like and simultaneously how the infant feels about her; thus the mother begins to initiate or maintain feelings, attitudes, and perceptions of her infant.

Two often conflicting forces are at play that influence the mother's perception of her infant. The first is the mother's initial reaction to her infant's temperament, behaviors, and physical appearance. The second and perhaps more rigid and bothersome is the mother's hopes and fears, which have tempered her preconception of what her infant should be like. This preconception is in a large part influenced by the socially valued "special" or "better-than-average" individual.

All these factors then influence the complex beginnings of interrelationships and the maternal-infant acquaintance process, in which two strangers are vulnerable while they get to know each other. The early perceptions and behaviors of a mother and infant can set the stage for future relationships by serving as a framework for the beginning of positive, nurturing interactions, or for the start of inappropriate and conflictual interpersonal interactions.

The initial reaction of a mother to her infant can be influenced by a variety of infant behaviors and interactions with her. For example, an infant who is generally content and seldom cries, has generally consistent behavioral responses, has usually predictable physiological functions, is not perceived as a problem eater (Fig. 4-1), and does not sleep all the time or stay

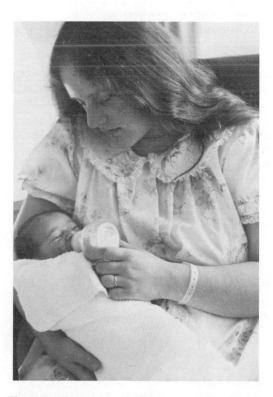

Fig. 4-1. The mother is asked to rate how much trouble she thinks her infant has in feeding at 3 days of age.

---

*From Broussard, Elsie R.: Personal communication, Feb., 1976.

awake for too long either so that the mother finds it rewarding to interact with the infant during his alert periods is more likely to be perceived by his mother in more positive ways. Any behavior can be perceived in a variety of ways, depending on when and where it occurs and what influenced its occurrence. For example, an infant who is in a deep sleep state during an expected feeding time and is difficult to awaken may be viewed by his mother as rejecting or not interested in her. However, the same infant may be viewed as content and pleasing if he goes into a deep sleep state after feeding.[3] An infant who does not cuddle consistently, cries when touched, vomits frequently, or refuses to suck because of sleepiness or other reasons can cause a mother to believe that her infant dislikes her.

As Kennedy[3] describes it, a positive maternal-infant acquaintance process is more probable when the mother is able to learn about the unique features and traits that make her infant an individual. Once a positive orientation begins, there is a greater likelihood for it to continue.

DEVELOPMENT OF THE NPI

In 1963 a longitudinal study was initiated by Broussard[1] for the purpose of identifying the interrelationship between the first-time mother's initial perceptions of her infant and the child's subsequent emotional developmental profile four and one half years later.

In keeping with the purposes of her doctoral dissertation, Broussard[1] developed the Your Baby and the Average Baby Perception Inventories. These inventories were designed to measure the mother's perceptions of her infant as compared to her concept of the average infant on six behavioral items, which include crying, spitting, feeding, elimination, sleeping, and predictability.

The long-term study phase began by asking 318 primiparas who delivered normal full-term infants to rate their babies at 1 to 2 days postpartum. At this first rating (Time I) they were asked to rate both the average baby and their own baby. On the second rating a month later (Time II), mothers of these same infants were asked to fill out the two inventories again. They also were asked to fill out another form that was designed to measure the degree of bother of an infant's behavior. The Degree of Bother Inventory assesses to what extent the six infant behaviors are perceived as problematic.

Results of study

The total scores for the 318 Your Baby and Average Baby Perception Inventories were examined to determine if mothers rated their infants as better than, less than, or the same as the average infant.

At the first rating on day 1 or 2 postpartum, it was found that 46.5% of the mothers rated their infants as better than average. The second rating by the mothers took place at 1 month of age. It was found that of the 318 women, 61.2% rated their infants as better than average, 13.2% rated their infants as equal to the average, and 25.6% rated their infants as less than the average baby.[4]

To test the hypothesis that the mother's perception of her 1-month-old infant was associated with the child's subsequent emotional development, Broussard[4] divided the original sample into two groups of high-risk and low-risk infants. The low-risk infants were those whose mothers had rated them as better than average at the end of 1 month. Those infants who had not been rated as better than average at 1 month comprised the high-risk sample, who were at risk for their later emotional development. Findings from the study suggest that almost 40% of the mothers had in all probability commenced unsatisfactory interactions with their infants.

The hypothesis that the mother's perception of her 1-month-old infant was associated with the child's emotional development was first tested when 85 of the original population of firstborns were assessed at 4½ years of age. When the 85 children were assessed independently by a clinician who did not know the original ratings of the children, 60% were diagnosed as having healthy responses. It is notable that 66% of the children originally rated as high risk were evaluated as needing intervention, whereas 20.4% of the children originally rated as low risk were found to be in need of therapy.

The proportion of children judged to be at high risk (not rated as better than average) in the original study and in the follow-up study four and one half years later was almost identical. The crucial variable associated most heavily with a child's later developmental or emotional problems correlated most highly with the mother's rating at 1 month, according to Broussard.[4] Thus the NPI shows predictive value for infants at high risk for later developmental problems.

Implications for an infant who is not perceived as better than average

One of the major considerations derived from the study centers around determining the implications for the infant of the mother who does not see her infant as better than average, who has a negative orientation to him, or who considers the infant as better than he is in the nursery setting. If the mother views the infant as not better than average, she may be inclined to treat him as less than average, and the infant's special and unique needs may go unmet. The infant may suffer from lack of the maternal attention he needs.§

Traditional concepts of what an infant is like, although they have been disproved, may also have a negative influence on the way a mother perceives her infant. If a mother does not think her infant will see, hear, or recognize another person until 6 months of age, the mother may not encourage or nurture more advanced behaviors. She may lose interest in the infant who, as a result, may not receive adequate, individualized sensory input, varied kinesthetic experiences, or enough predictable stimuli to encourage maturation, integration, and organization of the central nervous system. Thus cognition may not be activated regularly in an automatic way. This deprivation of the necessary and basic elements of kinesthetic, motor, and other sensory inputs may result in the infant's lack of progress in gaining mastery of himself and his environment, gaining in fine and gross motor skills, gradually advancing in personal-social skills, learning the pleasures of language development, and communicating in simple to more complex ways.§

At the same time the infant is being deprived, the mother may be suffering from feelings of inadequacy about her parenting behaviors, feel trapped, lose hope, and experience guilt and depression. The mother also may not be able to find alternative ways to respond to her infant that are advantageous to both of them in their early interactional patterns.§

A mother who does not rate an infant as better than average at 2 or 3 days of age and again at 1 month may in fact be asking for help for herself, although not on a conscious level. Her ratings for the infant are merely one indication that she too might be vulnerable; she may not perceive herself as adequate or competent. She may be overwhelmed or may be showing a number of signs that indicate a temporary inability to cope with the stress of parenting a new infant.§

In an as yet unpublished study, Broussard selected another population of 281 full-term, normal, healthy, firstborn infants in 1973. Based on the administration of the NPI, she identified a population at high risk and developed a pilot preventive program for infants at high risk. On the basis of her intensive clinical work with this population, she reports that "the mothers of infants at high risk seem to have very low self-esteem, lack confidence in themselves as individuals and as mothers, and have difficulty in understanding the infant's cues and responding to the infant's needs."*

Questions can be raised such as does the mother's low self-esteem precipitate a lack of self-confidence in responding to her infant? Does this low self-esteem encourage the mother to become more dependent on others around her? Can the mother ultimately learn to make optimum use of resources available to her?[5]

If a mother does not view herself as adequate, having strengths, being capable of changing from negative to positive behaviors, having other alternatives, or being the best resource for her infant, she may have a difficult time generating and maintaining appropriate and gratifying maternal behaviors toward her infant. Most mothers need to know and be supported for the fact that parenting is not easy the first time. The mother's behaviors may also be influenced by perceptions and attitudes she had of herself before the birth of her infant. It may not be easy for a new mother to see herself with strengths and as having the important assets of a woman, mother, and unique person. The mother can be helped to discover these important aspects about herself as she interacts with her new infant. Just as the mother's strengths need reinforcement, so do the infant's strengths need attention.§

Implications of study for child care professionals

Broussard and Hartner's[2] findings have implications for professionals in child health care.

§This symbol will appear throughout this chapter to indicate those ideas that were stimulated by the findings of Broussard's 1963 study.

*From Broussard, Elsie R.: Personal communication, Feb., 1976.

Essentially they need to be sensitive to what mothers are experiencing and remain in tune with the way mothers are receiving child care professionals' communications to them.[5] A non-judgmental attitude is critical if change in a mother's perception about her infant is to occur.

Parents usually know when problems exist between their infants and themselves, but they may need professional confirmation and permission to get help for themselves and their child so that the problems can be resolved. For this reason, continued surveillance by child care professionals is vital for intervention and collaborative efforts with the family.

The occurrence of an infant being rated as not better than average requires evaluation and action. Health care professionals must use their knowledge of the infant's development and their understanding of the parents and other possible family problems to make an assessment. Physicians, nurses, and those of other disciplines can evaluate the need for intervention and alternative means of helping the parent and infant. Health care professionals must abandon their optimistic tendency of believing that problems will disappear and that the child will outgrow any particular problems. As a result of Broussard and Hartner's 1963 longitudinal study, there is the suggestion that continued, prolonged, or repeated stress in parent-infant relationships due to parental perceptions can result in irreversible damage to the child. Stress in the parenting process inevitably leads to an interference with the child's capacity to learn and to develop sensorimotor skills, a sense of competence, and a capacity to relate to others in mutually satisfying interactions.§

Planning suitable interventions for mothers and infants

There are numerous and various models for interventions with mothers who do not perceive their infants as better than average.*

The infant's unique strengths deserve attention and need to be made concrete and visible to the mother in an empathetic and supportive way. The mother may benefit from an active listener who can help her sort out her concerns about herself and the infant. It is crucial that a mother begin to experience a positive orienta-

tion, to express positive attitudes, and to eventually express positive feelings about the infant's unique features.§

The mother might be receptive to differentiating positive features such as when the infant eats the best and most and when he prefers to eat. Any positive features of the infant that are pointed out by the mother can be reinforced and accentuated repeatedly. A mother may need reassurance that although a few activities did not get off to the start she had hoped, she has been able to work through her disappointments and her infant really does like her as is evident from the many positive ways he responds to her. A child care professional can remain sensitive to the mother's responses to positive comments about her infant in attempting to reverse the negative perceptions that exist. The mother may need to hear many favorable comments about her infant to help reorient herself to a new positive perspective of her infant. A mother may need reassurance on a continuing basis that the infant's behaviors which she considers most negative are temporary and transitory until the infant can adapt to his new environment. The mother may need a great deal of positive reinforcement from others that she alone is responsible for the positive changes that are occurring in the mother-infant acquaintance process. Her adeptness at problem solving, creativity, and approaches in promoting change in herself and her infant require affirmation to reinforce her continued efforts to maintain positive aspects of the mother-infant relationship.§

Mothers should probably be viewed as vulnerable if they rate their infants as not better than average. In a sense, they are asking for support because few mothers find it gratifying to perceive their infants as not better than average.§

Prompt intervention that is planned to meet a mother's needs and to help in her interactions with her infant on an ongoing basis may bring a resolution of stress and disturbances in the early mother-infant relationship, whereas failure to intervene may lead to irreversible changes for the mother and child. If a mother rates her infant as not better than average, it is a red flag to find out specifically what is disappointing her. A beginning point for intervention is consideration of the following salient questions: Is the problem the infant? What did she expect the infant to be like? Do the infant's physical features correspond to her expectations? To what degree do they differ? Is the infant 100% dif-

---

*It is important to note at this point that a mother would not be told the actual score her infant received from the NPI.

ferent than what she expected or only slightly different? What has she observed to be the most attractive features of the infant so far? What is the least appealing observation she has made? Elicit exact behavioral descriptions from the mother that give an accurate, clear picture of what she is seeing or perceiving. Can the mother talk about how disappointed she is and the fact that she is frustrated or discouraged? Would she like to discuss how she thinks the infant will develop? What is her principal worry? What does she think the infant will need most from her? What bothers her the most? What bothers her the least? Does she think the infant will change? What will change? When will it change? Where will it change? How does she think she will respond to a new change if it occurs?§

The discovery by observation and discussion that a mother is not capable of interacting optimally with her infant may suggest the need for using other care providers to meet the infant's needs. Broussard has used a specific technique of supplementary parenting through mother-infant group meetings with home visitation. As Broussard views it, supplementary parenting is valuable for the purpose of keeping the relationship of the primary mother and infant intact while supplementary parenting is provided. This technique takes place during group sessions and is carried out in a noncompetitive manner during the time the primary mother cannot meet the needs of her infant in a satisfactory manner. At the same time that supplementary parenting for the infant occurs, it provides an opportunity for helping the mother with her depression and poor self-esteem.[5] Broussard points out that "if professionals are to help mothers and infants in more effective ways, it is essential to be perceptive and aware of not just where the child is, but where the parent is developmentally—to be able to identify where the gaps were in the parents' own experiences with being parented and then provide assistance in these areas."[*] If optimal intervention is planned for the mother with a focus on her needs, there is a better chance she can meet her infant's needs later. Professionals can practice being more sensitive to the needs of mothers at difficult times and can learn to refrain from conveying to the mother that there is either something wrong with her or her infant.

---

*From Broussard, Elsie R.: Personal communication, Feb., 1976.

Regardless of the source of support or intervention, it is important that the mother begin to rely on her own values as she experiences them rather than on values imposed on her by others. It is vital that the mother learn to trust her own feelings more, accept them, and take responsibility for these feelings. An objective of significance for the parenting process now and in the future is the mother learning to trust herself and her infant and to accept change in both herself and her infant.[5] Child care professionals can reinforce a mother's appropriate, supportive responses to an infant. Critical approaches by health care professionals might lead to a further reduced self-esteem of the mother. A consistent, empathetic attitude toward the mother can be valuable when used with noncritical attitudes toward her behaviors and actions. Professionals can make themselves available to meet the mother's needs in a group setting in which the focus is the mother and her immediate feelings and needs.[5]

Such contacts with other mothers may give the mother a sense that there is continued interest in and concern for her. This in turn may help reduce the mother's feelings of self-blame or blame by the helping disciplines and thus permit her to use resources more effectively.

More emphasis can be placed on the mother's self-esteem before delivery.[5] It is important to find out what preparation she has made for the newborn. The mother's state of mind, emotional state, and fantasy levels can be determined, with this information as a baseline for preventive planning with the mother.

THE NPI

The major reasons for using the NPI are to determine a mother's baseline perceptions, determine priorities for intervention, and ensure that early preventive measures are implemented so that healthy, growth-fostering interactions are possible for both infant and mother, even though some beginning steps in the acquaintance process are commenced in less than optimal ways.

Administering the NPI

The NPI is easily and quickly administered by telling the mother the following: "We are interested in learning more about the experiences of mothers and their babies during the first few weeks after delivery. The more we can learn about mothers and their babies, the better we will be able to help other mothers with their

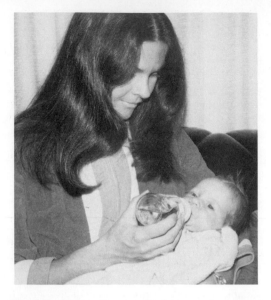

Fig. 4-2. The mother is asked to rate how much trouble she thinks her infant has in feeding at 1 month of age.

babies. We would appreciate it if you would help other mothers by answering a few questions."*

The procedures are identical for administering the Average Baby form of the NPI on the first or second postpartum day and the NPI at 1 month of age. The mother is handed the Average Baby form, shown on p. 89, while the individual administering the inventory says the following: "Although this is your first baby, you probably have some ideas of what most little babies are like. Will you please check the blank you *think* best describes what *most* little babies are like."*

The examiner, who remains with the mother during the entire procedure, waits until the mother has completed the Average Baby form, takes it from the mother, and then hands the mother the Your Baby form.

The procedure for administering the Your Baby forms of the NPI (pp. 89 and 90) is the same at Time I and Time II; however, the instructions given to the mother vary slightly to

take into account the time factor. At Time I the tester instructs the mother as follows: "While it is not possible to know for certain what your baby will be like, you probably have some ideas of what your baby will be like. Please check the blank that you *think* best describes what *your* baby will be like."*

At Time II, the tester gives the following instructions: "You have had a chance to live with your baby for a month now. Please check the blank you think best describes your baby."*

After the Average Baby and Your Baby Perception Inventories are administered, the mother is given the Degree of Bother Inventory, shown on p. 91, when the infant is 1 month old and is instructed as follows: "Listed below are some of the things that have sometimes bothered other mothers in caring for their babies. We would like to know if you were bothered by any of these. Please place a check in the blank that best describes how much you were bothered by your baby's behavior in regard to these."†

Method of scoring

Each behavioral item is scored on a five-point scale ranging from "a great deal," "a good bit," "a moderate amount," "very little," or "none." Numerical weights of 1 to 5 are assigned to each of the six single-item scales, beginning with 1 for "none" to 5 for "a great deal." The total scores for each perception inventory are obtained by adding the numerical scores for each of the items and then subtracting the total score of the Your Baby Perception Inventory from the total score of the Average Baby Perception Inventory. The difference between the two scores represents the NPI score. A positive score indicates a favorable perception of the infant, whereas a negative score indicates a less favorable perception by the mother. The criteria for determining an infant who is at risk for subsequent developmental problems are minus or zero scores. The infant is considered to be at low risk if the mother rates the infant as better than the average baby (a plus score).[1,2] For example, "Given a total Average Baby Perception Inventory score of 17 and a total Your Baby Perception Inventory score of 19, the NPI score is −2. Infants rated by their mothers as better than average (a plus score) at 1 month of age are

*From Broussard, Elsie R., and Hartner, Miriam Sergay Sturgeon: Further considerations regarding maternal perception of the first born. In Hellmuth, Jerome, editor: Exceptional infant: studies in abnormalities, vol. 2., New York, 1971, Brunner/Mazel, Inc., p. 446.

*Ibid., p. 446.
†Ibid., p. 448.

NEONATAL PERCEPTION INVENTORY I*

AVERAGE BABY

How much crying do you think the average baby does?

| a great deal | a good bit | moderate amount | very little | none |

How much trouble do you think the average baby has in feeding?

| a great deal | a good bit | moderate amount | very little | none |

How much spitting up or vomiting do you think the average baby does?

| a great deal | a good bit | moderate amount | very little | none |

How much difficulty do you think the average baby has in sleeping?

| a great deal | a good bit | moderate amount | very little | none |

How much difficulty does the average baby have with bowel movements?

| a great deal | a good bit | moderate amount | very little | none |

How much trouble do you think the average baby has in settling down to a predictable pattern of eating and sleeping?

| a great deal | a good bit | moderate amount | very little | none |

*Ibid., p. 442.

NEONATAL PERCEPTION INVENTORY I*

YOUR BABY

How much crying do you think your baby will do?

| a great deal | a good bit | moderate amount | very little | none |

How much trouble do you think your baby will have feeding?

| a great deal | a good bit | moderate amount | very little | none |

How much spitting up or vomiting do you think your baby will do?

| a great deal | a good bit | moderate amount | very little | none |

How much difficulty do you think your baby will have sleeping?

| a great deal | a good bit | moderate amount | very little | none |

How much difficulty do you expect your baby to have with bowel movements?

| a great deal | a good bit | moderate amount | very little | none |

How much trouble do you think that your baby will have settling down to a predictable pattern of eating and sleeping?

| a great deal | a good bit | moderate amount | very little | none |

*Ibid., p. 443.

NEONATAL PERCEPTION INVENTORY II*
AVERAGE BABY

How much crying do you think the average baby does?

| a great deal | a good bit | moderate amount | very little | none |

How much trouble do you think the average baby has in feeding?

| a great deal | a good bit | moderate amount | very little | none |

How much spitting up or vomiting do you think the average baby does?

| a great deal | a good bit | moderate amount | very little | none |

How much difficulty do you think the average baby has in sleeping?

| a great deal | a good bit | moderate amount | very little | none |

How much difficulty does the average baby have with bowel movements?

| a great deal | a good bit | moderate amount | very little | none |

How much trouble do you think the average baby has in settling down to a predictable pattern of eating and sleeping?

| a great deal | a good bit | moderate amount | very little | none |

*Ibid., p. 444.

NEONATAL PERCEPTION INVENTORY II*
YOUR BABY

How much crying has your baby done?

| a great deal | a good bit | moderate amount | very little | none |

How much trouble has your baby had feeding?

| a great deal | a good bit | moderate amount | very little | none |

How much spitting up or vomiting has your baby done?

| a great deal | a good bit | moderate amount | very little | none |

How much difficulty has your baby had in sleeping?

| a great deal | a good bit | moderate amount | very little | none |

How much difficulty has your baby had with bowel movements?

| a great deal | a good bit | moderate amount | very little | none |

How much trouble has your baby had in settling down to a predictable pattern of eating and sleeping?

| a great deal | a good bit | moderate amount | very little | none |

*Ibid., p. 445.

DEGREE OF BOTHER INVENTORY[*]

Crying				
	a great deal	somewhat	very little	none
Spitting up or vomiting				
	a great deal	somewhat	very little	none
Sleeping				
	a great deal	somewhat	very little	none
Feeding				
	a great deal	somewhat	very little	none
Elimination				
	a great deal	somewhat	very little	none
Lack of a predictable schedule				
	a great deal	somewhat	very little	none
Other (specify):				
_____	a great deal	somewhat	very little	none
_____	a great deal	somewhat	very little	none
_____	a great deal	somewhat	very little	none
_____	a great deal	somewhat	very little	none

[*]Ibid., p. 448.

---

considered at low risk. Those infants not rated better than average (minus or zero score) are at high risk for subsequent development of emotional difficulty."[*]

Based on the original study involving 318 primiparas delivering normal, full-term, single births, total scores range from 7 to 23 out of a possible score of 6 to 30, and differences between the scores range from +9 to -9. In addition, both inventories have shown both construct and criterion validity.[2]

The Degree of Bother Inventory is given to assess problems of infant behavior. It is administered when the infant is 1 month old. Values of 1 to 4 are assigned to each of the six items on the inventory. The score is calculated by totaling these values, with no attempt in weighting the items. Broussard[2] found that the range in scores is from 6 to 23 out of a possible range of 6 to 24. In addition, she found that the Degree of Bother Inventory has high face validity.

VALUE OF THE NPI IN PLANNING INTERVENTIONS

During the second or third day of life and again at 4 weeks of age, the NPI can be helpful in determining the interrelationship between

---

[*]Ibid., pp. 446-447.

the mother's perceptions and the infant's actual behaviors. This particular tool was designed to evaluate different aspects of a mother's perceptions or expectations of her infant's behavior. It specifically explores six behavioral dimensions: crying, feeding, spitting up, sleeping, bowel movements, and settling down.

If a mother rates her infant as not better than average in the feeding scale at 3 days and again at 4 weeks of age, it is recommended that every precaution be taken to rule out physical, physiological, and developmental delays. If a mother views her infant as not better than average, she should have an opportunity to discuss when she began to view the baby this way and the reasons that she views her baby as not better than average. She should also receive support for her ability to discuss this aspect of the baby's development.[§] Although it is sometimes difficult to discuss such issues as these, the mother may be relieved that she can bring it up. She can be questioned as to what she thinks would make it easier for her to feed the infant. In addition, she can be asked what she thinks would make it easier for the infant while eating. She can be queried as to what she had expected of her infant at this time and also what she has noticed about the infant's eating since she first started viewing it as a concern.[§]

The mother can be informed that it would be helpful to her if she would keep records of the infant's feeding behavior for 4 or 5 days and note the difficulties she experiences, the difficulties the infant experiences, how often they occur, how long the difficulties last, and what she does to alleviate the situation. The mother needs assurance that the child care professional has confidence in her ability to keep records, that her concerns are genuine and important, and that by examining the records she keeps with the health care professional, change is possible. It is important for health care professionals to avoid the use of "don't worry." In addition, it is important that child care professionals remind the mother that they are willing to discuss any further concerns which she may have regarding the feeding of her infant. Both observations of the feeding and the mother's records will serve as a basis for further encouragement, support, mutual problem solving, or referral to other sources for help, particularly if a central nervous system, metabolic, or major disease entity is suspected.§

The same principles of interviewing, guidance, and reassurance apply to the other five behavioral dimensions. If the mother perceives difficulties with the infant's crying; if the amount of spitting up is distressful to her; if the infant is not sleeping enough, sleeping too much, or sleeping differently from her expectations; if she perceives the infant's bowel movements as too often, not enough, or problematic; or if she continues to view the infant's patterns in settling down as unpredictable, not regular, and troublesome to her, then discussions and further collection of objective information can be helpful for supporting parents in their decision-making processes.§

The NPI can also serve as a useful guide in obtaining more in-depth descriptions from mothers about their infants and can easily be incorporated into interviewing techniques that assist mothers in anticipatory planning. As a screening device, it has unlimited value, with its major usefulness being the early identification of infants who will need ongoing surveillance in regard to parent-child interactions. It can be a useful reference and record for recommending families for preventive services within their community settings.

IMPLICATIONS OF THE NPI IN THE FIELD OF CHILD DEVELOPMENT

What are some implications of Broussard's hypothesis and her and Hartner's[2] findings for the field of child development? First, it is possible to study parent-infant interactions in a more objective way. The findings indicate clearly that by assessing a parent-infant relationship early in its existence, child care professionals can to a high degree predict the probability of outcomes for the parent and child. In addition, there is the exciting possibility that child care professionals may be able to predict early whether a given relationship between a mother and infant will promote or inhibit the child's individual developmental outcomes.§

Second, Broussard and Hartner's study is of great practical significance in that health care professionals now have some empirical facts concerning the essential elements that facilitate positive change in a parent-infant relationship.§

Finally, this inventory has significant implications for the education of those in the child care disciplines. The findings from the 1963 study by Broussard and Hartner[2] have far-reaching implications for those individuals working with parents and for the training of child care professionals. Because the NPI is a significant screening tool and instrument for prevention, child care professionals face the exciting possibility of being able to diagnose potential problems and work to prevent them, thus assuring more children of their right to healthy development.*

Broussard has provided child care professionals with the findings of her ten- and eleven-year outcome studies, which have significant implications for child care practices in the future.[6]

Outcome at 4½ years of age

The hypothesis that the mother's perception of her 1-month-old infant was associated with the child's subsequent emotional development was first tested when 120 of the original population of firstborns were evaluated at 4½ years of age by two child psychiatrists who had no knowledge of the children's predictive risk ratings.[2,3] Children categorized as low risk at 1 month of age had less emotional disorder at 4½ years of age than those categorized as high risk ($X^2 = 16.43$ P < .001). The mother's perception of the infant as measured by the NPI at Time I was not related to the child's development at 4½ years.[6]

---

*The NPI can be obtained by writing to Dr. Elsie R. Broussard, University of Pittsburgh, Graduate School of Public Health, Pittsburgh, Pa. 15261.

Outcome at 10 to 11 years of age

To determine to what extent the mother's perception of her infant continued to be predictive of the child's emotional development up to the preadolescent phase, 104 of the first-borns were evaluated when they ranged in age from 10 years 3 months to 11 years 9 months.

Except for racial distribution due to the loss of the 20 black subjects in the original population, the demographic data for the original population were comparable with the data for the present subpopulation. The proportion of children rated at high risk was almost identical in the original and follow-up groups (39% vs. 40.4%). There was no statistically significant difference between the groups with regard to other descriptive data (e.g., health of mother, type of delivery, etc.). With respect to these data, the 104 children were judged to be representative of the original 318.

As Broussard points out: The high prevalence of emotional disorder among these full-term, healthy, first-born children living for the most part within intact family units indicates the magnitude of the mental health problem. Our findings are in keeping with those of other investigators and point to the urgent need for the implementation of programs for the primary prevention of emotional disorders.

The critical variable associated with the child's emotional development in this study is judged to be the mother's early perception of him. This relationship appears to be independent of the educational level of either parent, father's occupation, changes in income, maternal age, type of delivery, family size, or occurrence of tonsillectomy.

The data indicate that *the association between the maternal perception of the neonate and the subsequent emotional development of the child has persisted over time and is predictive of the probability of mental disorder* at age 10/11 among our first-borns.*

---

*From Broussard, Elsie R.: Neonatal prediction and outcome at 10/11 years, unpublished paper presented at the 128th meeting of the American Psychiatric Association, Anaheim, Calif., May 8, 1975.

Because of the significance of the outcome studies on 10- and 11-year-olds who were originally in the sample, Broussard asserts that without a doubt, "The Neonatal Perception Inventory provides an easily administered screening instrument which can identify a population of newborns who are at much higher risk of developing emotional disorder than others."* Early identification alerts child care professionals to conduct a more comprehensive assessment to determine if intervention is indicated and affords a maximum opportunity for outlining and taking steps to assure a program of preventive intervention.

REFERENCES

1. Broussard, Elsie R.: A study to determine the effectiveness of television as a means of providing anticipatory counseling to primiparae during the postpartum period, unpublished dissertation, Graduate School of Public Health, University of Pittsburgh, 1964.
2. Broussard, Elsie R., and Hartner, Miriam Sergay Sturgeon: Further considerations regarding maternal perception of the first born. In Hellmuth, Jerome, editor: Exceptional infant: studies in abnormalities, vol. 2, New York, 1971, Brunner/Mazel, Inc.
3. Kennedy, Janet C.: The high-risk maternal-infant acquaintance process, Nurs. Clin. North Am. **8:**849-856, 1973.
4. Broussard, Elsie R., and Sturgeon, Miriam Sergay: Maternal perception of the neonate as related to development, Child Psychiatry Hum. Dev. **1:**16-25, Fall, 1970.
5. Broussard, Elsie R.: Personal communication, Feb., 1976.
6. Broussard, Elsie R.: Neonatal prediction and outcome at 10/11 years, unpublished paper presented at the 128th annual meeting of the American Psychiatric Association, Anaheim, Calif., May 8, 1975.

ADDITIONAL READING

Broussard, Elsie R.: Evaluation of televised anticipatory guidance to primiparae, unpublished paper presented at the meeting of the American Public Health Association, San Francisco, Calif., Nov. 3, 1966.

5

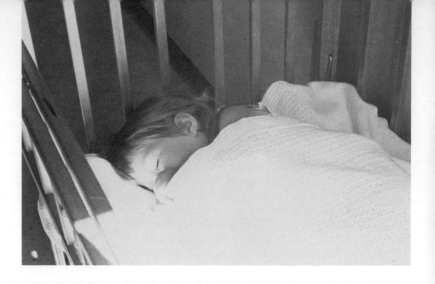

SLEEP

Sleep has been of interest to psychologists for a considerable period of time. The nature of sleep has not received proportionate or equal, systematic investigation by others in the health caring fields until recently.

The value of studying, describing, and observing sleep and its consequent helpfulness in planning care regimens, influencing newborn care scheduling such as feeding, and assisting parents anticipate what to expect in their infant's sleep behaviors at different developmental stages cannot be stressed enough.

Refined techniques are presently in use that have made objective study of sleep cycles, patterns, and states possible. Techniques of electrophysiology are increasingly being used to assist in reducing the mystery of sleep and basically to uncover significant relationships of sleep to behavior. Indices to progressive maturation of the central nervous system are accumulating with the advancement of understanding of sleep behavior.

QUIET AND ACTIVE SLEEP

Hartmann,[1] Parmelee and associates,[2] and Petre-Quadens[3] discuss the vast evidence that there are two qualitatively different sleep states. These are referred to as "non-REM sleep," and

"REM sleep."* Electrophysiological recording devices reveal distinct differences between non-REM and REM sleep states. Non-REM sleep, also known as synchronized, quiet, or orthodox sleep, is characterized by sleep spindles and slow waves on electroencephalography (EEG), a slow and regular pulse, lack of conjugate eye movements, partial relaxation of postural muscles, lack of body movements, regular respirations, and some chin electromyogram (EMG) activity.[1] REM sleep or desynchronized, dreaming, paradoxical, or active sleep, is characterized by low-amplitude EEG, many eye movements, total relaxation of postural muscles, irregular respirations, frequent small body movements, and absence of neck muscle tone. Sucking movements are observed in the newborn, as well as smiling.[3]

Active sleep is hypothesized by many investigators to be controlled by mechanisms in the pontine reticular system. Quiet sleep is thought to be a highly controlled state that requires intricate, complex feedback signals from the higher cerebral centers of the brain.

---

*"REM" refers to rapid eye movements, one of the characteristics differentiating the two sleep states.

Functions of sleep states

Hartmann[1] postulates that because of the distinct differences between the two sleep states, these states must have different functions. He concludes that there is a need for slow-wave sleep and that there is a relationship between anabolism and non-REM sleep, or, more specifically, macromolecule synthesis occurs during slow-wave sleep. He also hypothesizes that proteins are synthesized in the central nervous system during slow-wave sleep states.

Hartmann further postulates that desynchronized sleep has a relationship with restoration of ego functions, the ability to focus attention, and learning and memory mechanisms. In addition, he suggests that sleep has a role in memory storage and asserts that although the mechanism of the restorative function of sleep is unclear, it "makes sense to think of this as connecting recent information with old pathways or filing systems."[1]

Stages of sleep

Battle[4] has identified four different stages of sleep based on EEG studies for both adults and children. These stages are related specifically to depth of sleep. Stage I is characterized by an irregular and low-voltage alpha rhythm. A person who is awakened from stage I sleep may not recognize that he has been in a state of sleep. Stage I when associated with rapid eye movement is REM sleep and correlates with visual dreaming.

Stage II is characterized by sleep spindles (short bursts of sharply pointed alpha waves). These sleep spindles occur at intervals. An individual in stage II is more relaxed and can be awakened easily.

Stage III is characterized by the presence of delta waves. A wave pattern that is characterized by high voltage and low frequency occurs. Spindles are present. The person asleep is more relaxed. The vital signs change to decreased levels, and the person is less easily awakened.

The fourth stage is deep sleep, and delta waves are prominent.

Battle,[4] like other investigators, has described sleep cycles, which occur in each individual's sleep patterns. These cycles occur during the regular 7- to 8-hour sleep period. An adult descends from stage I to stage IV and then ascends back to stage I in cycles of 90 minutes. In a normal full-term neonate the average duration of a sleep cycle, which includes both a period of quiet sleep and active sleep, is usually 60 minutes. The duration of a cycle can range from 30 to 70 minutes.[5]

As the individual reascends to stage I, certain physiological differences are noted. Rapid eye movements, increase in respirations and pulse rates, and wide fluctuations in blood pressure occur. Most dreaming activity occurs in this REM period.[4]

After spending 10 to 15 minutes in stage I REM sleep, the person drops back to stage IV. The cycle repeats itself about three to five times during the night. Each time the sleeper returns to stage I REM sleep, he spends a longer period of time in this stage. Interestingly more time is spent in stage IV during the first half of the night, whereas the last third of the night is spent largely in stage I REM sleep.[4]

SLEEP PATTERNS OF THE NEWBORN

Like adults, children have cyclical fluctuations between quiet and active sleep periods. One of the most extensive studies of sleep of the newborn was reported by Parmelee and others[6] in 1961. Observation of 75 full-term infants during the first 3 days of life revealed a mean sleep length of 16.6 hours with a range of 10.5 to 23 hours.

The average total sleeping time for all 75 infants was 17 hours the first day. On the second day, 16.5 hours was the average sleeping time; and on the third day, 16.2 hours.

Parmelee and associates[6] reported that the average longest sleeping period for all the infants was 4.8 hours the first day, 4.2 hours the second day, and 4.5 hours the third day. It is notable that the longest uninterrupted sleep period for all 3 days occurred on the first day for 53.3% of the babies. The longest uninterrupted sleep period for 24% of the newborns occurred on the second day and for 22.7%, on the third day.

Metcalf[7] points out that within the first days of the newborn's life, key connections are established "between regulation of infant state and specific maternal cues, among which may be time characteristics of caretaking exchange." This information has been interpreted as an "indication possibly of these first hours as a time of key adaptation between caretaker and infant."[7] Metcalf further reports that the duration of awake states per 24 hours is greater during the first 3 days than at any time until the end of the first month of life.

Other investigators have extended their

studies of infant sleep duration to the first month of life.

Although in the study by Parmelee and associates,[6] the duration of periods of sleep and wakefulness during the first month of life was determined by record keeping on the part of mothers, the results were similar to studies of other investigators. The fact that the 75 infants were awake 7 to 8 hours a day, or 30% to 35% of a 24-hour period, is notable. During the remaining 65% to 70% of the day, the infants were asleep. It is also noteworthy that neither sleep nor awake periods were sustained for long periods of time.

The results of this study led Parmelee and co-workers[6] to hypothesize that the wide cyclical fluctuations of a newborn's sleep patterns are related to the inability of higher cerebral centers to sustain prolonged periods of sleep or wakefulness. Petre-Quadens[3] describes the rapid alternation of sleep and wakefulness as being progressively modified by circuits involving the cortex of the brain.

Petre-Quadens also reports that periodic awakening is likely influenced by necessities of feeding. She suggests that the total sleep cycle consists of quiet and active periods varying from 50 to 60 minutes and states that "this fundamental organization never disappears, but the periods lengthen, later on."[3]

According to Petre-Quadens, there is evidence suggesting that with increasing maturation, the infant's brain becomes able to sustain longer periods of behavioral inhibition, which is responsible for maintenance of both quiet and active sleep.

She reports that at the age of 1 month an infant has 21% to 22% active sleep per sleep cycle, and that the proportion of an infant's active sleep per sleep cycle corresponds to that of the adult. From 2 months of age, day sleep periods are shorter. In addition, at the age of 10 months, night sleep of the infant is similar in its organization to adult sleep.[3]

Petre-Quadens' data suggest that the newborn sleeps more during the day than at night and a higher proportion of REM stages are present during day sleep.[3]

An important and extensive investigation carried out by Stern and associates[8] in 1969 focused on sleep cycle characteristics in infants. Stern and associates concluded that the sleep-awake cycles of newborn infants are of shorter duration than those of adults, with the newborn awakening every 3 to 4 hours. His rest-activity

cycle within a sleep period is at least 30 minutes shorter than the adult's 90-minute cycle. They also recognized that the achievement of establishing a sleep-awake cycle that follows a diurnal pattern with a 24-hour periodicity is a major developmental task for infants.

The study showed that the length of time of the infant's sleep cycle increased from 47 minutes at term to 50.3 minutes at 8 months of age.[8] Full-term infants spent 38% of their time in active sleep, whereas 28% of their time was spent in quiet sleep. At 3 months of age, full-term babies were noted to spend 23% of the sleep cycle in active sleep, whereas quiet sleep was noted during 47% of the sleep cycle. Stern and co-workers also found that the amount of quiet sleep within a cycle increased with age, whereas the amount of active sleep tended to decrease.

These investigators reported that the amounts of quiet and active sleep are nearly equal at term, and by 3 months of age, quiet sleep unequivocally is twice the amount of active sleep.

As Stern and co-workers[8] pointed out, these age-related shifts in the proportion of quiet to active sleep are important indicators of maturation of the central nervous system. Parents and professional care providers can be observant of the behavioral clues that are associated with active and quiet sleep states. Active sleep, characterized by irregular respirations, irregular heart rate, frequent small body movements, and bursts of rapid eye movements, can be observed in infants. Quiet sleep, characterized by regular heart rate and the absence of body and eye movements, can also be observed without the necessity of an EEG.

SLEEP PATTERNS OF YOUNG INFANTS

Another extensive investigation by Parmelee and associates[9] focused on sleep-awake patterns of infants during their first 16 weeks of life. Parmelee and co-workers pointed out that sleep patterns of young infants can be a source of concern to parents, since an infant's sleep pattern is most often in conflict with that established by the adult. Parents' major concerns may focus on the need to be assured that an infant normally develops a night sleep pattern similar to that of the adult.

The investigation by Parmelee and associates[9] resulted in the following findings: the average amount of total sleep a day for the 46 infants under study was 16.32 hours in the first week; 16.25 hours of sleep in the second week, 15.43 hours in the fourth week, 15.42 hours in the eighth week, 15.11 hours in the twelfth week, and 14.87 hours in the sixteenth week.

They found that the average longest period of sleep a day was 4.05 hours in the first week, 4.41 hours in the second week, 6.47 hours in the eighth week, 7.67 hours in the twelfth week, and 8.48 hours in the sixteenth week. By the sixteenth week of age the average longest period of sleep had increased by 4.4 hours, or was double that of the second week of life.

The average longest period of wakefulness a day was 2.39 hours in the first week, 2.61 hours in the second week, 3.08 hours in the fourth week, 3.15 hours in the eighth week, 3.41 hours in the twelfth week, and 3.56 hours in the sixteenth week. Thus a major finding of the study was that although infants show increasing ability to sustain long periods of sleep, the increase in ability to sustain long periods of wakefulness is not as great.[9]

As these investigators pointed out,[9] the steady and rapid increase in the infant's ability to sustain prolonged periods of sleep in the first 16 weeks of life is reassuring to parents. Parmelee and associates noted the pleasure parents experience in observing changes in the infant's behavior as the infant begins to entertain himself when awake at about the twelfth week of life. They also reported that there is a dramatic decrease in crying during wakefulness after the sixth week of life and again at about 12 weeks of age.

Thus by the end of 12 to 16 weeks of life the infant is expected to sleep for prolonged periods, establishing definite diurnal cycles with more sleep at night (e.g., 7 PM to 7 AM) than in the daytime (e.g., 7 AM to 7 PM). As a result, the sleep pattern of the infant becomes more synchronized with that of its parents.[9]

For purposes of assessment, if a diurnal cycle is not established, further monitoring of sleep behaviors may be needed. There is a high correlation between the establishment of a diurnal cycle and progressive central nervous system maturation; thus the lack of such a pattern might indicate an index to problems with processing of sensory input, inhibitory functions of the cerebral cortex, or disorders of the central nervous system.

Results of a study by Parmelee and others[2] suggest that the premature infant of low gestational age spends the majority of sleep in a state that parallels REM active sleep. The amount of active sleep decreases as the premature infant approaches full-term gestational age.

SLEEP PATTERNS DURING THE FIRST TWO YEARS

Traisman and co-workers[10] reported the results of a longitudinal study of 530 infants and their sleep patterns during the first two years of life. They found that the total sleeping time for infants at 1 month of age was 17.31 hours a day. The total sleeping time at 8 weeks was reported to be 15.30 hours. During the next 10 months, only a minimal reduction in total sleeping time was found. Traisman and associates reported that the 1-year-old child slept an average of 1 hour less than the 8-week-old child. The number of naps over this same time period for these children decreased from three to two, and total nap time was reduced by about 4 hours, from 6.59 to 2.40 hours. The longest sleeping period increased from 8.71 hours in the 8-week-old infant to 11.94 hours in the 1-year-old child.

These investigators reported that the same trends occurring in the first year carried over to the second year with minimal differences. Total sleeping time became shorter, total nap time decreased by approximately 30 minutes, naps became less frequent, and the longest sleep period averaged 12 hours by 2 years of age.

SLEEP AND FUSSINESS

Metcalf[7] reports attempts to relate EEG developments to fussiness in the infant's first 3 months of life. It has been observed that infants at 4 to 5 weeks of age experience states of fussiness lasting for a period of a week or two. This fussy stage tends to diminish by the age of 3 months. The fussiness is postulated to be related to mechanisms for brain maturation.[7] According to Metcalf, after the age of 5 weeks, sensory input is processed in a different way than it was before 5 weeks. He suggests that at about the age of 6 weeks there is a gradual development of information-processing inhibitory capacity of the infant, whose sensory input begins to be "filtered."

Metcalf reports that at 2½ or 3 months of age, EEG tracings and behavioral parameters become disrupted again for a brief period. Periods of fussiness might be anticipated.

SLEEP AND ITS ADAPTIVE FUNCTIONS

Sander[11] discusses sleep and its adaptive functions. He suggests that the rhythmicity of sleep has a vital adaptive significance with regard to the relationship of timing of environmental cycles and the infant's own innate sleep-awake cycle. For example, Sander reminds us that how the infant's caregiver interprets the neonate's smile in the sleep-onset REM period can make a notable difference in the interruption or noninterruption of a sleep-awake epoch. The smile may occur as the infant is falling asleep; the parent may view it as a social clue and interpret it as an opportunity for social interaction, whereby a course of interactions is begun that stimulates and arouses the infant while he is falling asleep. Parents may be disappointed, confused, or frustrated by their attempts, as well as their inability to know when to refrain from interfering with something as simple and natural as the course of their infant's sleep-awake cycle.

IMPLICATIONS OF SLEEP STATES AND PATTERNS

The implications of different sleep states and patterns are numerous. Parents as well as child care professionals can learn to be more sensitive to the cues indicating the depth of sleep of the infant. Care providers can learn to refrain from trying to feed an infant in a deeper level of sleep, when and when not to handle, and definitely when not to interact.

Thus sleep, which is being recognized as an increasingly significant parameter in an infant's growth and development, has the following implications for observation, assessment, guidance, support, and reassurance for parents:

1. Parents can learn to observe behavioral differences in their infant's levels of sleep, that is, quiet as compared to active sleep.

2. Parents can be informed about the average amount of hours a newborn or infant spends in an actual sleep state per sleep period (the newborn is asleep 17 to 20 hours a day).

3. Parents can learn the average number of hours an infant sleeps during the day with increasing age.

4. Parents can learn the average amount of awake time the infant has with increasing age. After 3 months he should be sleeping 8 hours a day.

5. Parents can be informed about when the infant will begin to spend the majority of sleep time at night. The infant should be sleeping through the night by 5 months.

6. Parents can learn behavioral clues that signal the infant is going to sleep and not socially interacting.

7. Parents can learn to anticipate brief fussy periods, which correspond to maturation of the central nervous system.

8. Parents can learn to be more sensitive to the sleep cycles, rates, and patterns that the infant is establishing and base their care or interactions correspondingly. Parents can learn to feed the infant during awake rather than drowsy periods, even though they think it is time for nutrients.

9. Parents can learn that there are cycles that are intrinsic to infants and that each infant is unique; parents cannot change the infant's sleep cycles or states any more than they can change his temperament or the features of his face.

10. Parents can learn that the infant does not sleep all the time, that there are periods in which the infant is awake and alert, and that certain alert states correspond and are conducive to the ability to learn.

11. Parents can learn of the vital nature of awake states that occur during the first 3 days and their potential impact on later interpersonal relationships.

12. Short cycles of sleep, absence of cyclic organization, or long periods of sleep cycles may be clues to disorders or abnormalities in central nervous system maturation and may necessitate longitudinal objective records or in-depth investigations.

13. Parents in general can anticipate the newborn to be asleep for 17 to 20 hours a day. Sleep periods will be regular, lasting about 4 hours. The average amount of wakefulness is 7 to 8 hours out of 24 hours, with wakefulness sustained as long as 1 to 2 hours. At term, parents can anticipate that half of the newborn's sleep will be active REM sleep, whereas the remainder will be typified by non-REM or quiet sleep. The infant will be in both awake and quiet sleep states throughout the day and will be awake and active for as long as 1 to 2 hours during the day. Parents can learn that with an increase in age, the infant is expected to spend longer periods in sustained, quiet sleep.

14. If a sleeping concern is present, it is important to assess parental interactions or responses to what they describe as problematic, to consider their definition of the concern, to assess the sleeping environment, and to observe the child's own unique patterns and typical sleep characteristics.

REFERENCES

1. Hartmann, Ernest: Functions of sleep. In Jovanovic, U. J., editor: The nature of sleep: International symposium, Stuttgart, 1973, Gustav Fischer Verlog.
2. Parmelee, Arthur H., Wenner, Waldemer H., Akiyama, Yoshio, Schultz, Marvin, and Stern, Evelyn: Sleep states in premature infants, Dev. Med. Child Neurol. **9:**70-77, 1967.
3. Petre-Quadens, Olga: Sleep in the human newborn. In Petre-Quadens, Olga, and Schlay, John D., editors: Basic sleep mechanisms, New York, 1974, Academic Press, Inc.
4. Battle, Constance U.: Sleep and sleep disturbances in young children: sensible management depends upon understanding, Clin. Pediatr. **9:**675-682, 1970.
5. Dreyfus-Briseac, C.: Sleeping behavior in abnormal newborn infants, Neuropaediatrie **1:**354-366, 1970.
6. Parmelee, Arthur H., Schulz, Helen R., and Disbrow, Mildred A.: Sleep patterns of the newborn, J. Pediatr. **58:**241-250, 1961.
7. Metcalf, David: General discussion: significance of the sleep parameters in early behavioral development, In Petre-Quadens, Olga, and Schlay, John D., editors: Basic sleep mechanisms, New York, 1974, Academic Press, Inc.
8. Stern, Evelyn, Parmelee, Arthur H., Akiyama, Yoshio, and others: Sleep cycle characteristics in infants, Pediatrics **43:**65-70, 1969.
9. Parmelee, Arthur H., Wenner, Waldemer H., and Schulz, Helen R.: Infant sleep patterns: from birth to 16 weeks of age, J. Pediatr. **65:**576-582, 1964.
10. Traisman, Alfred S., Traisman, Howard S., and Gatti, Richard: The well baby care of 530 infants, J. Pediatr. **68:**608-614, 1966.
11. Sander, Louis W.: General discussion: significance of the sleep parameters in early behavioral development, In Petre-Quadens, Olga, and Schlay, John D., editors: Basic sleep mechanisms, New York, 1974, Academic Press, Inc.

6

ASSESSMENT OF INFANT TEMPERAMENT

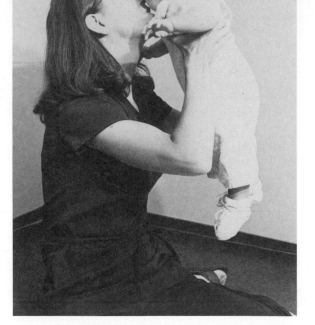

How many times has a professional in child care heard parents describe their infant as "so different" or "he demands so much" or "he gets upset so easily"? These are prime examples that different infants have different temperaments even within the same family. An infant's temperament requires adjustments by family members, particularly if the infant's temperament is opposite of what the parents expected or what they are used to. If parents are asked, they will tell you the differences between one child and another in their family. An infant's temperament can have lasting effects on his development. Infants who have temperamental qualities that are at extremes may even be at risk for having conflicts with their parents.

Child care professionals should recognize that differences in infants' temperaments are important. There is a growing body of literature that focuses on the individual differences of newborns, infants, and children. Brazelton[1] has unquestionably gone into more depth than other investigators in an attempt to define individual differences of infants in the newborn period and in the first month of life. Thomas and associates[2] developed a semistructured interview to

obtain descriptions of infants' behaviors in specific situations. These investigators studied nine categories of primary reactivity, or temperament. Buss and Plomin[3] developed a temperament questionnaire for research use, but reports are not yet available of its usefulness in clinical practice.

Some assessment tools such as those developed by Brazelton (Chapter 3) and Broussard (Chapter 4) focus on the infant during the first month of life, but few instruments are available that can be used to identify infant problems at a later stage, particularly the second half of the first year of life. One useful tool now available was developed by William Carey, a pediatrician. Carey was interested in knowing the effect an infant's temperament has on his present management and future development. The Carey Infant Temperament Questionnaire can be useful in planning an infant's care and management.

IMPORTANCE OF INFANT TEMPERAMENT

The Carey Infant Temperament Questionnaire, designed as a clinical screening instrument for detecting the temperament of infants between 4 and 8 months of age, is in increasing demand by child care professionals. Carey's questionnaire was adapted for pediatric use from the research interview of Thomas and co-workers.[2] The focus of these researchers' work was on temperamental differences in infants.

Carey[4] defines "infant temperament" as the emotional reactivity, or behavioral style (regardless of the origins), that is displayed by an infant in the early months of life. According to Carey, this temperament is an important variable in infant development and is deserving of further attention by child care professionals. With consistent assessment of infant temperament, the development of certain preventive health care models, which can enhance the well-being of both the infant and his parents, is possible.

The Carey questionnaire is intended as another means by which child care professionals can improve their assessment skills for determining an infant's temperament that will have an impact on an infant's parents and other caregivers.

OBJECTIVES OF THE CAREY INFANT TEMPERAMENT QUESTIONNAIRE

The primary objective of the questionnaire is to attain greater objectivity in identifying the temperament profile of the infant. This makes a more individualized approach possible for helping parents determine alternatives in handling, caring for, and interacting with their infant.

Carey[4] emphasizes the value of having ways to identify maternal concerns without placing the mother in a position of feeling guilty, responsible for the infant's temperament, or incompetent in dealing with an infant who is consistently fussy. He encourages health care professionals to be more sensitive to the needs of parents so that parents do not conclude that their infant's problem is one of parental mismanagement. Instead Carey demonstrates the significance of the use of the infant questionnaire to obtain a more individualized, in-depth profile of those temperamental characteristics which either accentuate parental distress and concerns or increase positive parental attitudes toward the infant.

Carey advocates that the infant's temperament be assessed on a continuing basis. Once

the infant's temperamental traits can be delineated, more valuable approaches for determining appropriate case management of infants and their parents are possible.

Management of the infant between 4 and 8 months of age is based on an accurate picture of the infant's unique characteristics rather than on what others think he is like. Carey stresses that parental biases about the infant's temperament can be minimized by the administration of his questionnaire, which is designed to measure an individual infant's style of reactions in many areas and avoids the mother's global impressions.

OVERVIEW OF THE CAREY INFANT TEMPERAMENT QUESTIONNAIRE
Mothers' answers to questionnaire

The questionnaire consists of seventy statements that are to be answered by the mother. Each statement has three choices from which the mother selects the best description of her infant's behavior. (See questionnaire, pp. 104 to 110.)

These statements relate specifically to sleep, feeding (Fig. 6-1), elimination patterns, and play behaviors. In addition, the questionnaire contains statements describing the infant's reactions to diapering (Fig. 6-2) and dressing; bathing; and care procedures such as nail cutting, hair brushing, taking medicines, and face and hair washing (Fig. 6-3). Also included are descriptions about the infant's reactions to visits to the physician; responses to illness; sensory reactions and adaptive behavioral mechanisms to stimuli such as light, sounds, and touch; and responses to persons, places, and situations. The seventy statements elicit the mother's general impression of her infant's temperament, her comparisons of her infant with other infants of the same age, and whether her infant's temperament is a problem to her.

After completing the statements, the mother is asked to provide both medical and social information about her family. Significantly, Carey also included a section in which the mother is asked to rate her infant's temperament as average, more difficult than average, or easier than average in general, as well as to compare her infant with other infants in each of the nine categories of temperament. This allows the rater to determine how realistically the mother views her infant.

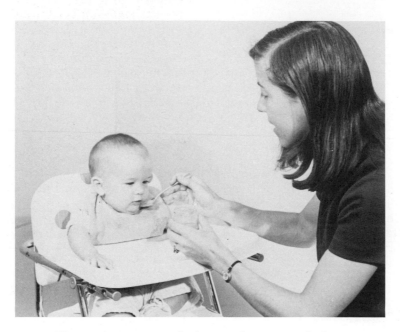

Fig. 6-1. Assessing an infant's general reactions to feeding.

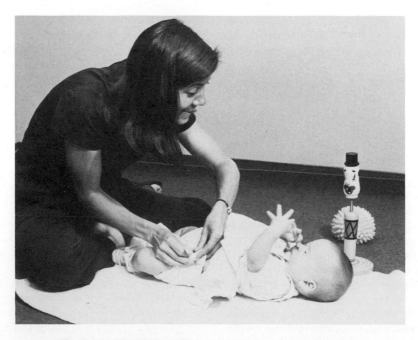

Fig. 6-2. Assessing an infant's temperament during diapering.

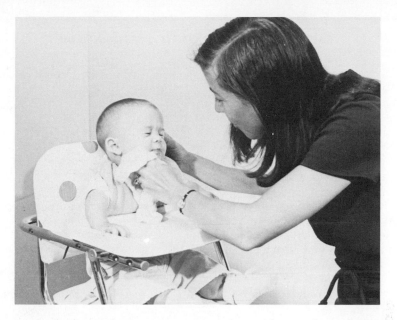

Fig. 6-3. Assessing an infant's temperament to care procedures such as washing face.

The questionnaire is aimed at obtaining descriptions about an infant's behaviors and particularly how each infant responds in specific situations. Mothers who complete the questionnaire are asked to select from three possible choices that best describe the infant's behaviors in each of nine categories of infant temperament. These nine categories include activity, rhythmicity, adaptability, approach, sensory threshold, intensity, mood, distractibility, and persistence.[5] For example, item 3 from the questionnaire is "(a) generally happy (smiling, etc.) on waking up and going to sleep; (b) variable mood at these times; (c) generally fussy on waking up and going to sleep."[6] The questionnaire seeks to obtain information on the infant's actual responses, not subjective interpretations of the infant's behavior. Thus the mother filling out the questionnaire chooses and circles either "a," "b," or "c" to represent the descriptive statement that accurately describes her infant.

Accompanying instructions state that if none of the descriptive statements is appropriate, no response is to be attempted. Furthermore, the mother is reminded that there are no good or bad or right or wrong answers, just descriptions that correspond to an infant's typical response.

THE CAREY INFANT TEMPERAMENT QUESTIONNAIRE

The questionnaire is presented on the following pages. It is preceded by the following letter given to mothers that includes some of the instructions for the questionnaire:

Dear Ms. _____

The purpose of the enclosed questionnaire is to determine the general pattern of your baby's response to his or her environment by getting specific information about many areas of functioning. You will also be asked some questions about that environment and about your general impressions of the baby. Please answer the questions without skipping about.

The temperament questionnaire itself consists of 70 statements about the baby, each with 3 choices. Please circle the letter "a," "b," or "c" before the choice that properly describes the baby. If none of the 3 possibilities is truly suitable, please do not circle any letter. For example, a baby may have no illness yet. If there has been a change in the baby, the answer should be what applies more recently. There are no good and bad or right and wrong answers, only descriptions of what the baby does. It will probably take 15 to 25 minutes.

Thank you very much for your participation. The results will be shared with you later if you are interested.[*]

[*]From Carey, William B.: Carey Infant Temperament Questionnaire, Media, Pa.

Text continued on p. 110.

CAREY INFANT TEMPERAMENT QUESTIONNAIRE*

Sleep

1. (a) Generally goes to sleep at about the same time (within half hour) night and naps.
   (b) Partly the same time, partly not.
   (c) No regular pattern at all. Times vary 1-2 hours or more.
2. (a) Generally wakes up at about same time, night and naps.
   (b) Partly the same times, partly not.
   (c) No regular pattern at all. Times vary 1-2 hours or more.
3. (a) Generally happy (smiling, etc.) on waking up and going to sleep.
   (b) Variable mood at these times.
   (c) Generally fussy on waking up and going to sleep.
4. (a) Moves about crib much (such as from one end to other) during sleep.
   (b) Moves a little (a few inches).
   (c) Lies fairly still. Usually in same position when awakens.
   With change in time, place or state of health:
5. (a) Adjusts easily and sleeps fairly well within 1-2 days.
   (b) Variable pattern.
   (c) Bothered considerably. Takes at least 3 days to readjust sleeping routine.

Feeding

6. (a) Generally wants and takes milk at about same time. Not over 1 hour variation.
   (b) Sometimes same, sometimes different times.
   (c) Hungry times quite unpredictable.
7. (a) Generally takes about same amount of milk, not over 2 oz. difference.
   (b) Sometimes same, sometimes different amounts.
   (c) Amounts taken quite unpredictable.
8. (a) Easily distracted from milk feedings by noises, changes in place or routine.
   (b) Sometimes distracted, sometimes not.
   (c) Usually goes right on sucking in spite of distractions.
9. (a) Easily adjusts to parents' efforts to change feeding schedule within 1-2 tries.
   (b) Slowly (after several tries) or variable.
   (c) Adjusts not at all to such changes after several tries.
10. (a) If hungry and wants milk, will keep refusing substitutes (solids, water, pacifier)
    for many minutes.
    (b) Intermediate or variable.
    (c) Gives up within a few minutes and takes what is offered.

NOTE: For scoring instructions and revised means, refer to the *Journal of Pediatrics,* **77:**188, 1970, and **81:**414, 1972, respectively.

EDITOR'S NOTE: Carey and McDevitt have revised the Infant Temperament Questionnaire[8] since the publication of the first edition of this book. There are now 95 items, which are scored on a 6-point frequency scale. Unfortunately it was not possible to obtain permission to reprint the entire new version here. However, a sample copy can be obtained by sending a check for $5.00 to Dr. William B. Carey, 319 West Front St., Media, Pa. 19063. Unlimited photocopying of the forms is permissible. (Reference: Revision of the Infant Temperament Questionnaire, Pediatrics **61:**735-739,1978.) Two questionnaires for older children are available on the same terms from different sources: 1. Toddler Temperament Scale (1- to 3-year-old children) developed in 1978 by W. Fullard, S. C. McDevitt, and W. B. Carey. Write to William Fullard, Ph.D., Department of Educational Psychology, Temple University, Philadelphia, Pa. 19122. 2. Behavioral Style Questionnaire (3- to 7-year-old children)[9] developed in 1975 by S. C. McDevitt and W. B. Carey. Write to Sean C. McDevitt, Ph.D., Devereux Center, 6436 E. Sweetwater, Scottsdale, Ariz. 85254. Reference: The measurement of temperament in 3- to 7-year-old children, J. Child Psychol. Psychiatry **19:**245-253, 1978. A fourth questionnaire, for 8- to 12-year-old children, is nearing completion and will soon be ready for distribution.

CAREY INFANT TEMPERAMENT QUESTIONNAIRE—cont'd

11. (a) With interruptions of milk or solid feedings, as for burping, is generally happy, smiles.
    (b) Variable response.
    (c) Generally cries with these interruptions.
12. (a) Always notices (and reacts to) change in temperature or types of milk or substitution of juice or water.
    (b) Variable.
    (c) Rarely seems to notice (and react to) such changes.
13. (a) Suck generally vigorous.
    (b) Intermediate.
    (c) Suck generally mild and intermittent.
14. (a) Activity during feedings—constant squirming, kicking, etc.
    (b) Some motion: intermediate.
    (c) Lies quietly throughout.
15. (a) Always cries loudly when hungry.
    (b) Cries somewhat but only occasionally hard or for many minutes.
    (c) Usually just whimpers when hungry, but doesn't cry loudly.
16. (a) Hunger cry usually stopped for at least a minute by picking up, pacifier, putting on bib, etc.
    (b) Sometimes can be distracted when hungry.
    (c) Nothing stops hunger cry.
17. (a) After feeding baby smiles and laughs.
    (b) Content but not usually happy (smiles, etc.) or fussy.
    (c) Fussy and wants to be left alone.
18. (a) When full, clamps mouth closed, spits out food or milk, bats at spoon, etc.
    (b) Variable.
    (c) Just turns head away or lets food drool out of mouth.
19. (a) Initial reaction to new foods (solids, juices, vitamins) acceptance. Swallows them promptly without fussing.
    (b) Variable response.
    (c) Usually rejects new foods. Makes face, spits, out, etc.
20. (a) Initial reaction to new foods pleasant (smiles, etc.), whether accepts or not.
    (b) Variable or intermediate.
    (c) Response unpleasant (cries, etc.), whether accepts or not.
21. (a) This response is dramatic whether accepting (smacks lips, laughs, squeals) or not (cries).
    (b) Variable.
    (c) This response mild whether accepting or not. Just smiles, makes face or nothing.
22. (a) After several feedings of any new food, accepts it.
    (b) Accepts some, not others.
    (c) Continues to reject most new foods after several tries.
23. (a) With changes in amounts, kinds, timing of solids, does not seem to mind.
    (b) Variable response. Sometimes accepts, sometimes not.
    (c) Does not accept these changes readily.
24. (a) Easily notices and reacts to differences in taste and consistency.
    (b) Variable.
    (c) Seems seldom to notice or react to these differences.
25. (a) If does not get type of solid food desired, keeps crying till gets it.
    (b) Variable.
    (c) May fuss briefly but soon gives up and takes what offered.

Continued.

CAREY INFANT TEMPERAMENT QUESTIONNAIRE—cont'd

Soiling and wetting

26. (a) When having bowel movement, generally cries.
    (b) Sometimes cries.
    (c) Rarely cries though may get red in face. Generally happy (smiles, etc.) in spite of having b.m.
27. (a) Bowel movements generally at same time of day (usually within 1 hour of same time).
    (b) Sometimes at same time, sometimes not.
    (c) No real pattern. Usually not same time.
28. (a) Generally indicates somehow that is soiled with b.m.
    (b) Sometimes indicates.
    (c) Seldom or never indicates.
29. (a) Usually fusses when diaper soiled with b.m.
    (b) Sometimes fusses.
    (c) Usually does not fuss.
30. (a) Generally indicates somehow that is wet (no b.m.).
    (b) Sometimes indicates.
    (c) Seldom or never indicates.
31. (a) Usually fusses when diaper wet (no b.m.).
    (b) Sometimes fusses.
    (c) Usually does not fuss.
32. (a) When fussing about diaper, does so loudly. A real cry.
    (b) Variable.
    (c) Usually just a little whimpering.
33. (a) If fussing about diaper, can easily be distracted for at least a few minutes by being picked up, etc.
    (b) Variable.
    (c) Nothing distracts baby from fussing.

Diapering and dressing

34. (a) Squirms and kicks much at these times.
    (b) Moves some.
    (c) Generally lies still during these procedures.
35. (a) Generally pleasant (smiles, etc.) during diapering and dressing.
    (b) Varied.
    (c) Generally fussy during these times.
36. (a) These feelings usually intense: vigorous laughing or crying.
    (b) Varied.
    (c) Mildly expressed usually. Little smiling or fussing.

Bathing

37. (a) Usual reaction to bath—smiles or laughs.
    (b) Variable or neutral.
    (c) Usually cries or fusses.
38. (a) Like or dislike of bath is intense. Excited.
    (b) Variable or intermediate.
    (c) Like or dislike is mild. Not very excited.
39. (a) Kicks, spashes and wiggles throughout.
    (b) Intermediate—moves moderate amount.
    (c) Lies quietly or moves little.
40. (a) Reaction to very first tub (or basin) bath. Seemed to accept it right away.
    (c) At first protested against bath.

CAREY INFANT TEMPERAMENT QUESTIONNAIRE—cont'd

41. (a) If protested at first, accepted it after 2 or 3 times.
    (b) Sometimes accepted, sometimes not.
    (c) Continued to object even after two weeks.
42. (a) If bath by different person or in different place, readily accepts change first or second time.
    (b) May or may not accept.
    (c) Objects consistently to such changes.

Procedures—nail cutting, hair brushing, washing face and hair, medicines
43. (a) Initial reaction to any new procedure—generally acceptance.
    (b) Variable.
    (c) Generally objects; fusses or cries.
44. (a) If initial objection, accepts after 2 or 3 times.
    (b) Variable acceptance. Sometimes does, sometimes does not.
    (c) Continues to object even after several times.
45. (a) Generally pleasant during procedures once established—smiles, etc.
    (b) Neutral or variable.
    (c) Generally fussy or crying during procedures.
46. (a) If fussy with procedures, easily distracted by game, toy, singing, etc.—and stops fussing.
    (b) Variable response to distractions.
    (c) Not distracted; goes on fussing.

Visits to doctor
47. (a) With physical exam, when well, generally friendly and smiles.
    (b) Both smiles and fusses: variable.
    (c) Fusses most of time.
48. (a) With shots cries loudly for several minutes or more.
    (b) Variable.
    (c) Cry over in less than a minute.
49. (a) When crying from shot, easily distracted by milk, pacifier, etc.
    (b) Sometimes distracted, sometimes not.
    (c) Goes right on crying no matter what is done.

Response to illness
50. (a) With any kind of illness much crying and fussing.
    (b) Variable.
    (c) Not much crying with illnesses. Just whimpering sometimes. Generally his usual self.

Sensory—reactions to sounds, light, touch
51. (a) Reacts little or not at all to unusual loud sound or bright light.
    (b) Intermediate or variable.
    (c) Reacts to almost any change in sound or light.
52. (a) This reaction to light or sound is intense—startles or cries loudly.
    (b) Intermediate—sometimes does, sometimes not.
    (c) Mild reaction—little or no crying.
53. (a) On repeated exposure to these same lights or sounds, does not react so much any more.
    (b) Variable.
    (c) No change from initial negative reaction.
54. (a) If already crying about something else, light or sound makes crying stop briefly at least.
    (b) Variable response.
    (c) Makes no difference.

Continued.

CAREY INFANT TEMPERAMENT QUESTIONNAIRE—cont'd

Responses to people

55. (a) Definitely notices and reacts to differences in people: age, sex, glasses, hats, other physical differences.
    (b) Variable reaction to differences.
    (c) Similar reactions to most people unless strangers.
56. (a) Initial reaction to approach by strangers positive, friendly (smiles, etc.).
    (b) Variable reaction.
    (c) Initial rejection or withdrawal.
57. (a) This initial reaction to strangers is intense: crying or laughing.
    (b) Variable.
    (c) Mild—frown or smile.
58. (a) General reaction to familiar people is friendly—smiles, laughs.
    (b) Variable reaction.
    (c) Generally glum or unfriendly. Little smiling.
59. (a) This reaction to familiar people is intense—crying or laughing.
    (b) Variable.
    (c) Mild—frown or smile.

Reaction to new places and situations

60. (a) Initial reaction acceptance—tolerates or enjoys them within a few minutes.
    (b) Variable.
    (c) Initial reaction rejection—does not tolerate or enjoy them within a few minutes.
61. (a) After continued exposure (several minutes) accepts these changes easily.
    (b) Variable.
    (c) Even after continued exposure, accepts changes poorly.

Play

62. (a) In crib or play pen can amuse self for half hour or more looking at mobile, hands, etc.
    (b) Amuses self for variable length of time.
    (c) Indicates need for attention or new occupation after several minutes.
63. (a) Takes new toy right away and plays with it.
    (b) Variable.
    (c) Rejects new toy when first presented (won't grasp it or drops it right away).
64. (a) If rejects at first, after short while (several minutes) accepts new toy.
    (b) Variable.
    (c) Adjusts slowly to new toy.
65. (a) Play activity involves much movement—kicking, waving arms, etc. Much exploring.
    (b) Intermediate.
    (c) Generally lies quietly while playing. Explores little.
66. (a) If reaching for toy out of reach, keeps trying at it for 2 minutes or more.
    (b) Variable.
    (c) Stops trying in less than ½ minute.
67. (a) When given a toy, plays with it for many minutes.
    (b) Variable.
    (c) Plays with one toy for only short time (only 1-2 minutes).
68. (a) When playing with one toy, easily distracted by another.
    (b) Variable.
    (c) Not easily distracted by another toy.
69. (a) Play usually accompanied by laughing, smiling, etc.
    (b) Variable or intermediate.
    (c) Generally fussy during play.

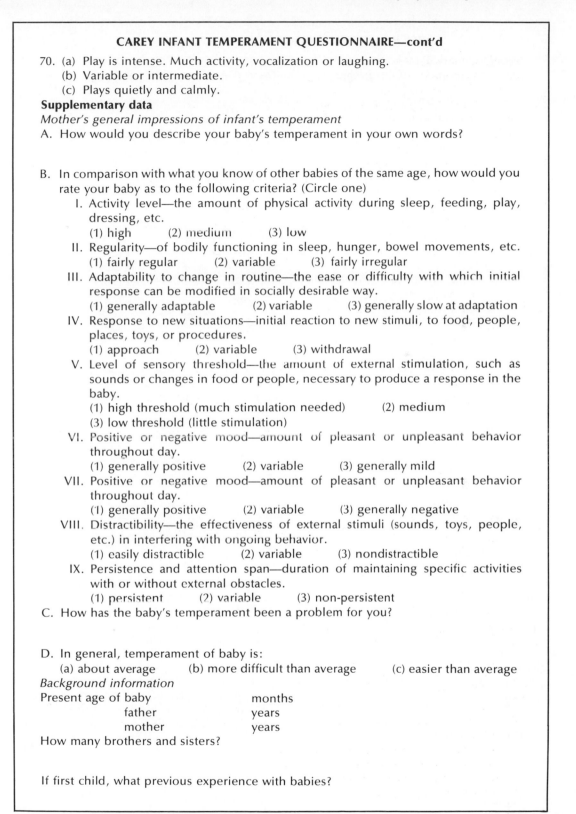

CAREY INFANT TEMPERAMENT QUESTIONNAIRE—cont'd

70. (a) Play is intense. Much activity, vocalization or laughing.
    (b) Variable or intermediate.
    (c) Plays quietly and calmly.

Supplementary data

Mother's general impressions of infant's temperament

A. How would you describe your baby's temperament in your own words?

B. In comparison with what you know of other babies of the same age, how would you rate your baby as to the following criteria? (Circle one)
    I. Activity level—the amount of physical activity during sleep, feeding, play, dressing, etc.
       (1) high   (2) medium   (3) low
    II. Regularity—of bodily functioning in sleep, hunger, bowel movements, etc.
       (1) fairly regular   (2) variable   (3) fairly irregular
    III. Adaptability to change in routine—the ease or difficulty with which initial response can be modified in socially desirable way.
       (1) generally adaptable   (2) variable   (3) generally slow at adaptation
    IV. Response to new situations—initial reaction to new stimuli, to food, people, places, toys, or procedures.
       (1) approach   (2) variable   (3) withdrawal
    V. Level of sensory threshold—the amount of external stimulation, such as sounds or changes in food or people, necessary to produce a response in the baby.
       (1) high threshold (much stimulation needed)   (2) medium
       (3) low threshold (little stimulation)
    VI. Positive or negative mood—amount of pleasant or unpleasant behavior throughout day.
       (1) generally positive   (2) variable   (3) generally mild
    VII. Positive or negative mood—amount of pleasant or unpleasant behavior throughout day.
       (1) generally positive   (2) variable   (3) generally negative
    VIII. Distractibility—the effectiveness of external stimuli (sounds, toys, people, etc.) in interfering with ongoing behavior.
       (1) easily distractible   (2) variable   (3) nondistractible
    IX. Persistence and attention span—duration of maintaining specific activities with or without external obstacles.
       (1) persistent   (2) variable   (3) non-persistent
C. How has the baby's temperament been a problem for you?

D. In general, temperament of baby is:
    (a) about average   (b) more difficult than average   (c) easier than average

Background information

Present age of baby   months
                father   years
                mother   years
How many brothers and sisters?

If first child, what previous experience with babies?

Continued.

CAREY INFANT TEMPERAMENT QUESTIONNAIRE—cont'd

Supplementary data—cont'd

Any complications of this pregnancy or delivery? (Describe)

Any complication for baby in newborn nursery? (Describe)

Any illness in baby so far? (Describe)

Is present housing arrangement adequate for your present needs?

Father's and mother's educational achievements. (Circle number)

Father's   *Mother's*
   1. Graduate professional training completed   1.
      (M.A., Ph.D., etc.)
   2. 4 year college completed   2.
   3. Partial college training   3.
   4. High school graduate   4.
   5. Partial high school   5.
   6. Junior high school completed   6.
   7. Less than 7 years of school   7.
Anything else significant about the baby's surroundings at present?

Date completed_____

METHOD OF SCORING

The mother's completed questionnaire is rated according to each of the nine categories of temperament on a separate scoring sheet. (See Fig. 6-4, pp. 112 and 113.) Scoring is accomplished by transposing the mother's response on each of the seventy statements to the nine category columns on the scoring sheet. Each of the nine columns of scores is then totaled.

After the scores for each of the nine categories have been calculated, an infant is assigned one of four diagnostic clusters: difficult, intermediate, high or low, or easy, which are defined as follows:

A difficult baby is defined as one who has 4 or 5 difficult-easy category scores on the difficult side of the mean (irregular, low in adaptability, initial withdrawal, intense, and predominantly negative mood) with at least two of these more than one standard deviation from the mean. Easy babies have no more than two difficult category ratings, neither being

greater than one standard deviation. Intermediate infants (high and low) fall in between.[*]

Carey[5] was able to obtain seventy-six ratings on the nine categories of infant reactivity (six of the seventy items given points in two categories). Each infant receives nine reactivity scores. Carey explains how he obtained the mean scores for each of the nine categories of infant reactivity as follows:

The total ratings at the three levels in each category were then multiplied by 0, 1, and 2, e.g., the total of intense ratings was multiplied by 0, variable by 1, and mild by 2. These products were added and that sum divided by the total number of completed items in the category. This yielded a mean score between 0 and 2,

---

[*]From Carey, William B.: Clinical applications of infant temperament measurements, J. Pediatr. **81:** 824, 1972.

Table 6-1. Means and standard deviations for nine temperament categories by questionnaire technique*

Category	Mean ± SD	For scoring questionnaire	
		Slightly to moderately difficult	*Very difficult*
Activity	0.49 ± 0.31		
Rhythmicity	0.55 ± 0.47	0.56-1.02	1.03-2.00
Adaptability	0.34 ± 0.26	0.35-0.59	0.60-2.00
Approach	0.47 ± 0.33	0.47-0.79	0.80-2.00
Threshold	1.09 ± 0.38		
Intensity	1.06 ± 0.31	0.76-1.05	0.00-0.75
Mood	0.41 ± 0.23	0.41-0.63	0.64-2.00
Distractibility	0.54 ± 0.31		
Persistence	0.71 ± 0.41		

*From Carey, William B.: Measuring infant temperament, J. Pediatr. **81:**414, 1972.

representing the infant's typical reaction for that category.*

In comparing his mean scores with those obtained by Thomas and associates[6] for infants about the same age, Carey[5] reports that "on the basis of the numerical score alone, i.e., using 1 as the midpoint, one could conclude that by both techniques the average baby at four to eight months is active, regular, adaptable, high in initial approach, low in threshold, mild, predominantly positive in mood, distractible, and persistent."*

Carey's original base sample of 101 subjects was extended to 200 for standardization purposes.[4] The population sample subjects were reported to have the following ratings: 14% were rated as difficult, 47.5% were designated as intermediate (24 were high and 71 were low), and 38.5% were rated as easy babies.

With the standardization sample increased to 200 subjects, Carey[7] recomputed the means and standard deviations for the nine categories of temperament. The revised scores are presented in Table 6-1.

USEFULNESS OF THE QUESTIONNAIRE

The Carey Infant Temperament Questionnaire is viewed as easy to administer and simple and quick to score. The usual time for this procedure is 8 to 10 minutes. The mother has the option of completing it at home. The questionnaire is of little care value unless pro-

fessional feedback is given to the mother.

Used for the purpose for which it was designed, the Carey Infant Temperament Questionnaire is a valuable adjunct in planning, implementing, and fostering more effective interactions between infants and parents. The three principal uses of the questionnaire are as follows:
1. To serve as a basis for general discussion of an infant's temperament
2. To serve as a basis for discussing an individual infant's needs
3. To help with clinical problems of which infant temperament can be a part

Determining an infant's temperament lessens haphazard guessing on the part of the child care professional about what the infant is like or what the parents may be experiencing with the infant's behavioral responses in the home environment.

Perhaps most importantly the Carey tool fills an assessment gap both in terms of subject and age period. Few tools have heretofore concentrated on either temperamental characteristics or the critical 4- to 8-month development period. Even fewer instruments have offered the validity of baseline data or have indicated intervention and management strategies on an ongoing basis.

IMPLICATIONS OF THE QUESTIONNAIRE FOR PARENTS AND CHILD HEALTH PROFESSIONALS

Based on clinical observations, in my opinion it is important to determine how the mother has interpreted the tool's language. What do the terms mean to her, and how do they apply to

*From Carey, William B.: A simplified method for measuring infant temperament. J. Pediatr. **77:**190, 1970.

Activity (H M L)	Rhythmicity (R V I)	Adaptability (A V N)	Approach (A V N)	Threshold (H M L)	Intensity (I V M)	Mood (P V N)	Distractibility (D V N)	Persistence (P V N)
4 a b c	1 a b c	5 a b c				3 a b c	8 a b c	
	2 a b c	9 a b c						
	6 a b c							
	7 a b c							
13 a b c			19 a b c	12 c b a	15 a b c	11 a b c	16 a b c	10 a b c
14 a b c					18 a b c	17 a b c		
	27 a b c	22 a b c		24 c b a	21 a b c	20 a b c		25 a b c
		23 a b c		28 c b a	26* a b a	26* c b a		
						29 x b a		
				30 c b a	32 a b c	31 x b a		
34 a b c		35* a b c			36 a b c	35* x b a	33 a b c	
39 a b c					38 a b c	37 a b c		

40			41 a b c	40 a x c	42* a b c	48 a b c	45 a b c	46 a b c	
			42* a b c	43 a b c			47* a b c	49 a b c	
			44 a b c						
			47* a b c						
50			53 a b c	56* a b c	51 a b c	52 a b c	50 c b a	54 a b c	
					55 c b a	57 a b c	56* a b c		
						59 a b c	58 a b c		
60	65 a b c		61 a b c	60* a b c			60* a b c		62 a b c
			64 a b c	63 a b c			69 a b c	68 a b c	66 a b c
						70 a b c			67 a b c

Fig. 6-4. Carey Infant Temperament Questionnaire scoring sheet. Responses on the questionnaire are transposed to this score sheet, providing a total score of high, medium, or low for each category of temperament. x = no score; * = score in two categories. (From Carey, William B. In Westman, Jack D., editor: Individual differences in children, New York, 1973, John Wiley & Sons, Inc.)

her infant? Such information can be elicited by asking her some of the following questions: "What is a normal infant like?" and "How does your infant differ from this?" The mother can further describe what her infant's activity is like. What would she like to see different in her infant's activity? When specifically would she like to see change? What does she perceive as average for rhythmicity of biological functions? How long has she observed these differences? How long has she desired a change in her infant's behaviors? How does an average infant adapt to change in routine? What is her own infant's response to new routines? (Give examples of specific routines.) Can she give direct observational data? Will she keep records of when she thinks her infant either adapts to change or fails to adapt to change? What does she do to make it easier for the infant to change? Do her methods help? What else has she thought of? Would she describe how her infant either approaches or withdraws in a new situation? What bothers her the most about her infant's behaviors? Have other people agreed with her own observations? How long has she noticed these behaviors in her infant? How long has it been a source of discomfort to her?

Would she describe the baby's intensity of response? How does her infant compare with other infants and to what extent is her infant similar or different? Would she describe some behaviors and specify precisely what she means?

Has she noticed that the infant's mood is always the same? How many times can she remember the infant as having the same mood? Is there any time when the infant's mood is different? Does her behavior influence the infant's mood? How does her behavior specifically influence the mood of her infant?

How distractible is the average infant? How does her infant compare to the average infant in distractibility? How long does she expect the infant to maintain his attention? What is the longest time and the shortest time for maintaining his attention? Would she describe how often in the last 3 days her infant has been distractible? What could she do to respond differently to the infant's distractibility?

Does she equate "different" with being "bad"? Does she ever see the infant changing his characteristics? When does she anticipate he will change?

Has she noticed her infant being persistent?

How does she define persistent? When is the infant persistent? (Describe when she last saw him persistent.) Does she wish him to change this trait? What does she prefer to do to alter persistence? Will she be comfortable with persistence to some activities? By asking some of these questions, a mother is encouraged to participate in a mutual problem-solving process with the child care professional.

As Carey[4] indicates, it is important that mothers gain a more objective view of infant temperament and behaviors so that more effective counseling, support, advice, and reassurance can be offered to those who describe or indicate concerns about interacting with, caring for, and providing for their infant's needs. Carey suggests that this tool has potential value for the nurse and physician in assessing and exploring implications for parents of an infant who is either extremely distractible, persistent, very active, or inactive or who has a "slow to warm up" style.

The questionnaire has equally significant implications for child care professionals to encourage mothers or fathers to define precisely what they mean when they use descriptive adjectives like "difficult," "active," "slow," "average," or others. It also suggests the need for collaboration between parents, nurses, and physicians.

In my opinion, the questionnaire automatically serves as a base on which to begin mutual problem solving and to teach parents about intervention techniques and their role in changing their infant's behavior or responding to his unique temperamental traits.

As Carey[4] points out, infants who display various temperaments also differ in their rates of development. For example, he found that very active infants walked sooner than the inactive ones. Infants found to be persistent used two words with meaning significantly more frequently than nonpersistent infants at one year of age.

As a result of these findings, parents may need assistance in learning about the impact of temperament on development. The findings also suggest that parents' expectations about their infant's development need examining so that their expectations can be formulated on a more realistic basis.

Carey's data[4] suggest that the difficult temperament syndrome of an infant, a low sensory threshold, or both are among the intrinsic factors associated with colic in infancy. Thus if a difficult temperament is involved, parents might be helped to anticipate and prevent further problems. Those parents who have difficult, irritable infants also need support for the energies they invest in attempting to console an infant.

These findings suggest that the Carey Infant Temperament Questionnaire has tremendous implications for parents and professionals in child health care. By being able to screen for temperamental qualities, individual differences of the infant, and his adaptations to significant persons in his environment, there is a better possibility of planning anticipatory care and implementing child care strategies that optimize development of the infant and interactions between him and his care providers.

REFERENCES

1. Brazelton, T. Berry: The Neonatal Behavioral Assessment Scale, London, 1973, William Heinemann Ltd., and Philadelphia, 1973, J. B. Lippincott Co.
2. Thomas, Alexander, Chess, Stella, Birch, H. G., Hertzig, M. E., and Korn, S.: Behavioral individuality in early childhood, New York, 1963, New York University Press.
3. Buss, Arnold M., and Plomin, Robert: A temperament theory of personality, New York, 1975, John Wiley & Sons, Inc.
4. Carey, William B.: Clinical applications of infant temperament measurements, J. Pediatr. **81:**823-828, 1972.
5. Carey, William B.: A simplified method for measuring infant temperament, J. Pediatr. **77:**188-194, 1970.
6. Carey, William B.: Measurement of infant temperament in pediatric practice. In Westman, Jack D., editor: Individual differences in children, New York, 1973, John Wiley & Sons, Inc.
7. Carey, William B.: Measuring infant temperament, J. Pediatr. **81:**414, 1972.
8. Carey, William B., and McDevitt, S. C.: Revision of the Infant Temperament Questionnaire, Pediatrics **61:**735-739, 1978.
9. McDevitt, S. C., and Carey, William B.: The measurement of temperament in 3- to 7-year-old children, J. Child Psychol. Psychiatry **19:**245-253, 1978.

ADDITIONAL READINGS

Carey, William B.: Night waking and temperament in infancy, J. Pediatr. **84:**756-758, 1974.
Carey, William B., Lipton, Willa L., and Meyers, Ruth A.: Temperament in adopted and foster babies, Child Welfare **53:**352-359, 1974.
Chess, Stella: Individuality in children, its importance to the pediatrician, J. Pediatr. **69:**676-684, 1966.
Escalona, S. K.: The roots of individuality, Chicago, 1968, Aldine Publishing Co.
Korner, A. F.: Individual differences at birth: implications for early experience and later development, Am. J. Orthopsychiatry **41:**608-619, 1971.
Riciuti, H. N.: Social and emotional behavior in infancy, Merrill-Palmer Q. Behav. Dev. **14:**82, 1968.
Rutter, M., and others: Genetic and environmental factors in the development of "primary reactor patterns," Br. J. Soc. Clin. Psychol. **2:**161, 1963.
Thomas, A., Chess, S., and Birch, H. G.: Temperament and behavior disorders in children, New York, 1968, New York University Press.

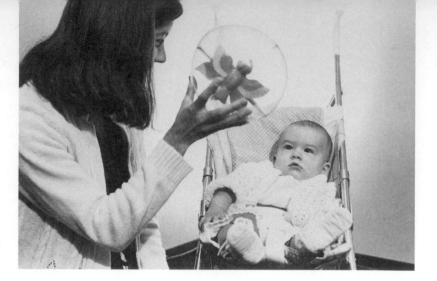

7

GUIDE FOR
ASSESSMENT OF THE INFANT'S
ANIMATE AND INANIMATE ENVIRONMENT

An infant's early adaptation and subsequent mastery of behaviors and skills in information processing, development of fine and gross motor skills, socialization, and language production can be vastly influenced by the quality and quantity of stimuli that are available and offered within his learning environment. Thus it is important that stimuli be provided for each infant and that these be neither excessive nor deficient for his individual needs.

It is vital that direct observations be made of the environmental stimuli that are offered and the infant's response to them. Observations of the variety, range, timing, amount, and frequency of efforts made by the infant's caregiver are necessary for assuring appropriate quality and quantity of stimuli.

Parents exercise a vital role in providing, regulating, and judging appropriate stimulation for their children from the newborn period on. It is important that parents interact with their infants to stimulate learning, cognitive functioning, personal-social adaptations, and language development.

To meet the individual needs of an infant, one must have knowledge and baseline information about the infant's environment and whether it is responding to his unique and changing needs.

Generally, data indicate that infants and young children are vulnerable to both nurturing and depriving environments. There are hazards to beginning stimulation too early or too late and in providing too much or too little stimulation. Carefully planned programs of early infant stimulation and social interaction can assist the growth and development of infants and children.

Attention in the child care field has focused on measuring the infant's growth and developmental progress at different time periods. Tools have been designed and standardized and are used in routine evaluations of a child's growth and development. Less attention has been invested in development and standardization of tools that measure the environment in which the child grows and develops.

The environment, which nurtures or impedes the processes of development for any child, merits further examination (Fig. 7-1). As discussed in the following section, certain observations are made to obtain baseline data on an infant's environment.

ASSESSMENT OF AN INFANT'S ENVIRONMENT

Essentially the child care professional is looking for excessive or inadequate provision of stimuli for an infant; it is also important that monitoring for developmentally appropriate stimulation be initiated. Observations should be carried out on the following developmental tasks, stimuli, and environments that are provided for infants, as well as on mother-infant interactions and mothers' assessments of infants' stimulation.

A. Opportunities to develop head control
1. What is infant's favorite position to be held?
2. How often is position changed (number of times)?
3. What position is infant placed? Different?
4. Is infant held in front, back, or side of parent?
5. Is infant pulled to sitting position? How often?
6. Is infant placed on abdomen? How often? On back? How often?
7. How long is infant held once picked up?

B. Visual accommodation
1. Are there varied opportunities to see? From different heights such as on floor, sofa, chair, crib?
2. What is available to see?

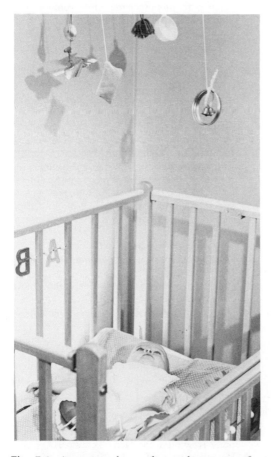

Fig. 7-1. Assessing the quality and quantity of an infant's inanimate environment. The infant is attending to the different visual stimuli in her line of vision.

3. Is light varied?
4. Are objects varied?
5. How much face-to-face contact is there? Does infant follow faces and inanimate objects? What is length of time infant attends to object, face, toy, or activity?
6. Are visual objects complex? Simple? Colorful? Bright or dull?
7. Is infant placed in different rooms throughout the day?
8. Does mother look directly at infant's eyes and face? Does infant focus on mother's eyes and face?

C. Motor control
1. Is there evidence of infant play with hands, fingers, and feet?
2. Is there evidence of encouragement and opportunity to develop head and chest control? How many times a day?
3. Does parent place infant in a position to turn freely?
4. Is infant ever briefly placed in standing position for weight bearing?
5. Does mother encourage movement of infant's arms and legs while he is bathed, dressed, and fed?
6. Are infant's movements restricted? Does mother interfere with or stop an activity that infant begins? Verbal restrictions (number of times)? Physical restrictions (number of times)?
7. Does clothing or blankets impede movement?

D. Feeding
1. How often is infant touched and mode?
2. Is infant held in horizontal or up position?
3. How much time is required for feeding?
4. Does mother smile or talk? Does her affect change? Does infant's affect change?
5. How close is infant held to mother, or if not held, what is mother's proximity while infant is being fed?
6. Does mother hold infant, or does another person?
7. Is infant propped?
8. Is there evidence of face-to-face or eye-to-eye contact?
9. Does mother observe infant's reactions?
10. What is mother's behavior in response to infant (talking, smiling, touching, etc.)?
11. Is technique of feeding varied (i.e., does mother offer nipple to each side of infant's mouth so that he gets opportunities to grasp it on right and left side of mouth, not just one side)?
12. When is spoon-feeding begun? What is mother's technique? Infant's reaction?
13. Is there evidence of oral-sensory stimulation?

E. Language
1. Is there eye-to-eye contact?

2. Is there face-to-face contact? How near is mother to infant usually when verbalizing or making sounds?
3. Does mother repeat sounds that infant makes?
4. Does infant's activity change in response to sounds he hears?
5. Does mother talk spontaneously while washing, feeding, holding, dressing, playing, and walking around with infant?
6. What sounds are heard? What is content of what is being said?
7. When does infant make sounds and how often?
8. What is total number of maternal vocalizations to infant during observation period?

F. Sleeping environment
1. Is crib changed to different positions in room?
2. Is surface stimulation varied? Weight of covers varied?
3. Is room temperature varied?
4. What is position in which baby is placed to sleep?
5. How much time does infant spend sleeping or lying on back?

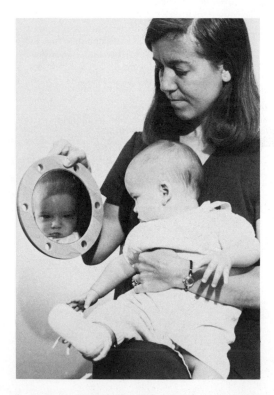

Fig. 7-2. Determining an infant's reaction to an inanimate stimulus that is offered within her developmental environment. The mother has provided a mirror for the infant to attend to. The infant is purposefully attending to the bright object.

6. How often is infant on side or abdomen?
7. How much freedom of movement does infant have?
8. Where does infant sleep?
9. Are patterns of sleep similar from day to day, changing, or inconsistent?

G. General stimuli available in infant's environment
1. How much stimulus is available for baby to see (e.g., presence of mobiles)?
2. Are covers soft, silky, smooth, velvety, furry, rough, fuzzy, colorful, and clean?
3. What is intensity and variability of noise levels in rooms (e.g., quiet, loud, consistent)?
4. What is number, size, shape, and appropriateness of toys selected? Are they different textures, shapes, sizes, colors, in crib, offered at appropriate times, or handed to him? What is infant's ability to reach, grasp, and hold onto toys? Are toys alternated?

H. Tactile stimuli
1. When held, is infant in actual contact with mother's trunk, chest, shoulders, head, and/or face?
2. What is frequency of touching, rubbing, patting, kissing, bouncing, rocking, and holding?
3. How long is infant usually left alone? How much time in playpen, infant seat, crib, or swing?
4. Are specific efforts made to attend to infant while he is quiet and amusing himself?
5. Are infant's head, neck, trunk, and extremities supported steadily when held?
6. How consistent is mother in her approaches to picking up and holding?
7. Is infant moved about quickly, slowly, abruptly, or gently and held closely and firmly?
8. How often does mother present a toy or object?
9. Does infant experience different positions in space (e.g., lifted up, turned around, and moved in different rhythms)?

I. Movement pattern
1. How often does infant move?
2. What objects or persons does infant move away from?
3. What objects or persons does infant move toward?
4. How many different places does infant move to and from?
5. How frequently does infant move head, chest, trunk, arms, and legs?
6. Do activity levels change in different environmental settings or with different care providers?

J. Provision of activities for infant
1. Does mother hold attention of infant by either nonverbal efforts, body movements, or use of toys? How often for each?
2. Does mother hold or attempt to entertain infant by verbal attempts?
3. If infant does not attend to mother's verbal or

physical efforts, what is her response (i.e., continuation or termination of effort to get infant to respond)?

4. Does mother offer verbal or nonverbal stimuli at a time when infant appears in an alert and attending state?
5. Does mother respond to infant's state of alertness by providing stimulation?
6. Does mother respond to inactive state, fatigue, or sleepy states by reducing efforts at stimulation? Is novelty of stimuli available?

K. Bathing
1. How often is infant bathed? Length of time of bath?
2. Who bathes infant?
3. What is infant's reaction?
4. What is mode and place?
5. Are diapers changed? How often? By whom?

L. Dressing
1. What is weight of clothes?
2. Are they loose or tight?
3. Are they dry and clean?
4. How often are clothes changed?
5. Is there variety in textures and colors of clothing?

M. Consoling
1. What is mother's definition of "fussiness," "irritated," and "distressed," and what explanation does she give for infant's crying?
2. What is mother's method of consoling infant when fussing and/or crying?
3. Does mother verbalize to infant? For how long?

4. Does mother touch infant? Where?
5. Does mother pick infant up?
6. Once picked up, does mother move, touch, stroke, caress, or rock infant?
7. Does mother talk to infant while holding?
8. Does mother distract with toys when fussing or crying occurs?
9. At what point of fussing or crying does mother attempt to console infant? How long does it take before crying or fussiness stops?
10. Does mother offer pacifier?
11. Does mother offer food?
12. Is infant placed in bed? Infant seat? Another location?
13. Does mother attend at onset of fussing?
14. When does infant begin to demonstrate signs of being consoled?
15. What is mother's response?
16. What is average number of times mother consoles infant a day?

N. Mother's assessment of infant's stimulation
1. Has mother thought of ways to promote head control, visual development, motor control, infant feeding, language, and appropriate patterns of sleep?
2. What has mother noted about infant's reactions to her attempts?
3. Has mother observed changes in infant's behavior?
4. How does mother view infant's development for his age? Is infant meeting mother's expectations?

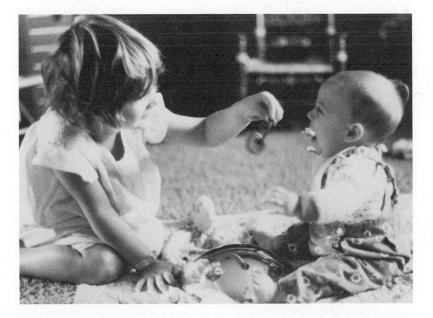

Fig. 7-3. Assessing an infant's interactions and responses to both an animate stimulus (child) and inanimate stimulus (bell).

5. What behaviors of infant are most satisfying to mother? What are least satisfying?

6. Has mother begun to consider next steps of development and ways to promote advances in infant's behavior?

7. Does mother express positive statements about infant's growth and development and her efforts at influencing infant's behavior?

IMPORTANCE OF SUPPORTIVE FEEDBACK TO PARENTS

Most parents like to feel a sense of adequacy about the appropriateness of the environment for their infant's development. It is important to encourage and reinforce parental sensitivity to the developmental needs of an infant and to an environment that is most suitable to the infant's changing needs. The child care professional should encourage parents in the following areas:

- Resourcefulness in trying methods
- Consistency of approach
- Appropriateness of efforts
- Consideration of alternative ideas and methods

Are parents offered verbal support, and are observations that are made of their efforts to provide appropriate animate and inanimate stimuli shared with them?

Health care professionals and parents may find it helpful to use the Parent-Infant Care Record to record the number of times the infant's environment has changed, how much consoling is necessary, and the frequency and duration of interactions in general. The record, kept by one of the parents, can be useful as a reference for discussing concerns, problems, or lack of both. The Parent-Infant Care Record can be useful to a child care professional who may use it to offer supportive feedback concerning the effectiveness of parents to foster a nurturing, developmental environment that corresponds to their infant's needs.

THE PARENT-INFANT CARE RECORD

The Parent-Infant Care Record is designed in the form of a clock face to help record both day and nighttime care activities (Fig. 7-4). Parent-infant care activities, including feeding, diapering, sleeping, holding, consoling, parent play, environment change, position change, and checking, and baby's and parent's mood changes are recorded over a 24-hour period. Recording begins from the start and finish line as indicated in Fig. 7-4. Care information and baby's or mother's mood are recorded within 15-minute time periods as shown on the clock form.

Instructions

Following are the instructions to the mother:

1. There are nine circles within the clock face, each circle corresponding to a care activity. The type of care given, time care occurred, number of times care was given, and length of time care was provided are recorded in the appropriate circle. The wider, outermost circle is used for indicating both the baby's and mother's corresponding mood changes.

2. Three different symbols are used for recording care, length of care activity, and the mood of both baby and mother. These are an X, an arrow, and a happy or unhappy face.

3. Use a pencil for recording daytime information and a pen for nighttime records. If similar activities occur at the same time during the day or night, simply record appropriate symbols side by side in the same circle.

4. Begin the daytime record at 7:30 AM in the clock face and the nighttime record at 7:30 PM.

5. Place an X in appropriate circles to indicate each time that the baby was either diapered or checked by the mother or when infant's position was changed. "Change" refers to placing the baby on his left side after being on the right side, placing the baby on his stomach after being on his back, and other similar changes.

6. Draw complete arrows to show when the following activities begin, continue, or stop: feeding, parent play, consoling infant for fussing or crying, picking up and holding baby, all the baby's sleep periods (no matter how short), and changes in the baby's environment (e.g., if the infant is placed on the couch or bed after being removed from the bassinet or crib, if moved from the bedroom to infant seat in the kitchen, or if moved from a higher place like the kitchen table to a blanket on the floor).

7. To show perceived mood changes of the baby or mother during day, night, morning, or evening, draw these figures to indicate a happy ☺ or unhappy ☹ face. Draw the mother's face to the right within the outermost circle, and draw the infant's face to the left within the outermost circle. Draw the mother's face next to the infant's face to indicate corresponding mood changes or lack of change in mood. The mother's face should be drawn proportionately larger than the infant's face to distinguish between them.

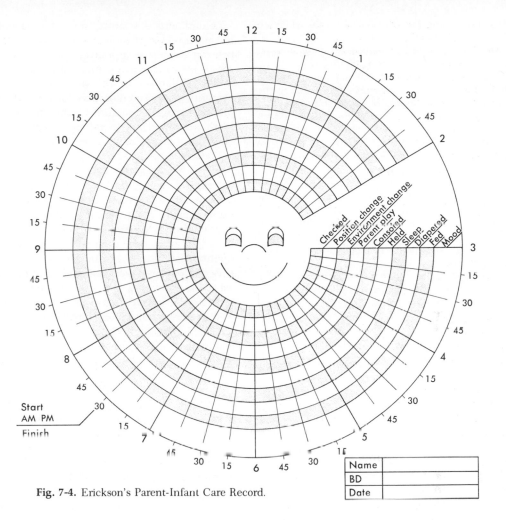

Fig. 7-4. Erickson's Parent-Infant Care Record.

Name	
BD	
Date	

8. Please comment if there is anything unusual.

Some mothers may wish to keep records on only selected activities contained in the Parent-Infant Care Record, which is permissible.

Example of a case record

The mother of a 6-day-old newborn recorded parent-infant care and activities for 24 hours. The data when analyzed revealed the following information.

The mother had checked her infant eight times during the day and four times during the night. She changed the infant's position seven times during the day and two times during the night. She recorded a change in the infant's environment six times during the day and three times during the night.

The mother played with the infant twice during the day. She consoled the infant six times during the day for crying and three times during the night. A total of 2 hours 7 minutes was recorded for consoling the infant. The average consolation periods occurred for 15 minutes at a time. Twice as much time was spent in consoling the infant during the daytime as compared to nighttime. The daytime consoling activities were noted to be shorter but more frequent than nighttime consoling periods.

She held her infant five times during the day and four times during the night. The mother perceived holding as nondemanding of her, and she reported that she enjoyed the opportunity of holding the infant. The mother held the infant for long periods at night while the infant slept. The longest period of night holding was 1 hour 22 minutes.

The mother recorded nine sleep periods during the daytime and three sleep periods during the night. A total of twelve sleep periods were noted, and the infant slept for a total of 16 hours 52 minutes. The mother was reassured her infant's duration of sleep was average.

The mother diapered the infant eight times during the day and four times during the night.

The mother noted that she fed the infant five times during the day and three times during the night. A total of 4.2 hours was spent in feeding during the 24-hour period. The mother accounted for one lengthy feeding period at night as enjoyable. This feeding period lasted from 3:15 AM to 4:15 AM and was described as pleasant for the mother.

Moods as recorded by the mother revealed that there were no periods when she was unhappy and the infant was happy. She did record four periods in which she was happy and the infant was unhappy. The infant had nine happy faces as contrasted to seven brief unhappy times. The mother seemed pleased that her infant was happy more often than it was unhappy.

The mother stated that the record was helpful to her in having what she thought she was observing validated by her own recordings. Because of the number of times the mother was up during the night, she was queried as to whether she was getting enough sleep for herself. She responded that she was appreciative of the nurse's concern for her but was making up for any loss of sleep at night by short naps throughout the day.

This mother remarked that the record was useful in helping her pay more attention to her infant and that she had enjoyed discussing it with a supportive nurse.

IMPLICATIONS OF THE PARENT-INFANT CARE RECORD

The Parent-Infant Care Record is valuable in obtaining accurate data so that objective, preventive care approaches can be offered. It is a helpful adjunct in conveying appropriate empathetic support to mothers, particularly during the early mother-infant acquaintance process and as the infant makes changes in early developmental patterns.

The record, if used as designed, offers child care professionals a systematic approach to being more sensitive to needs that infants have as well as the ongoing needs of parents.

Information of importance to the mother and child health professional can be gained, shared, and explored on an objective basis. For example, the Parent-Infant Care Record can help determine the length of time the mother spends in feeding an infant, the longest and shortest periods of time between feedings, the longest and shortest periods of time spent in feeding, the average number of feedings during the daytime and nighttime, and the average number of feedings in a 24-hour period.

In addition, the mother may find it helpful to keep a record of the longest periods of happiness an infant has in a given day; the hours in which he seems most content, and whether the infant is happier in the morning, afternoon, evening, after feedings, play, or after environmental changes that the mother makes. The mother can find out the infant's average periods of happiness an hour, as well as his average periods of happiness a day. It can be helpful to explore whether the infant's happy periods correspond to the mother's positive periods. If a mother has perceived her infant as fussy, it can be helpful to have concrete data to examine to orient her to the infant, who may have longer periods of happiness than she describes, or she might learn that the infant has more happy periods than fussy periods a day. The mother is asked to draw in a happy or unhappy face to indicate the infant's mood or temperament, as well as her own mood in response to the baby's needs. Most mothers experience a more positive perception and orientation when they can actually observe and document their infant's and their own moods in an objective way.

A mother can find it helpful to keep track of the infant's fussy periods too. The record can serve as a valuable means of pointing out the shortest periods of fussiness, the longest periods of fussiness, and the average number of fussy periods in an hour, day, or week. Sometimes mothers become subjective in their estimations of the infant's fussy periods. By keeping records, a mother can be helped to look objectively at the occurrence of fussiness. Perhaps she can learn the infant is not as fussy as she thought or for shorter periods of time than she thought. At the same time, the record can be useful as a frame of reference to explore the mother's reactions to fussy periods and her mood changes, which might correspond to the infant's crying or fussy periods. Perhaps she can express her views on how frustrating it is to try to console the infant. Her effective efforts at consoling the infant can be acknowledged as well.

Results of the record can serve to increase the child care professional's sensitivity to the mother's needs as well as the infant's needs. A record kept by a mother offers important clues about her experiences, efforts, and interactions that might warrant further in-depth consideration.

As a result of keeping records of position changes, environmental changes, or parent play, objective feedback can be offered to a mother who is committed to providing both appropriate animate and inanimate stimuli in an environment that best responds to her infant's needs.

If a mother keeps an accurate record of the number of times the infant is consoled and the length of time it takes to quiet her infant, a concrete reference is established for validating the mother's concern of fussiness and the actual amount of time she is consoling the infant. A record of the amount of time needed for consoling the infant is necessary before the mother can accurately and objectively participate in more effective problem-solving methods. Perhaps she can try other ways of consoling her infant. The mother can be asked what she thinks will be most effective and least effective if changes are planned by her.

The record a mother keeps of the amount of time spent in holding an infant is important. Being held offers kinesthetic stimuli, which is important sensory input for the infant. The amount of time an infant is held may serve as an indicator of whether the mother likes to hold the infant and does it spontaneously or if the infant is held as a result of crying. It might be important from the standpoint that the mother does not hold the infant frequently because she describes the infant as resistive to being held. Some mothers interpret certain behaviors of the infant as clues indicating that he "doesn't like being held." If a mother wants to hold her infant and enjoys touching and holding, she may be frustrated or disappointed to have an infant whom she describes as not wanting to be held. These data would merit further observations and in-depth supportive discussions with the mother about her views of the infant's behavior and what it means to her and perhaps a further exploration of other clues that signal the need for obtaining an in-depth picture of the infant's temperament and interactional styles with other people or activities.

Records are valuable for determining patterns and changes in sleep behavior. At birth the normal infant spends an average of 17 hours a day in sleep.[1] By 12 to 14 weeks of age, the infant's sleep cycles and patterns have changed, with the infant establishing a diurnal cycle or sleeping through the night.[2] If the infant is not sleeping through the night after 3 months of age, a more extensive examination is indicated. Sleep patterns are increasingly being recognized as an index of maturation, integration, and organization of the central nervous system.[3]

The longest period of sleep a day can be recorded and explored with the mother. Also the mother can learn what the shortest periods of sleep are for her infant. The average sleep periods a day can be estimated by the records the mother keeps. She may subjectively think that her infant is sleeping too much or too little but may learn that the infant is sleeping the appropriate amount of time for his age period. This information that her infant's sleep is well within normal limits can be a source of relief or reassurance to the mother. If the infant's sleep patterns are not indicative of normal patterns, further exploration can occur. In addition to the average sleep periods a day, the average number of hours the infant sleeps during the daytime can be calculated. The average number of hours of sleep a night can also be recorded.

The record can be a source of support for the mother, can help in validating her concerns about her baby, and, more importantly, can help the child care professional give more appropriate responses to a mother who is unhappy, getting up during the night, exhausted, or showing other needs during the time she is getting to know her infant and during the time she is involved in his care.

Both mothers and health care professionals can gain information from records that are kept on a systematic basis. The following information can be obtained:

1. Longest periods of sleep a day
2. Shortest periods of sleep a day
3. Average sleep periods a day
4. Average number of hours of sleep during the daytime
5. Average number of hours of sleep during the night
6. Longest periods between sleep
7. Shortest periods between sleep
8. Longest periods of feeding
9. Shortest periods of feeding
10. Average number of feedings during the daytime
11. Average number of feedings during the night
12. Longest periods between feedings
13. Shortest periods between feedings
14. Longest periods of the infant's happiness
15. Shortest periods of happiness
16. Most likely hours or periods of happiness
17. Average number of happiness periods throughout the day
18. Average periods of fussiness

19. Average number of the fussy periods during the daytime
20. Average number of fussy periods during the night
21. Longest periods of fussiness (daytime or night)
22. Shortest periods of fussiness (daytime or night)
23. Number of times the mother checks the infant (daytime or night)
24. Average number of times the mother checks the infant
25. Number of times the mother changes the infant's position (daytime or night)
26. Number of times the mother changes the infant's environment (daytime or night)
27. Number of times the infant is consoled (daytime or night)
28. Average length of time needed for consoling the infant (daytime or night)
29. Most effective mode of consoling the infant
30. Number of times the infant is held during the daytime
31. Number of times the infant is held during the night
32. Average number of times the infant is held in a 24-hour period
33. Average number of diaper changes during the daytime or night
34. Number of happy or positive times the mother experiences during the daytime or night
35. Average number of times the mother is awake and attending the needs of the baby during the night

The Parent-Infant Care Record, kept for a period of 5 to 7 days, can be helpful in determining objective patterns of mother-infant care. It can be effective in obtaining objective data about mother-infant care activities occurring during a day or over a specified period of time. The child care professional can find it useful in offering appropriate counseling, guidance, and assistance to parents once or on a serial basis.

USES OF THE PARENT-INFANT CARE RECORD

The following list contains suggested uses of the Parent-Infant Care Record:

- Be given to mothers who are rooming in to keep track of activities and infant care occurring during the day and evening while in the hospital
- Be used in detecting early clues of difficulty

occurring between infant and mother before they are discharged from the newborn setting by serving as a useful reference for anticipatory guidance for problems concerning sleep, feeding, or consoling

- Be used in encouraging mothers from the beginning that their observations are accurate and are *important*
- Be the foundation for identifying teaching needs of parents with newborns and infants
- Serve to indicate the need for further observations by other health care professionals
- Be used as part of the infant's early baby book and the record that the mother keeps during the first week
- Become an integral part of the infant's hospital record for reference in later comparisons
- Be used as baseline information for parents and professionals and serve in many ways as an objective, reliable reference from which to make more accurate comparisons of infant and parental progress toward selected objectives
- Be used in teaching mothers to look for patterns of behavior, to record when activities begin and end, and to become accustomed to objective ways to describe their interactions rather than relying on global terms
- Serve as a valuable source in acquainting the mother with actual infant behaviors

If the mother is not able to or does not keep records when asked during the newborn period or early phases of infancy, the following implications should be considered:

1. The mother may be uncomfortable with observations.
2. She may not be able to sort out one behavior from another.
3. She may not understand the directions.
4. She may not be psychologically ready to make observations.
5. She may not feel the need for observations.

Nurses and physicians can become more sensitive and can convey appropriate responses and interest in what parents are observing and doing, how parents are responding to their infant's needs, and how parents are trying to effect change. Looking at the parents' records affords an opportunity to acknowledge the parents' identification of concerns, their problem-solving abilities, and their strengths in beginning and continuing efforts to effect and evaluate change in the early acquaintance process between parents and infants.

SUMMARY

The Parent-Infant Care Record has been designed to assist clinical practitioners to improve their observations, record keeping, and problem-solving approaches with mothers of newborns, young infants, or children. The use of the Parent-Infant Care Record relies on a mother keeping a daily record of selected activities usually for a period of a week. The data obtained can be a foundation for anticipatory guidance, emotional support, reassurance, identification of problems, and mutual participation in problem solving and decision making with parents, nurses, physicians, or other child care professionals.

REFERENCES

1. Parmelee, Arthur H., Schulz, Helen R., and Disbrow, Mildred: Sleep patterns of the newborn, J. Pediatr. **58:**241-250, 1961.
2. Parmelee, Arthur H., Wenner, Waldemar H., and Schulz, Helen R.: Infant sleep patterns: from birth to 16 weeks of age, J. Pediatr. **65:**576-582, 1964.
3. Stern, Evelyn, Parmelee, Arthur H., Akiyama, Y., and others: Sleep cycle characteristics in infants, Pediatrics **43:**65-70, 1969.

ADDITIONAL READINGS

Caldwell, Bettye M.: The fourth dimension in early childhood education, In Hess, Robert, and Bear, Roberta, editors: Early education, Chicago, 1968, Aldine Publishing Co.

Caldwell, Bettye M., and Richmond, Julius B.: The Children's Center in Syracuse, New York. In Dittman, Laura L., editor: Early child care: the new perspectives, New York, 1968, Atherton Press.

Denenberg, V. H.: Critical periods, stimulus inputs, and emotional reactivity: a theory of infantile stimulation, Psychol. Rev. **71:**335-351, 1964.

Deutsch, Cynthia, and Deutsch, Martin: Brief reflections on the theory of early childhood enrichment programs, In Hess, Robert, and Bear, Roberta, editors: Early education, Chicago, 1968, Aldine Publishing Co.

Ellis, Richard: Prekindergarten education for the disadvantaged child. In Hellmuth, Jerome, editor: Disadvantaged child, vol. 1, Seattle, 1967, Special Child Publications of the Seattle Sequin School, Inc.

Gordon, Ira J.: Baby learning through baby play: a parent's guide for the first two years, New York, 1970, St. Martin's Press, Inc.

Hellmuth, Jerome, editor: Exceptional infant: the normal infant, vol. 1, Seattle, 1967, Bernie Traub & Jerome Hellmuth Co., Publishers.

Hess, Robert, and Bear, Roberta, editors: Early education, Chicago, 1968, Aldine Publishing Co.

LeLouis, M. R.: An experimental program to increase sitting-up skills in infants twelve to sixteen weeks of age, unpublished master's thesis, University of Washington, 1966.

Murphy, Lois B.: Spontaneous ways of learning in young children, Children **14:**210-216, Nov.-Dec., 1967.

Murphy, Lois B.: Individualization of child care and its relation to environment, In Dittman, Laura L., editor: Early child care: the new perspectives, New York, 1968, Atherton Press.

Painter, G.: Infant education, San Rafael, Calif., 1968, Dimensions Publishing Co.

Provence, Sally: The first year of life: the infant. In Dittman, Laura, L., editor: Early child care: the new perspectives, New York, 1968, Atherton Press.

Provence, Sally: The Yale Child Study Center project. In Dittman, Laura L., editor: Early child care: the new perspectives, New York, 1968, Atherton Press.

Provence, Sally, Palmer, Francis H., Gordon, Ira J., Schaefer, Earl S., and Robinson, Halbert: Children under three—finding ways to stimulate development; some current experiments, Children **16:**53-62, March-April, 1969.

Robinson, Halbert: The Frank Porter Graham Child Development Center. In Dittman, Laura L., editor: Early child care: the new perspectives, New York, 1968, Atherton Press.

Yarrow, Leon: Conceptualizing the early environment. In Dittman, Laura L., editor: Early child care: the new perspectives, New York, 1968, Atherton Press.

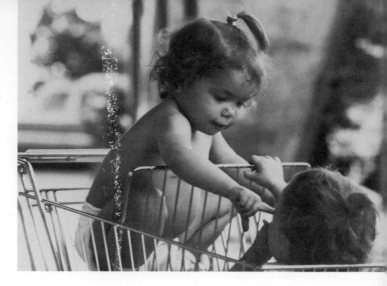

8

ASSESSMENT OF
THE CHILD'S ENVIRONMENT

A great deal of attention has been focused in recent years on standardizing tools that accurately assess growth and development of children. Less attention has been directed at assessing the animate and inanimate aspects of the child's environment that either foster or impede a child's growth and developmental processes. There is more concern for ways to assess the quality and quantity of social, emotional, and cognitive support that is available in a young child's environment. Although there have been almost no tools available that permit the precise measurement of the child's developmental and learning environment, this trend is changing.

Dr. Bettye M. Caldwell has been doing research for many years to develop hypotheses about the nature of the environment and how it best meets the needs of children. Over the past decade she formulated the view that it is not the social status or family structure that necessarily predicts a child's subsequent cognitive outcomes. She hypothesized that what was most important were various characteristics of the environment that could predict a child's developmental outcomes. This theoretical view stimulated her and her associates to devise a tool by which the subtle aspects of the young

child's environment could be measured to determine which specific features were most likely to influence the child's development. They endeavored to create a measure of the home environment that could warn of developmental risk before age 3 years.

Based on clinical observations and observations in the home, an inventory was developed that was intended to tap the environmental characteristics of a child from birth to 3 years of age that might be associated with favorable developmental outcomes for the child. This instrument is called the Home Observation for Measurement of the Environment (birth to three). The inventory endeavors to measure the following six subscales: (1) the emotional and verbal responsivity of the mother, (2) avoidance of restriction and punishment, (3) organization of the physical and temporal environment, (4) provision of appropriate play materials, (5) maternal involvement with the child, and (6) opportunities for variety in daily stimulation.

Caldwell also developed the Home Observation for Measurement of the Environment (three to six). This inventory is intended to tap the changing environment of the older child between 3 and 6 years of age. This inventory endeavors to measure the following seven subscales: (1) provision of stimulation through equipment, toys, and experiences; (2) stimulation of mature behavior; (3) provision of a stimulating physical and language environment; (4) avoidance of restriction and punishment; (5) pride, affection, and thoughtfulness; (6) masculine stimulation; and (7) independence from parental control.

The Home Observation for Measurement of the Environment (referred to as the HOME), developed by Caldwell and associates over the past fifteen years, is one of the first major tools of its kind to focus on the environment.

Because of Caldwell's research, means of providing substantive feedback to parents about the way they regulate their child's environment and how to effect environmental changes that best facilitate their child's growth and development are available. Such feedback can also be used to help parents meet their own needs for assuring their child an appropriate environment at different stages of development.

As an infant or child progresses in his adaptive functioning, there are corresponding needs for the developmental environment to change simultaneously. Parents may experience the need for help in creating and sustaining an environment that is most suitable for their child or may need reassurance that the environment is regularly and consistently providing appropriate input both in terms of timing and frequency that enhances the child's growth and development. Nurses, physicians, and early child educators can respond in more appropriate ways by expanding their roles in terms of developmental assessment and management of infants and children, as well as assessment of the child's developmental environment. By doing so, such professionals can improve their ability to provide counseling and guidance within a preventive framework.

Both inventories (birth to three and three to six) offer a valuable framework for systematically and objectively collecting information about the subtle aspects of a child's environment that can be used for the mutual benefit of both the child and his parents. The HOME may be used to assess not only the home environment but any environment in which the child spends time. It can be administered to the mother or any other primary caregiver. (It should be noted that the instruction manual relates only to the birth to three inventory.)

Although extensive standarization data are not available, both inventories measure inanimate and animate qualities and quantities and the variation and complexity of the child's environment.

Caldwell[1] states that the purpose of the HOME is to obtain samples of certain aspects of the quantity and quality of social, emotional, and cognitive support available to a young child within his home.

The selection of items has been guided by empirical evidence of the importance of certain types of experience for nourishing the behavioral development of the child. Included were such things as the importance of the opportunity to form a basic attachment to a mother or mother substitute; an emotional climate characterized by mutual pleasure, sensitive need gratification, and minimization of restriction and punishment; a physical environment that is both stimulating and responsive, offering a variety of modulated sensory experience; freedom to explore and master the environment; a daily schedule that is orderly and predictable; and an opportunity to assimilate and interpret experience within a consistent cultural milieu.[*]

Indices of health and nutritional status are not included in the inventory. As Caldwell asserts:

The development of this Inventory represents a conviction that such a gross structural designation as social class is insensitive to the cumulative transactions that occur daily between the infant and his environment and that an attempt to describe and measure these transactions will not only provide a more accurate description of the learning environment but will in addition help to pin-point areas in which intervention is needed.[†]

She further states:

The original intention was that all items should be based on direct observation of the interaction between caretaker (usually the mother) and the child. A large pool of items was generated, all of which required actual observation of mother-child behavior. But a conceptual examination of the items suggested that many important areas of infant experience were unfortunately excluded with this restriction on the type of items. Accordingly, with succeeding versions of the Inventory (the present is the fourth revision), items requiring interview data were added.[†]

---

[*] From Caldwell, Bettye M.: Instruction manual inventory for infants (Home Observation for Measurement of the Environment), Little Rock, Ark., 1970, p. 1.
[†] Ibid., p. 2.

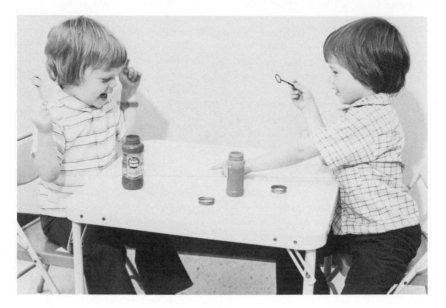

Fig. 8-1. The environment is assessed for provision of appropriate play materials for children.

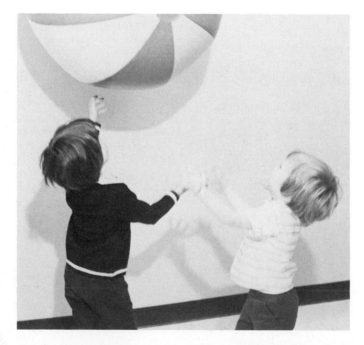

Fig. 8-2. Assessing the environment for toys or equipment that involve gross and fine motor skills.

Caldwell[1] suggests that prior to use, observation, and scoring of the HOME, the observer should be reasonably familiar with the content of each individual item.

The HOME can be of significance in the following ways:

1. Determining the frequency of contacts between adult caregivers and children
2. Determining that the child is in an environment that is both stimulating and responsive to his needs
3. Helping determine whether the emotional climate is positive or negative in nature
4. Helping determine if there is provision for sensory experiences that are neither understimulating nor overstimulating to the child
5. Helping determine the adequacy of novelty and range of contacts with others
6. Helping identify areas of strengths and weaknesses in a family
7. Planning appropriate guidance for a family
8. Identifying developmental risk before a child is 3 years of age
9. Planning intervention strategies when weaknesses or deficits are observed

One of Caldwell's original goals in developing the HOME was to have information gained from observations available for family guidance. It was her intent to be able to identify areas of strength and weaknesses in a family. She emphasizes that if the caregiving disciplines could profile a family's patterns, then those working with families could determine those areas which were in need of extra efforts by professionals in child health.

The HOME (birth to three) measures forty-five items in six major categories (pp. 130 to 132). The HOME (three to six) measures eighty items in seven major categories (pp. 133 to 137).

GENERAL INSTRUCTIONS FOR THE HOME

The HOME is administered by a person who goes into the home at a time when the child is awake and can be observed in his normal routine for that time of day. The entire procedure in the home generally takes about an hour.[1]

Making arrangements for the visit

The visit should never be made without careful advance arrangements; otherwise the mother might be led to think that an attempt is being made to catch her "off guard" (e.g., when her

Text continued on p. 137.

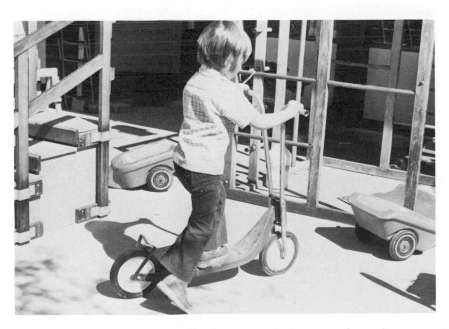

Fig. 8-3. This child has a scooter in the play environment to foster muscle coordination, posture, and balance.

HOME OBSERVATION FOR MEASUREMENT OF THE ENVIRONMENT

BIRTH TO THREE

Date of interview _____

Child designee _____
  Name   Age   Sex   Ethnicity

Child's birthday _____ Birth order _____

Mother's name _____ Father's name _____

Address _____

Categories	Raw scores	Percentile scores
I. Emotional and verbal responsivity of mother	_____	_____
II. Avoidance of restriction and punishment	_____	_____
III. Organization of physical and temporal environment	_____	_____
IV. Provision of appropriate play materials	_____	_____
V. Maternal involvement with child	_____	_____
VI. Opportunities for variety in daily stimulation	_____	_____
Totals	_____	_____

I. Emotional and verbal responsivity of mother

	Yes	No
1. Mother spontaneously vocalizes to child at least twice during visit (excluding scolding).		
2. Mother responds to child's vocalizations with a verbal response.		
3. Mother tells child the name of some object during visit or says name of person or object in a "teaching" style.		
4. Mother's speech is distinct, clear, and audible.		
5. Mother initiates verbal interchanges with observer—asks questions and makes spontaneous comments.		
6. Mother expresses ideas freely and easily and uses statements of appropriate length for conversation (e.g., gives more than brief answers).		
*7. Mother permits child occasionally to engage in "messy" type of play.		
8. Mother spontaneously praises child's qualities or behavior twice during visit.		
9. When speaking of or to child, mother's voice conveys positive feeling.		
10. Mother caresses or kisses child at least once during visit.		
11. Mother shows some positive emotional responses to praise of child offered by visitor.		
Subscore		

From Caldwell, Bettye M.: Home Observation for Measurement of the Environment (birth to three), 1970.
*Items that may require direct questions.

HOME—cont'd

BIRTH TO THREE—cont'd

II. Avoidance of restriction and punishment

	Yes	No

12. Mother does not shout at child during visit.

13. Mother does not express overt annoyance with or hostility toward child.

14. Mother neither slaps nor spanks child during visit.

*15. Mother reports that no more than one instance of physical punishment occurred during the past week.

16. Mother does not scold or derogate child during visit.

17. Mother does not interfere with child's actions or restrict child's movements more than three times during visit.

18. At least ten books are present and visible.

*19. Family has a pet.

Subscore

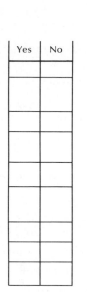

III. Organization of physical and temporal environment

	Yes	No

20. When mother is away, care is provided by one of three regular substitutes.

21. Someone takes child into grocery store at least once a week.

22. Child gets out of house at least four times a week.

23. Child is taken regularly to doctor's office or clinic.

*24. Child has a special place in which to keep his toys and "treasures."

25. Child's play environment appears safe and free of hazards.

Subscore

IV. Provision of appropriate play materials

	Yes	No

26. Child has some muscle activity toys or equipment.

27. Child has a push or pull toy.

28. Child has stroller or walker, kiddie car, scooter or tricycle.

29. Mother provides toys or interesting activities for child during interview.

30. Provides learning equipment appropriate to age—cuddly toy or role-playing toys.

31. Provides learning equipment appropriate to age—mobile, table and chairs, high chair, play pen.

32. Provides eye-hand coordination toys—items to go in and out of receptacle, fit together toys, beads.

*Items that may require direct questions.

Continued.

HOME—cont'd

BIRTH TO THREE—cont'd

IV. Provision of appropriate play materials—cont'd	Yes	No
33. Provides eye-hand coordination toys that permit combinations—stacking or nesting toys, blocks or building toys.		
34. Provides toys for literature and music.		
Subscore		

V. Maternal involvement with child	Yes	No
35. Mother tends to keep child within visual range and to look at him often.		
36. Mother talks to child while doing her work.		
37. Mother consciously encourages developmental advance.		
38. Mother invests "maturing" toys with value via her attention.		
39. Mother structures child's play periods.		
40. Mother provides toys that challenge child to develop new skills.		
Subscore		

VI. Opportunities for variety in daily stimulation	Yes	No
41. Father provides some caretaking every day.		
42. Mother reads stories at least three times weekly.		
43. Child eats at least one meal per day with mother and father.		
44. Family visits or receives visits from relatives.		
45. Child has three or more books of his own.		
Subscore		

HOME OBSERVATION FOR MEASUREMENT OF THE ENVIRONMENT

THREE TO SIX

Date of interview _____

Child designee _____
              Name   Age   Sex   Ethnicity

Child's birthday _____ Birth order _____

Mother's name _____ Father's name _____

Address _____

_____

Categories	Raw scores	Percentile scores
I. Provision of stimulation through equipment, toys, and experiences	_____	_____
II. Stimulation of mature behavior	_____	_____
III. Provision of stimulating physical and language environment	_____	_____
IV. Avoidance of restriction and punishment	_____	_____
V. Pride, affection, and thoughtfulness	_____	_____
VI. Masculine stimulation	_____	_____
VII. Independence from parental control	_____	_____
Totals	_____	_____

I. Provision of stimulation through equipment, toys, and experiences

1-12 The following are present in home and either belong to child subject or he is allowed to play with them:

	Yes	No
1. Toys to learn colors, sizes, shapes—typewriter, pressouts, play school, peg boards, etc.		
2. Toy or game facilitating learning letters (e.g., blocks with letters, toy typewriter, letter sticks, books about letters, etc.).		
3. Three or more puzzles.		
4. Two toys necessitating some finger and whole hand movements (crayons and coloring books, paper dolls, etc.).		
5. Record player and at least five children's records.		
6. Real or toy musical instrument (piano, drum, toy xylophone or guitar, etc.).		
7. Toy or game permitting free expression (finger paints, play dough, crayons or paint and paper, etc.).		
8. Toys or game necessitating refined movements (paint by number, dot book, paper dolls, crayons and coloring books).		
9. Toys to learn animals—books about animals, circus games, animal puzzles, etc.		
10. Toy or game facilitating learning numbers (e.g., blocks with numbers, books about numbers, games with numbers, etc.).		

From Caldwell, Bettye M.: Home Observation for Measurement of the Environment (three to six), 1976.

Continued.

I. Provision of stimulation through equipment, toys, and experiences—cont'd

	Yes	No
11. Building toys (blocks, tinker toys, Lincoln logs, etc.).		
12. Ten children's books.		
13. At least ten books are present and visible in the apartment.		
14. Family buys a newspaper daily and reads it.		
15. Family subscribes to at least one magazine.		
16. Family member has taken child on one outing (picnic, shopping excursion) at least every other week.		
17. Child has been taken out to eat in some kind of restaurant three-four times in the past year.		

18-20 Child has been taken by a family member to the following within the past year:

	Yes	No
18. Airport		
19. A trip more than 50 miles from his home (50 miles radial distance, not total distance).		
20. A scientific, historical, or art museum.		
21. Child is taken to grocery store at least once a week.		
Subscore		

II. Stimulation of mature behavior

22-29 Child is encouraged to learn the following:

	Yes	No
22. Colors		
23. Shapes		
24. Patterned speech (nursery rhymes, prayers, songs, TV commercials, etc.)		
25. The alphabet		
26. To tell time		
27. Spatial relationships (up, down, under, big, little, etc.)		
28. Numbers		
29. To read a few words		
30. Tries to get child to pick up and put away toys after play session—without help.		
31. Child is taught rules of social behavior which involve recognition of rights of others.		
32. Parent teaches child some simple manners—to say, "Please," "Thank you," "I'm sorry."		
33. Some delay of food gratification is demanded of the child, e.g., not to whine or demand food unless within ½ hour of meal time.		
Subscore		

III. Provision of a stimulating physical and language environment
(observation items, except **45)

	Yes	No
34. Building has no potentially dangerous structural or health defect (e.g., plaster coming down from ceiling, stairway with boards missing, rodents, etc.).		
35. Child's outside play environment appears safe and free of hazards (no outside play area requires an automatic "No").		
36. The interior of the apartment is not dark or perceptibly monotonous.		
37. House is not overly noisy—television, shouts of children, radio, etc.		
38. Neighborhood has trees, grass, birds—is esthetically pleasing.		
39. There is at least 100 square feet of living space per person in the house.		
40. In terms of available floor space, the rooms are not overcrowded with furniture.		
41. All visible rooms of the house are reasonably clean and minimally cluttered.		
42. *Mother uses complex sentence structure and some long words in conversing.		
43. Mother uses correct grammar and pronunciation.		
44. Mother's speech is distinct, clear, and audible.		
**45. Family has TV and it is used judiciously, not left on continuously (no TV requires an automatic "No"—any scheduling scores "Yes").		
Subscore		

IV. Avoidance of restriction and punishment
(observation items, except **51 and **52)

	Yes	No
46. Mother does not scold or derogate child more than once during visit.		
47. Mother does not use physical restraint, shake, grab, pinch child during visit.		
48. Mother neither slaps nor spanks child during visit.		
49. Mother does not express over-annoyance with or hostility toward child—complain, say child is "bad" or won't mind.		
50. Child is not punished or ridiculed for speech.		
**51. No more than one instance of physical punishment occurred during the past week (accept parental report).		
**52. Child does not get slapped or spanked for spilling food or drink.		
Subscore		

*Throughout interview this refers to *mother* OR other *caregiver* who is present for interview.

Continued.

HOME—cont'd

THREE TO SIX—cont'd

V. Pride, affection, and thoughtfulness

(observation items, except **53, **54, **55, **56, **57, **58, **59)

	Yes	No
**53. Parent turns on special TV program regarded as ''good'' for children (*Captain Kangaroo, Magic Toy Shop,* Walt Disney, *Flipper, Lassie,* educational TV, etc.).		
**54. Someone reads stories to child or shows and comments on pictures in magazines fives times weekly.		
**55. Parent encourages child to relate experiences or takes time to listen to him relate experiences.		
**56. Parent holds child close ten to fifteen minutes per day, e.g., during TV, story time, visiting.		
**57. Parent occasionally sings to child, or sings in presence of child.		
**58. Child has a special place in which to keep his toys and ''treasures.''		
**59. Child's art work is displayed some place in house (anything that child makes).		
60. Mother introduces interviewer to child.		
61. Mother converses with child at least twice during visit (scolding and suspicious comments not counted).		
62. Mother answers child's questions or requests verbally.		
63. Mother usually responds verbally to child's talking.		
64. Mother provides toys or interesting activities or in other ways structures situation for child during visit when her attention will be elsewhere. (To score ''Yes'' mother must make an active guiding gesture or suggestion to structure child's play.)		
65. Mother spontaneously praises child's qualities or behavior twice during visit.		
66. When speaking of or to child, mother's voice conveys positive feeling.		
67. Mother caresses, kisses, or cuddles child at least once during visit.		
68. Mother sets up situation that allows child to show off during visit.		
Subscore		

VI. Masculine stimulation

	Yes	No
69. Child sees and spends some time with father or father figure four days a week.		
70. Child eats at least one meal per day, on most days, with mother (or mother figure) and father (or father figure). (One-parent families get an automatic ''No.'')		

HOME—cont'd

THREE TO SIX—cont'd

VI. Masculine stimulation—cont'd

	Yes	No

71-73 The following are present in home and either belong to child subject or he is allowed to play with them:

71. Ride toy (tricycle, scooter, wagon, bike with or without training wheels).

72. Medium wheel toys—trucks, trains, doll carriage, etc.

73. Large muscle toy (jump rope, swing, ball, climbing object, etc.).

Subscore

VII. Independence from parental control

	Yes	No

74. Child is encouraged to try to dress himself.

75. Child is permitted to choose some of his clothing to be worn except on very special occasions.

76. Child is permitted some choice in lunch or breakfast menu.

77. Parent lets child choose certain favorite food products or brands at grocery store.

78. Child is permitted to go to another house to play without having the caregiver accompany him.

79. Child can express negative feelings without harsh reprisal.

80. Child is permitted to hit parent without harsh reprisal.

Subscore

Total score

---

house is not clean or she is not tidy). Caldwell[1] advises that advance contact may be made either by letter or telephone, making certain that the mother being contacted knows the following: (1) whom the interviewer represents and what kind of information he needs, (2) how much time she should allow for the visit, (3) that it is important for the child to be present and awake, and (4) that the mother will be giving something of value to the interviewer, the group he represents, and to all people who are concerned about how young children grow and develop.

Caldwell suggests that in making the contact the interviewer might wish to use the following speech, with appropriate changes made:

I am from the Center for Early Development and Education at Kramer School. We are interested in seeing what your child does when he is in his home territory—how he occupies his time, what he likes to play with, whether he plays by himself or with someone else, etc. Because of this we will want to come at a time when he is likely to be awake and going about his usual routine. My visit will last about an hour. I would very much appreciate the opportunity to visit with you.*

It is crucial that the home visit be made at a time when the child is awake (at least for part of the visit). If after an appointment has been carefully arranged the interviewer makes a trip to the home and finds that the child has just

---

*From Caldwell, Bettye M.: Instruction manual inventory for infants (Home Observation for Measurement of the Environment), Little Rock, Ark., 1970, p. 20.

gone to sleep, it is probably wise to forego that visit and make another appointment (preferably for later the same morning or afternoon). This inconvenience to the interviewer is necessary, since scoring on at least one third of the items is predicated on interactions between the mother and child during the visit. However, if the child is asleep when the interviewer arrives but is expected by the mother to awaken any moment, it is all right to go ahead and begin the

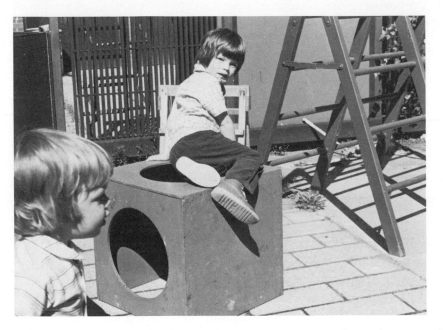

Fig. 8-4. Children have play equipment to climb on to encourage muscle coordination, problem solving, and development of posture and balance.

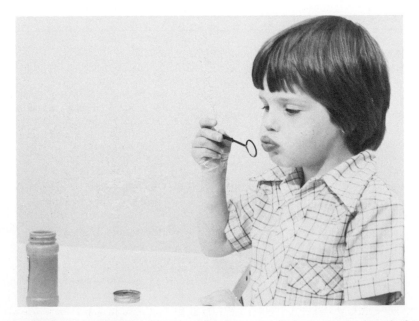

Fig. 8-5. The child's environment is assessed for play materials that are appropriate for his age.

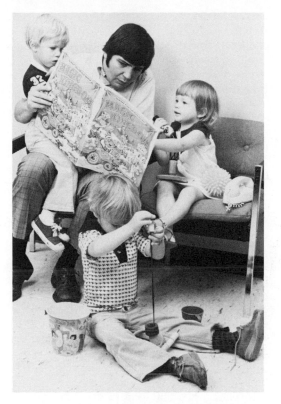

Fig. 8-6. Children's environment is assessed for opportunities for variety in daily stimulation. The father is involved in some play activities.

visit with the mother. The interviewer should save all items that require observation of the mother and child together and go on to items that rely on the interview.[1]

The interview

Caldwell does not recommend a standard interview for eliciting the information necessary to score those items which require information that cannot be obtained by observation (e.g., whether the child is taken to the grocery store). She does, however, recommend one standard feature—good interviewers. As defined by Caldwell:

A good interviewer is a person who can be at ease herself or himself in the situation, can put the mother or caregiver at ease, can easily adjust subsequent questions to answers given by the mother, and can ask questions in such a way as to avoid putting the informant on the defensive and thereby trying to second guess the interviewer as to what is the "right" or "expected" response.*

The interviewer's goal is to be objective and accepting as opposed to approving or disapproving. This is essential if the interviewer is to find out how the mother feels and what she does with the child rather than what she may think

*Ibid, p. 20

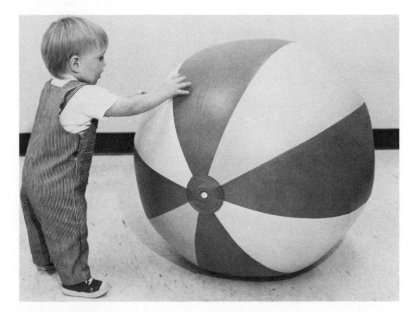

Fig. 8-7. The child's environment is assessed for provision of push toys that encourage mastery of fine and gross motor skills, problem solving, and learning about different sizes, shapes, and colors.

you want her to say. It is highly recommended that if at all possible an observer accompany a person already trained in the use of the inventories prior to initiating the interview all alone.

Caldwell suggests an appropriate technique for beginning the interview and for helping the mother to relax. This is to ask her to describe a typical day in the home, using the following statement or something similar:

You will remember that we are interested in knowing the kinds of things your infant (child) does when he is at home. A good way to get a picture of what his days are like is to have you think of one particular day—like [today]— and tell me everything that happened to him as well as you can remember it. Start with the things that happened when he first woke up. It is usually easy to remember the main events once you get started.*

If the mother cannot get started, help her with questions like "Was he the first one to wake up?" or "Where did he eat his breakfast?"[1]

Caldwell[1] cautions that the interviewer must be careful not to ask questions in a threatening or seemingly judgmental manner. For example, rather than ask, "Do you ever read stories to your child?" (item 44 on the birth to three HOME), it is preferable to ask, "Do you ever manage to find time to sit down and read to him?" If the mother answers affirmatively, the interviewer can explore further by inquiring, "How often does he like you to do that?"

Almost all the items in sections I and II of both inventories require observation only and must not be based on verbally supplied information.

Caldwell suggests that it is advisable to complete the coding of the HOME before leaving the house. The interviewer must *not* trust his memory. Before the interviewer leaves the home, he should have placed a check in either the Yes or No column for every item.

Caldwell reinforces the concept that ". . . *the intent of the assessment procedure is to get a picture of what the child's world is like from his perspective—i.e., from where he lies or sits or stands or moves about and sees, hears, smells, feels, and tastes that world."*†

The inventory is attempting to assess the home environment from the perspective of the child, and Caldwell[1] reminds the interviewer not to think in terms of the respondent's

"passing" or "failing" HOME items or the HOME as a whole. Caldwell also discourages conveying that the respondent is passing or failing in his answers.

The interviewer is reminded too that not everything unfolds exactly according to the assessment guide. The interviewer may be in observing items section I and observe or note an important interaction or event in section III of the HOME.

Scoring

Observations that are made and answers that are given by the mother or primary caregiver to a semistructured interview administered within the home serve as the basis of scoring.

All items on the HOME receive binary scores —Yes or No—and no attempt is made to rate finer gradations. In clinical use of the instrument, however, interviewers are encouraged to make notes on the form and to jot down their general impressions after each home visit. It is also important to keep in mind the fact that all observation items refer to the contemporary situation, that is, to conditions prevailing at the time of the visit.[1]

It is suggested that a judgment of "not applicable" be avoided; instead, interpret the item in terms of reasonable limits of the child's age and score accordingly even if a rating of No seems unfair for a baby whose mother does not read to him at 3 months. Each item is to receive a Yes or No.

Caldwell relates that the score for a given home consists of the total number of items marked Yes. In scoring the inventories, special care should be taken to interpret correctly those items in which failure to act in a given way identifies the behavior assumed to be facilitative to development. For example, item 14 on the HOME (birth to three) states, "Mother neither slaps nor spanks child during visit." If neither occurs, then this should be marked in the Yes rather than in the No column. This seemingly awkward procedure is preferable to the even more awkward alternative of having to remember to subtract from the total score those Yes responses that correlate negatively with the total score.[1]

The HOME yields subscores for each of the subscales and a total score. At the end of each set of items belonging to a given subscale, space is provided for recording the total score for that particular subscale. On the cover sheet, space is provided for transcribing all raw scores for the

---

*Ibid., p. 22.
†Ibid., p. 30.

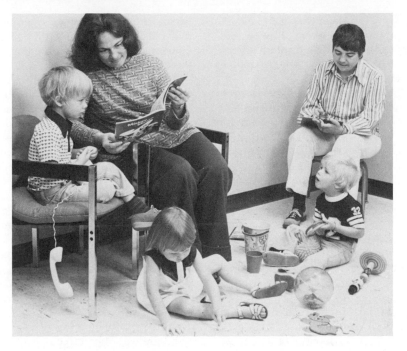

Fig. 8-8. The emotional and verbal responsivity of the mother to a child is assessed using the HOME.

subscales and then computing the total raw score.

Training

In lieu of formal training by the developers of the instrument, the best procedure is to have people work in pairs on at least a dozen home visits. On the first two visits they should alternate serving as interviewers and score jointly, with each giving reasons for his decisions whenever there is disagreement. Both should consult with each other frequently to clarify scoring for individual items. The next ten interviews should be scored independently, although all scoring differences should be discussed and clarified. If these two persons agree on their coding for 90% of the items on each of the last ten inventories administered, then both should be able to administer the inventory individually.[1] It is reported that raters can quickly be trained to achieve a 90% level of agreement.

PREDICTIVE VALUE OF THE HOME

Elardo and associates[2] designed a study using the HOME with 77 mothers and infants. Their purpose was to explore the inventory's ability to predict later mental test performance. Data were collected on all the infants by using the Mental Development Index (MDI) of the Bayley

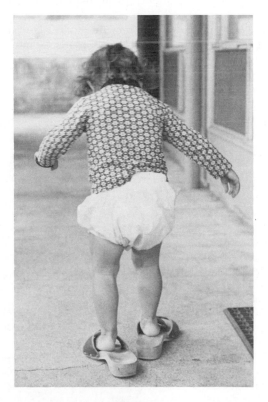

Fig. 8-9. A child's environment is assessed for evidence that the parent provides role-playing toys.

Scales of Infant Development at 6 and 12 months of age and scores from the Stanford-Binet scale at 36 months. Each infant's home environment was assessed at 6, 12, and 24 months with the HOME.

Results of the study indicate that measures of the home environment when the infant is 6 months old do not correlate highly with the infant's performance on the MDI at 6 or 12 months of age; however, the correlation between measures of the home environment at 6 months of age and Stanford-Binet performance at 3 years of age is extremely significant.[2] The correlation between home environment measured at 12 and 24 months and Stanford-Binet performance is also significant. The investigators found that during the first year of life, the HOME subscales relating to organization of the physical and temporal environment and, to a lesser extent, opportunity for variety in daily stimulation seem most highly related to mental test performance. Elardo and co-workers point out that beginning at 12 months of age, provision of appropriate play materials to and maternal involvement with the child seem to show the strongest relationships to mental test performance.

The data generated from the study showed that the most enriching environments for children in the study sample were those in which a mother or other primary caregiver provided an infant with a variety of age-appropriate learning materials and at the same time promoted developmental advances by attending, talking, and positively responding to the child.[2]

A major result of this study was to maintain and strengthen the predictive value of the HOME. The inventory was also scrutinized for reliability as the study was carried out.

Because of its predictive aspects, the HOME has major diagnostic and management possibilities for all child care professionals.

Although the concept and objectives of the inventories have been accepted as valid from the beginning, the tool has undergone many revisions primarily in an attempt to make it applicable to almost any child's environment and usable by a variety of professional observers, with a scale that is valid, reliable, and easy to administer. Throughout the vigorous testing period, the HOME has emerged as one of the best means of assessing the subtler aspects of the quality and quantity of social, emotional, and cognitive support that is available to a young child within his home environment.

IMPLICATIONS OF ENVIRONMENTAL ASSESSMENT FOR THE CHILD

It is universally recognized that optimal development can be achieved when there is emphasis on assessment of the child's environment. Changes in a child's development may depend

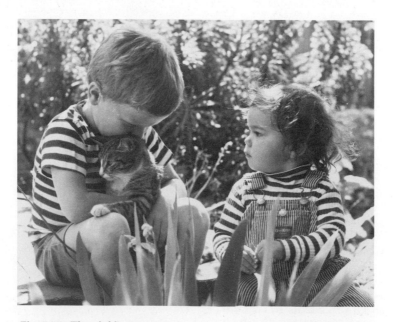

Fig. 8-10. The child's environment is assessed for the presence of a pet.

on both the quality and quantity of kinesthetic, auditory, visual, and other sensory inputs he receives from his environment. A child may be receiving too little or too much change or novelty. His environment may not be organized, predictable, or nurturing, or it may be supportive and sensitive to his needs for consistency, trust, dependability, and organization. It may be introducing change at a rate compatible with the child's pace of assimilating change, or it may be one in which there is not too much pressure to succeed. On the other hand, the environment may be nurturing. It may provide optimal amounts and timing of social, emotional, and cognitive support for the child. There may be sufficient feedback, appropriate kinds of attention for appropriate kinds of behavior, and a consistency in feedback and responsiveness pro-

vided by parents that fosters all facets of the child's changing needs.

A child is potentially vulnerable for being at risk in his present and subsequent development if he is not receiving adequate, individualized, and variable sensory inputs of an animate or inanimate nature that direct the way a child processes information. An adequate environment will influence the extent and timing of a child's gains in mastery of himself and his environment and how he progressively makes gains in fine motor, gross motor, personal-social, and language skills. At the same time, if a child is deprived of the ingredients that are necessary for the acquisition of social, emotional, cognitive, personal-adaptive, and motor skills, his parents may not feel adequate about their ability to provide what is best for their child. These

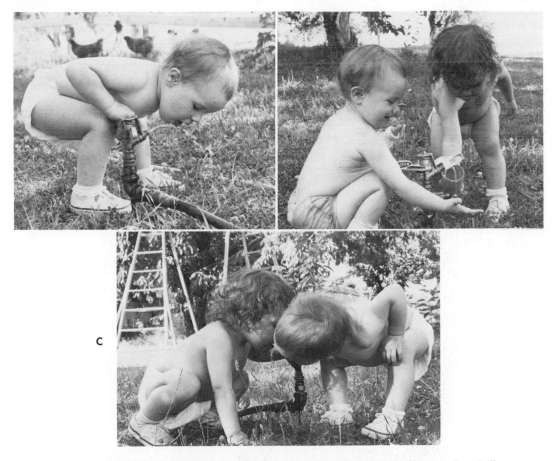

Fig. 8-11. A, The child's environment is assessed for evidence that parents provide toys that challenge the child to develop new skills. **B,** The child's environment provides opportunities for new learning experiences. **C,** The child's environment fosters social interactions.

same parents may lack adequate support systems themselves. A child whose environment is deficient may correspond to a parent who is also suffering a lack of environmental stimuli.

IMPLICATIONS OF ENVIRONMENTAL ASSESSMENT FOR PARENTS

Just as fulfilling a child's environmental needs is important for a healthy continuum of change, parents too need reassurance, support, guidance, and opportunities to discuss their perceptions of providing an environment that meets their child's needs. In addition, a parent's need to know "Am I doing the right things for my child?" must be met.

Parents who are responsive to their child's needs and are attempting to offer substantial input or refrain from too much stimuli deserve acknowledgment of the ways they have elected to create a healthy, appropriate, nurturing environment.

Sometimes parents try too hard, expect too much of themselves, and tend to go to extremes in doing the right thing for their child at exactly the right time. Parents may need support to relax their efforts, to take the pressure off themselves, and to give themselves credit for the appropriate environment they have created and maintained for their child.

A systematic assessment of the child's environment can be a reference for feedback to parents. This feedback is characterized by giving the parents specific examples of observations that were made about the child's environment. If an environment is found lacking, excessive, or deficient in particular stimuli, the parents can participate in discussing change. Naturally the strengths of the environment are described first. Parents can be queried whether they have any questions or concerns or if they have thought about the way they select toys, provide opportunities for variety, or respond when their child initiates a conversation with them.

The parents' observations of the environment can be a significant point of reference for discussion purposes. They can be asked specifically if their observations concerning activities and interactions and their descriptions of a typical day are congruous with what the assessment guide revealed. Is there anything about the environment that they wish to change? Of all the aspects of the environment they would change, what would their first priority be? How would they begin to initiate change? Do they think this change would be an advantage to the child (or children) or themselves. What disadvantages do they see? Have they thought of ways in which the environment could be altered for the benefit of the child? Have they thought of ways of changing the environment that would make it more positive for themselves or other family members? Is there anything that they would change, for example, to make it easier for them and their child to communicate better in words? Is there any way that parents might make it easier for their child to pay attention, get interested in, or play with a toy in a different way?

HELPING PARENTS SET LIMITS FOR THEIR CHILDREN

Many parents need to know that setting limits for children is an extremely important concern. Most parents need reassurance that all parents at some time are confronted with setting limits and that they may find it easier to achieve their goals by trying something different than what they have tried before. For example, if spanking or yelling does not seem to work, is there another way that parents can get the child to conform to their expectations? It is important to convey to parents that they have tried a variety of methods, some of which seem to be working, whereas others are not as successful for them in achieving the results they desire. At the same time, parents may need to hear that it must be tiresome and even frustrating to keep trying something that does not work. Some parents need to hear from an astute observer and an active listener that maybe they are preferring a change. It is important to check with this perception. Is either of the parents in fact saying, "Yes, I would like to see a change in the way I set limits"? Parents need to realize that changing everything at once is not possible or even desirable. What one single change might the parents consider necessary? After the parents have set a realistic goal and have discussed the ways they would initiate change and evaluate its effectiveness, their ability to solve problems, to make choices, and to make decisions should be acknowledged.

USEFULNESS OF THE HOME FOR TEACHING PARENTS

There is increasing awareness and sensitivity to the need to use the HOME for teaching parents. As a teaching tool, it serves to foster more appropriate interpersonal interactions between parents and children. It can help parents feel more potent and confident about their parental abilities to provide an environment that is most responsive to their child's individual needs, as well as their own. Used properly the inventories can be valuable in reassuring parents about their unique capabilities to determine the child's readiness for new or different stimuli. It can be a helpful guide in selecting appropriate learning experiences that correspond with the child's level of development. Used for the purpose for which it was created, the HOME can focus on both the child's changing needs, as well as the parents' resourcefulness in meeting these ongoing needs.

This tool in combination with other developmental assessment tools can serve as a reliable index to assist parents with anticipatory guidance, to prevent problems, to diminish those that are present, to help parents in an educational process of change, to assist them in setting reachable objectives and individualized goals, and to facilitate better communication between parent and child. The results of an environmental assessment can serve as a reference for discussing a mother's or father's concerns, can serve as a framework for giving reinforcement to parents for efforts to promote an environment that responds to their child's needs, and help to differentiate concerns and priorities of change. Most importantly, the HOME offers a reliable framework for determining which parts of the environment merit change. An overall assessment does not necessarily correspond to overall change. Parts of the environment may require special attention to best meet the needs of the child based on his different developmental rates.

CONSIDERATIONS FOR THE OBSERVER

A unique facet of the HOME is that the observer rates the interactions that he sees; he does not make judgments or conclusions about his interactions with a child or mother but rather the interactions that occur between the mother and child.

Like other tools, the HOME relies on beginning interrater reliability. Caldwell suggests that observers work in pairs on the first twelve home visits to increase objectivity of assessment and to decrease subjective interpretations.

One assessment in the home can never be considered sufficient to determine adequacy of the environment. The HOME is best used in combination with selected developmental assessment tools.

If change of the environment is recommended for meeting the needs of the child or parent, it is suggested that the tool be used on a routine basis. The first record would serve as baseline information against which subsequent assessments of the environment could be compared.

By using the inventories on a serial basis, changes in the environment can be observed in a systematic and reliable manner. Parents can be offered valuable feedback on a more objective, concrete basis and can be assisted in seeing the changes they were able to implement. Changes in the child's development can be documented as well.

The nurse, physician, and early child care professional could benefit from using objective methods in their continuing observations of the stability of change or lack of it. Subsequent and systematic observations are made possible by the structure of the HOME.

SUMMARY

The HOME gives sensitive indicators of appropriate kinds and amounts of animate-inanimate stimulation an infant or child may need at one time compared with another time. This inventory offers a valid way of observing the structure of the environment and the consistency or inconsistency of stimuli presented to or thrust at a child; it gives a profile of what a day is like within a specific home environment; it presents objective information about who helps or does not help with selected aspects of caregiving; it gives a picture of what activities or events a child can predict or expect; and it offers a way of determining both the positive and negative aspects of the environment and how these meet the needs of a child. Most importantly, the HOME inventories are designed to evaluate the environment from the child's point of view.

In their endeavors to meet the challenge of promoting optimal development in young children, child care professionals have one more instrument that enables them to measure the subtle aspects of a child's environment, which are crucial in the formative period of life.* It is

---

*Copies of the HOME and the HOME instruction manual may be obtained from Dr. Bettye M. Caldwell at the Center for Early Development and Education, University of Arkansas, 814 Sherman Street, Little Rock, Ark. 72202.

clear that Caldwell's research has helped develop reasonably reliable, sensitive, and predictive measures of those aspects of the environment that influence a child's outcome. These measures are based on objectively discriminable animate and inanimate aspects of a child's environment. Studies with HOME have produced significant findings such as the not surprising finding that an optimal environment in the child's first year of life has a dramatic influence on cognitive performance at 3 years of age.

REFERENCES

1. Caldwell, Bettye M.: Instruction manual inventory for infants (Home Observation for Measurement of the Environment), Little Rock, Ark., 1970.
2. Elardo, Richard, Bradley, Robert, and Caldwell, Bettye M.: The relation of infants' home environments to mental test performance from six to thirty-six months: a longitudinal analysis, Child Dev. **46:**71-76, 1975.

ADDITIONAL READINGS

Caldwell, Bettye M.: Daily program II—a manual for teachers, Washington, D.C., 1965, Office of Economic Opportunity.

Caldwell, Bettye M.: What is the optimal learning environment for the young child? Orthopsychiatry **37:**8-21, 1967.

Caldwell, Bettye M.: On designing supplementary environments for early child development, BAEYC Rep. **10:**1-11, 1968.

Caldwell, Bettye M.: The rationale for early intervention, Except. Child. **36:**717-726, 1970.

Caldwell, Bettye M.: A timid giant grows bolder, Saturday Review, Feb. 20, 1971, pp. 47-66.

Caldwell, Bettye M.: Day care: pariah to prodigy, AACT Bull. **24:**1-6, 1971.

Caldwell, Bettye M.: Impact of interest in early cognitive stimulation. In Rie, Herbert, editor: Perspectives in psychopathology, Chicago, 1971, Aldine-Atherton.

Caldwell, Bettye M.: Do early childhood programs represent a new invasion of the domain of the family? Young Child. **28,** 1972.

Caldwell, Bettye M.: Infant day care—fads, facts, and fancies. In Elardo, R., and Pagan, B., editors: Perspectives on infant day care, Orangeburg, S.C., 1972, Southern Association on Children under Six.

Caldwell, Bettye M.: Kramer school—something for everybody. In Braun, S. J., and Wards, E. P., editors: History and theory of early childhood education, Worthington, Ohio, 1972, Charles A. Jones Publishing Co.

Caldwell, Bettye M., and Elardo, Richard: Innovative opportunities for school psychologists in early childhood education, School Psychol. Dig. **1:**8-16, 1972.

Caldwell, Bettye M., Hersher L., Lipton E. L., Richmond, J. B., Stern, G. A., Eddy, E., Drachman, R., and Rothman, A.: Mother-infant interaction in monomatric and polymatric families, Am. J. Orthopsychiatry **33:**653-664, 1963.

Caldwell, Bettye M., and Richmond, Julius B.: The Children's Center in Syracuse, New York. In Dittman, Laura L., editor: Early child care: the new perspectives, New York, 1968, Atherton Press.

Caldwell, Bettye M., and Smith, Lucille E.: Day care for the very young—prime opportunity for primary prevention, Am. J. Public Health **60:**690-697, 1970.

Caldwell, Bettye M., Wright, Charlene M., Honig, Alice S., and Tannenbaum, Jordan: Infant day care and attachment, Am. J. Orthopsychiatry **40:**397-412, 1970.

9

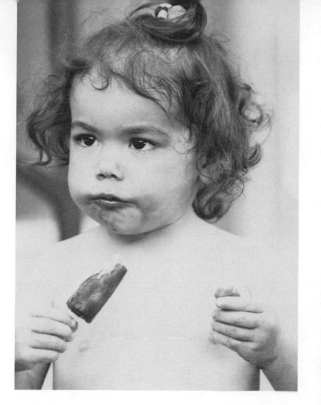

ASSESSING FOOD AND NUTRIENT INTAKE

Peggy L. Pipes, M.A., M.P.H.[*]

Parents receive advice about what and how to feed their children from many professionals such as dietitians, nurses, physicians, and nutritionists and from friends and relatives. Much of the advice is conflicting, and some is without a sound theoretical basis.[1] "It worked for my child" or "That's the way I've always done it" are commonly heard pronouncements.

The varieties of foods, formulas, and milk from which parents may select a diet for their children are many, and the effect of advertising on the child's food preference is great.

Infants and preschoolers have grown adequately and have ingested an adequate nutrient intake by consuming many different varieties and combinations of food, milk, and formulas. There are many views about appropriate ages and stages of development at which to add foods to an infant's diet, and there are multiple approaches of dealing with the child who does not eat the quantities of food the parents think he should. As a result, many parents are left in a total state of confusion about who to believe and whose advice to follow. They need help in

---
[*]Assistant Chief, Child Development and Mental Retardation Center, and Lecturer, School of Home Economics, University of Washington, Seattle, Washington.

selecting appropriate foods and vitamin and mineral supplements for their infants and young children. The child care professional has an important role to play in nutrition assessment and counseling.

PURPOSE OF ASSESSMENT

The purpose of assessing food intake is three-fold: (1) to acquaint the child care professional with the food and feeding practices of parents in regard to their children, (2) to obtain baseline data on the calorie and nutrient intake of a specific child from which a plan of therapy can be designed and progress can be measured, and (3) to permit parents to express their concerns and questions about foods, nutrients, and feeding behaviors.

OBTAINING INFORMATION

As a part of total health surveillance, child care professionals routinely elicit information about what and how much the infant or child is fed, as well as the parents' feeding practices. When permitted to do so, parents will usually express their concerns about the appropriateness of the child's food intake. With this input, the child care professional may identify previously unrecognized areas of concern also.

It is important to remember that most parents

have been exposed to a considerable amount of nutrition information and misinformation. Feeding a child is a most important aspect of parenting. Parents in their efforts to prove themselves good parents or to please the professional report a food intake which they feel will please her. The validity of food intake information may be questioned when there are multiple feeders (siblings, father, other relatives, baby sitters, and friends), and the informant in reality does not know exactly what or how much the child eats. Once preschoolers attain mobility and can walk and help themselves to food, the parents may simply not know how much the child is eating even though they may know what foods are available for snacks.

As in all interviews, leading questions, such as "When does the child first have something to eat?" or "Do you add anything to the cereal?" will elicit more accurate information than direct questions such as "When does the child eat breakfast?" or "How much sugar and cream do you put on his cereal?"

During the interview, one may find that the child is indeed receiving an appropriate nutrient intake and that parents have knowledge of nutrition and appropriate feeding practices. The interviewer can then proceed to other areas of concern. On the other hand, the child care professional may decide that the child is at nutritional risk and that more precise information is needed to evaluate the child's nutrient intake and adequately counsel the parents.

Following is an outline indicating those children at nutritional risk:

    I. Infants or children who have an inappropriate rate of weight gain
      A. Lack of sufficient weight gain: failure of the infant to gain at a rate in weight and/or length less than that appropriate for an infant in his percentile since the infant's last clinic visit
      B. Very rapid rate of weight gain
      C. Gross discrepancy between length and weight
    II. Infants whose parents prepare formula improperly or who use excessively expensive formula
      A. Formulas that are prepared to yield greater than or less than 20 calories per ounce unless therapeutically prescribed; concentrated formulas are offered to some infants because of the following reasons:
        1. Parents do not understand concentrated versus ready-to-feed formula

        2. Parents do not add sufficient water to concentrated formula
        3. Parents add additional formula powder to the water
      B. Calorically dilute formulas that are prepared as a result of the following:
        1. Parents do not understand method of formula preparation
        2. Lack of financial resources cause parents to add additional water to formula to extend the available food
        3. Parents feed skim milk due to lack of understanding
        4. Parents feed sugar water rather than milk because they do not understand the need for milk in infancy
    III. Infants or children who consume greater than 32 ounces or less than 16 ounces of milk a day
    IV. Infants whose parents lack skills in feeding technique and/or use equipment that makes it difficult for the infants to consume formula
      A. Parents who feed the infant on a schedule that offers the infant formula at intervals of less than 2 hours or more than 5 hours on more than one or two occasions during the day
      B. Parents who prop the bottle
      C. Breast-feeding infants who nurse for inappropriate long periods at each feeding
      D. Infants who are not appropriately burped
      E. Young infants who consistently fall asleep before completing an acceptable caloric intake whose parents are using firm nipples and have not adjusted the holes for the infant
    V. Infants less than 60 days old who consume greater than 145 calories per kilogram or less than 110 calories per kilogram
    VI. Infants of breast-feeding mothers who have the following problems
      A. Restrict their intake of food or a group of foods that contribute appreciably to the increment for nutrients during lactation
      B. Have questions about scheduling and the use of supplementary feedings
      C. Have infants who refuse the breast or bottle
      D. Are concerned about not having sufficient milk for their babies
    VII. Infants of parents who *appear* to have a lack of concern about feeding (e.g., prop the bottle or do not know what to feed)
    VIII. Children whose parents are overanxious about about what and how their children eat
    IX. Infants or children who receive inappropriate nutrient supplements
      A. Lack of use of necessary vitamin supplements
      B. Use of excessive amounts of vitamin supplements or of high-potency vitamin supplements

C. Use of unnecessary vitamin supplements

D. Use of unnecessarily expensive vitamin supplements

X. Children who are offered inappropriate kinds of semisolids and table food
  A. Additions of semisolids to the milk
  B. Lack of addition of sufficient amounts of iron-containing foods at appropriate levels of growth
  C. Excessive use of semisolids, which distorts the milk intake
  D. Addition of excessive quantities of high-carbohydrate foods or alcoholic beverages (e.g., beer, wine, carbonated beverages, cookies, crackers, potato chips, french fries)
  E. Addition of excessive quantities of high-calorie semisolids (e.g., meats, egg yolks, cookies)
  F. Use of infant and junior dinners to replace meat

XI. Infants or children who refuse an entire group of foods

XII. Children of parents who have questions regarding what or how much to feed

XIII. Children whose parents do not use food to support developmental progress
  A. Finger foods (when the infant reaches out for food [approximately 6 to 7 months], finger foods that will not splinter and cause choking should be added)
  B. Appropriate progress in texture and consistency (when finger foods are introduced, the progression to soft mashed table foods can be begun; when strained meats are refused, finely chopped meat from the table can be offered)
  C. Progression of bottle to cup (when the infant is developmentally 9 to 12 months of age, experience with a cup should be offered)

XIV. Children whose parents follow food faddist rules or who have questions about food fads or diets
  A. Feed sugar water or herb tea instead of milk
  B. Feed raw cow's or goat's milk
  C. Refuse vitamin supplements

XV. Infants or children with physical handicaps that influence the child's ability to ingest food (e.g., poor suck, cleft lip or palate, tongue thrust)

XVI. Children of parents who lack skill in home management
  A. Time and money management
  B. Housekeeping
  C. Food purchasing and procurement

XVII. Children of families who do not take advantage of the resources available to them to aid and improve the nutrition of their children (e.g., food stamps, supplemental food program, school lunch)

XVIII. Children who have specific therapeutic dietary problems

A 3- or 7-day record of the child's food intake can provide precise quantifiable information about his food intake, provided the parent is motivated to measure and record everything the child consumes. Most parents are willing to keep these records, provided they know the reasons for the request. Parents are sufficiently consistent in both the amount and type of food they feed their infants so that an average of 3 days of food consumed will provide sufficiently precise baseline data on which decisions for counseling can be made. There is, however, sufficient day-to-day variability in the appetite and food consumption of the older child to require an average of 7 days of food consumed if decisions about the adequacy of the child's food intake are to be made.

To achieve accuracy in recording food intake, the recorder should be instructed to record the time of day the food was consumed, the type of food, the method of preparation, and household measures (fractions of measuring cups, level teaspoons, or tablespoons) of food consumed. Recipes for mixed dishes should accompany the food records. Vitamin and mineral supplements should also be recorded.

The instructions for recording the Seven-Day Food Record used at the Child Development and Mental Retardation Center at the University of Washington in Seattle, Washington, are shown in Fig. 9-1.

ASSESSING AND CALCULATING THE FOOD INTAKE

Requests for records of food intake are made in response to a specific concern of the parent and child care professional about nutrient or calorie intake. How the record is assessed depends on the initial concern, the types and amounts of food that appear on the record, and the child's past and present rate of growth. A nutritionist can be of invaluable help to the child care professional in determining the nutrients, calories, or both that must be calculated from tables of food values, as well as those which are obviously consumed in appropriate amounts. This determination is made on the nutritionist's knowledge of foods as sources of nutrients and the appropriateness of the child's rate of growth. It is unnecessary to calculate the amount of vitamin C intake, for example, when

Date _____   Day of week _____

Weight _____

Time	Food	Amount	How prepared

INSTRUCTIONS

1. Record *all* food or beverages immediately *after* they are eaten or drunk.

2. Measure the amounts of each food carefully in terms of standard measuring cups and spoons. Record meat portions in ounces or as fractions of pounds, for example: 8 ounces of milk; one medium egg; ¼ pound of hamburger; one slice of bread, white; ½ small banana.

3. Indicate method of preparation, for example: medium egg, fried; ½ cup baked beans with two-inch slice salt pork; four ounces steak, broiled.

4. Be sure to include any condiments, gravies, salad dressings, butter, margarine, whipped cream, relishes, etc., for example: ¾ cup mashed potatoes with 3 tablespoons brown gravy; ¼ cup cottage cheese salad with two olives, ½ cup cornflakes with 1 teaspoon sugar and ⅓ cup 2% milk.

5. Be sure to include all between meal foods and drinks, for example: coffee with 1 ounce of cream; 12 ounces of coke; four sugar cookies; one 10¢ candy bar (list brand).

6. If you eat away from home, please put a little symbol * beside the foods.

Fig. 9-1. Seven-Day Food Record. (From Nutrition Department, Child Development and Mental Retardation Center, University of Washington, Seattle, Wash., 1975.

it is known that the child has a glass of orange juice every day. It seems important, however, to calculate calories if the amounts of food consumed appear to be minute and if the child has not gained weight in the past 6 weeks.

Decisions concerning the adequacy of the infant's calorie and nutrient intake as well as the need for additional counseling should be made on the basis of the nutrients provided by the formula or milk, vitamin supplements, and semisolids consumed and on the mother's use of food to support developmental progress.

Infants can receive all the nutrients they need to grow adequately and to be well nourished from currently used proprietary formulas (Enfamil, Similac, or SMA), provided they consume formulas that contain iron and in amounts which support normal growth. Growth can be assessed by use of growth grids, observations of channels of growth, and percentile relationships of height to weight.

Infants who are breast-fed need supplementary vitamin D (400 IU per day). Those who consume an evaporated milk formula, 2% milk, or homogenized milk need 35 mg of vitamin C daily. Infants consuming breast milk, evaporated milk formula, 2% milk, or homogenized milk, should receive a food source or supplement of iron.

FOODS AS SOURCES OF CALORIES

The child's calorie needs depend on his basal metabolic rate, rate of growth, activity pattern, fecal loss of calories, and specific dynamic action.[2] Each child has his own rate of growth, activity pattern, and basal requirement for calories. The larger, more rapidly growing child obviously requires a greater number of calories than does the small, slower growing child. Any assessment of calorie intake should be made on the basis of size, that is, calories per kilogram, not total calories consumed.

The major portion of calories received by the young infant is derived from formula. As the infant grows older and parents offer larger amounts and greater varieties of semisolids and other foods, the calorie content of these foods become more and more important.

Studies by Foman and others[3] have shown that volume is the determining factor in the quantity of food consumed by the infant who is fed ad libitum for the first 41 days. Thereafter total calories appear to be influenced by the amount and type of food offered.

Commercial formulas can be purchased powdered, concentrated, or ready to feed. Powdered formulas are prepared by mixing one level tablespoon of powder with 2 ounces of water and concentrated formulas by mixing 1 ounce of the concentrate with 1 ounce of water. Ready-to-feed formula needs no dilution. Pooled human milk, properly prepared formulas, and homogenized milk provide 20 calories per ounce. Dilution of formulas by addition of extra water "because the baby spits" or to extend the milk or use of nonfat milk in early infancy can adversely affect the baby's growth. Feeding the baby formulas of higher than 20 calories per ounce concentration because parents do not understand the need to add water or because the parents think that an extra tablespoon of powder or a little extra concentrated formula will provide additional nutrients to produce a bigger and finer baby may result in an inappropriately rapid rate of growth, weight gain, or both and may also result in obesity in the infant.

As the infant grows older and is fed greater amounts of strained or blended foods, the selection of foods can modify the infant's calorie intake. Strained dinners and vegetables contain fewer calories per ounce than milk. Cereal mixed with formula, strained meats, fruits, and desserts contain greater numbers of calories per ounce than formula or milk (Table 9-1).

Discrepancies in height and weight as plotted on growth grids indicate to the child care professional that the growth rate needs to be monitored in relation to the child's food intake. Discrepancies in height and weight that increase between clinic visits indicate the need for assessing food intake of the child, feeding practices, and attitudes of the parents.

Feeding the infant can be reinforcing to parents. Overweight and obesity in infancy and early childhood is not uncommonly related to the pleasurable experience of offering food to the infant. Because the infant enjoys eating, parents or others may feed the child a little extra or an extra meal. As the child begins to reach out, pick up foods, and mouth them, many inappropriate and high-calorie foods such as cookies, candy, crackers, potato chips, ice cream, and others may be offered not only by parents but also by siblings, aunts, grandmothers, and others in the child's feeding environment.

Overfeeding and resulting excessive amounts of adipose tissue may be to the detriment of the child. Some studies indicate that overweight

Table 9-1. Nutrient allowances* and selected foods as sources of nutrients for infants†

Age in years	Kcal	Protein (gm)	Iron (mg)	Vitamin A (IU)	Vitamin D (IU)	Vitamin C (mg)
0 to ½	Kg × 117	Kg × 2.2	10	1,400	400	35
½ to 1	Kg × 108	Kg × 2.0	15	2,000	400	35

Calories	Protein (gm)	Iron (mg)	Vitamin A (IU)	Vitamin D (IU)	Vitamin C (mg)
Human milk 23/oz	Human milk 0.3/oz	Iron-fortified dry cereal‡ 1.1/Tbsp	Whole cow's milk 1,370/qt	Whole cow's fortified milk 400/qt	Orange juice 25/2 oz
Whole cow's milk 20/oz	Whole cow's milk 1.1/oz	Strained liver 2.2/½ jar	Evaporated milk 1,310/ 13 oz can	Evaporated milk 400/16 oz	Infant juice (assorted flavors) 24/2 oz
Evaporated milk 44/oz	Evaporated milk 2.2/oz	Strained beef 0.9/½ jar	Strained carrots 7,573/ ½ jar		Tomato juice 10/2 oz
2% milk 17/oz	Strained egg yolk 4.9/½ jar	Strained high meat dinner 0.49 to 1.09/ ½ jar	Sweet potato 3,372/ ½ jar		Vitamin C–fortified fruit drink 30 to 80/ 2 oz
Skim milk 10/oz	Strained meat 6 to 7/ ½ jar	Strained egg yolk 1.6/½ jar	Mixed vegetables 2,592/ ½ jar		
Karo syrup 120/oz	Strained high meat dinner 3.5 to 4/ ½ jar	Strained dinner 0.17 to 2.17/ ½ jar	Spinach 1,650/ ½ jar		
Strained egg yolk 87 to 107/ ½ jar (3½ Tbsp)	Strained dinner 1.2 to 1.9/ ½ jar		Peas 205/ ½ jar		
Meat 45 to 76/ ½ jar (3½ Tbsp)			Apricots 456/ ½ jar		
Dry infant cereal 9/Tbsp; dry weight			Peaches 141/ ½ jar		
Strained high meat dinner 41 to 55/ ½ jar (4½ Tbsp)			Fruit dessert 61/ ½ jar		
Strained dinner 25 to 47/ ½ jar (4½ Tbsp)					
Strained vegetables 18 to 46/ ½ jar					
Strained fruit 48 to 66/ ½ jar					

NOTE: Portion sizes are not equal but are portions most often reported by mothers as those consumed at a feeding.

*Modified from Food and Nutrition Board, National Academy of Sciences—National Research Council: Recommended dietary allowances, ed. 8, Washington, D.C., 1974, The Academy.

†Based on data from Foman, S. J.: Infant nutrition, Philadelphia, 1974, W. B. Saunders Co., and Professional Relations Department: Nutritive value of Gerber baby foods, Freemont, Mich., 1972, Gerber Products Co.

‡Check ingredient list for form of iron in the individual cereal.

and obesity in early childhood may be one factor in overweight and obesity in later life.[4-6] Whether this is related to the deposition of an excessive number of adipose cells during a critical period of development or to learned attitudes about food and eating practices has not yet been clearly defined.

Clinically, obesity has been seen to interfere with the acquisition of gross motor skills in the infant. Obesity also may be responsible for ridicule of the preschooler and school-age child by his peers, which can interfere with normal development of self-esteem.

Assessing the child's food intake can offer definitive information to parents about the child's source of calories and can give the child care professional clues to the etiology of the feeding problem. Excessive calorie intake may result from unusually large quantities of milk, an abundance of high-calorie finger foods, the use of a large number of high-calorie infant foods, or snacks offered by parents and friends between meals. Efforts should be directed toward reducing the child's rate of weight gain, not toward reduction in weight.

One factor responsible for the lack of appropriate gain in weight is an insufficient intake of calories and nutrients. The child may be unable to consume an adequate nutrient intake because of lack of oral motor skills or may refuse to consume appropriate amounts of food because of conflict with his parents about food and the feeding environment. In addition, he may be offered dilute formula, an excessive amount of low-calorie infant foods, or insufficient amounts of food. An assessment of the child's food intake can be valuable in determining the reason for an inappropriately slow rate of weight gain. The counselor should offer the parents information about methods of feeding their child, as well as selection of foods and formula preparation. Infants who continue to show a retarded rate of weight gain should be referred for medical evaluation.

FOODS AS SOURCES OF IRON

Iron deficiency anemia has been reported to be the most prevalent nutrition problem in the United States, occurring most frequently in premature infants and infants and children from low socioeconomic families.[7]

An infant's iron requirement is dependent on his iron reserves at birth, his rate of growth and resulting increase in blood volume, the percentage of iron absorbed from the food pre-

sented to him, and gastrointestinal or other blood loss from desquamation of cells.

It is important that attention be focused not only on the quantity but also the form and percentage of absorption of the iron offered to the infant or child.

The percentage of iron absorbed by the individual infant or child depends on the state of his iron nurture, the presence or absence of compounds or factors that inhibit or enhance absorption, and the form and amount of iron consumed.

Iron reserves depend on the child's initial endowment at birth, as well as his nutritional history of iron intake. The child who is deficient in iron absorbs a greater percentage of iron than his well-nourished peer. The presence of phytates generally inhibits absorption, and the presence of cellulose in vegetables is felt to reduce the percentage of iron absorbed from these foods.

Reducing agents and organic acids generally enhance iron absorption; this is the reason parents have been encouraged to offer iron supplements with orange juice.

A higher percentage of iron is absorbed from animal foods than from vegetables.[8] Iron in eggs is thought not only to be poorly absorbed, but the presence of eggs may reduce the percentage of iron absorbed from other food sources as well.[9]

Many cereals, flours, baked products, and infant formulas are fortified with iron salts. The amount of iron available to the child depends on the form of iron used to fortify the product, as well as the manufacturing process. Iron-fortified formulas contain ferrous sulfate, and this iron is reported to be well absorbed.[10] Iron in phosphate salts is reported to be poorly absorbed.[11]

A higher percentage of reduced iron is absorbed than iron in phosphate salts. The percentage of absorption of reduced iron depends on the particle size, the surface area, and porosity of the salt. The manufacturing process thus influences the percentage absorption.[12]

Infant cereals are fortified with metallic iron. Cereals for the older child are fortified with reduced or iron phosphate compounds.

In assessing the infant's or child's iron intake, one must be aware of the forms in which the iron is presented to the child. Parents also need this information so that nutrition labeling will not lead them to a false sense of security about the adequacy of their child's iron intake.

Table 9-2. Nutrient allowances and selected foods as sources of nutrients for preschool-age children*

Age in years	Kcal	Protein (gm)	Iron (mg)	Vitamin A (IU)	Vitamin D (IU)	Vitamin C (mg)
1 to 3	1,300	23	15	2,000	400	40
4 to 6	1,800	30	10	2,500	400	40

	Calories	Protein (gm)	Iron (mg)	Vitamin A (IU)	Vitamin D (IU)	Vitamin C (mg)
Dairy						
	Whole milk—½ cup — 80	Milk—½ cup — 4.4		Whole milk—½ cup	Whole milk—½ cup — 175	
	2% milk—½ cup — 68	Cheddar cheese—1 oz — 7.5		Cheddar cheese—1 oz	Cheddar cheese—1 oz — 350	
	Skim milk—½ cup — 44			Ice cream—¼ cup	Ice cream—¼ cup — 175	
	Cheddar cheese—1 oz — 120					
	Ice cream—¼ cup — 70					
Cereal/bread						
	Enriched bread—½ slice — 35	Enriched bread—½ slice — 1.1	Enriched bread—½ slice — 0.3			
	Enriched rice, macaroni noodles—½ cup — 100	Enriched rice, macaroni—½ cup — 2	Enriched cereal—½ cup — 0.6			
	Ready-to-eat cereal—¾ cup — 70	Ready-to-eat cereal—¾ cup — 2.1				
	Cooked cereal—½ cup — 55	Cooked cereal—½ cup — 2				
	Saltine cracker—1 — 15					
Meat						
	Meat, poultry, or fish—1 oz — 80	Meat, poultry, or fish—1 oz — 7	Lean meat—1 oz — 1			
	Peanut butter—1 Tbsp — 87	Peanut butter—1 Tbsp — 4.2	Liver—1 oz — 2.6			
			Peanut butter—1 Tbsp — 0.3			
Egg						
	Egg—1 medium — 80	Egg—1 medium — 6.5	Egg—1 medium — 1.2	Egg—1 medium	Egg—1 medium — 590	
Fruit/vegetable						
	Legumes—¼ cup — 90	Legumes—¼ cup — 1.7	Legumes—¼ cup — 1.5	Carrots—¼ cup — 5,250		Spinach—¼ cup — 14
	Potato chips—5 each — 55		Spinach—¼ cup — 1.1	2 medium sticks — 3,700		Cabbage—¼ cup — 16
	Baked or boiled potato—1 (2-inch diameter) — 93		Fruit—½ cup — 0.3	Spinach—¼ cup — 4,050		Broccoli—¼ cup — 34
	Green beans—¼ cup — 6		Vegetable—¼ cup — 0.3	Winter squash—¼ cup — 2,100		Tomato juice—½ cup — 16
	Carrots—¼ cup — 15			Corn—¼ cup — 300		Baked or boiled potato—1 small — 10
	2 medium sticks — 14			Tomato juice—½ cup — 800		Orange—1 small — 50
	Apple—1 small — 48			Cantaloupe—⅛ (6-inch diameter) — 2,600		Orange juice—½ cup — 50
	Banana—1 small — 84			Peach—½ medium — 650		Strawberries—5 each — 30
	Orange—1 small — 49			Orange—1 small — 200		Cantaloupe—⅛ (6-inch diameter) — 25
	Orange juice—½ cup — 45					Vitamin C–fortified fruit drinks—2 oz — 30–80
Other						
	Sugar, jelly, or jam—1 tsp — 20			Butter or margarine—1 tsp	Butter or margarine—1 tsp — 165	
	Butter, margarine, oil, or mayonnaise—1 tsp — 35					
	Cookies—each — 96					

*Based on data from Church, C. F., and Church, H. N.: Food values of portions commonly used. ed. 12, Philadelphia, 1975, J. B. Lippincott Co.

The Academy of Pediatrics has recommended that every infant receive an iron-fortified formula or a supplement of ferrous sulfate during the first year of life as a preventive measure.[13] Few parents, however, are willing to continue feeding their infants formula after they are 5 to 6 months of age. If the formula is discontinued and cereals fortified with reduced iron have not previously been introduced to and accepted by the infant, there are few foods likely to appear in his diet that offer appropriate sources of iron for infants.

Preschool children rarely consume greater than 5 to 8 mg of iron a day because they rarely consume greater than 1,000 to 1,200 calories daily. Most preschoolers lack the ability to chew fibrous meat well. One to two ounces of meat providing an average of 1 to 2 mg of iron is a generous portion for most preschoolers. In addition, many cereals contain a form of iron that is poorly absorbed. It appears that if iron deficiency anemia is to be prevented in the preschool-age child, efforts must be begun in infancy. Iron absorbed during infancy can be stored and then made available during the preschool years when iron intake can be predicted to be less than 8 mg a day in most children.

Table 9-1 shows iron sources for infants, and Table 9-2 shows iron sources for preschoolers.

Parents counseled to provide cereals and formulas that contain iron should be told why the selection of these foods is important. If more parents knew why iron-fortified foods were important in infancy, fewer would discontinue their use when their children were 5 to 6 months old.

WATER

Under usual conditions the water requirement of normal infants is met if they are fed breast milk or one of the commonly used formulas that has been properly prepared.[14] Water intake may become a problem when concentrated formulas are not mixed with equal amounts of water or when parents do not properly measure powdered formula or misunderstand the proportions of powder to water.

In very warm climates, evaporative water loss increases. It may be important to counsel parents to offer additional water under these conditions. Infants who lose additional water because of diarrhea or fever should be referred to a physician.

DEVELOPMENTAL ASPECTS OF FEEDING

Many aspects of the child's development influence his eating. As the infant matures, oral motor development enables him to progress from a liquid to a semisolid diet to a diet of table food. The trunk, arms, hands, and even psychosocial processes play a significant role in the maturation of patterns of eating. When the infant begins to sit up and can reach out for food, he learns to take finger foods to his mouth and to bite and chew them. He learns to feed himself first with his fingers, then with utensils. When he becomes mobile, he learns to walk and get food for himself.

The normal newborn sucks involuntarily. He coordinates sucking, swallowing, and breathing. During sucking, the tongue surrounds the lower half of the nipple and moves up and down. Milk is drawn out of the nipple by rhythmic lip contractions and the partial vacuum that results from the action of the tongue and lower jaw. As the infant matures, a backward and forward movement of the tongue develops. This movement produces a projection of the tip of the tongue over the lower lip. In some instances, the tongue projection is so marked that it is difficult to put a spoon in his mouth. When semisolid foods are fed, the tongue may push the food out of the mouth.[15]

The addition of semisolid foods during the early developmental stage of tongue projection often leads the parents to believe that the baby does not like the food presented to him. Since there is no nutritional advantage (other than acquainting the infant with iron-containing foods) to the early addition of semisolids, it seems reasonable to counsel the parents to delay the introduction of these foods.

Some parents, however, believe that acceptance of semisolid foods is a developmental landmark for their child. Others are convinced that as soon as the baby eats cereal, he will sleep through the night. If parents think that they must feed the infant semisolid food, permitting the baby to suck the food off the spoon rather than inserting it into his mouth is often more successful. Some attention should also be paid to posture. A semireclining position, such as in an infant seat, seems more favorable for the action of gravity than an upright position.

As the involuntary tongue projection diminishes and tongue movements that move the food in the mouth develop, the child begins munching movements. The ability to chew follows the disappearance of the tongue thrust reflex. This stage has been defined by Illingworth and Lister[16] as the critical or sensitive period for learning to eat solids. They suggest that if children are not offered solid foods shortly after they have learned to chew, there may be considerable difficulty in getting them to take solids later. They may refuse solid foods, refuse to chew them, or vomit them.

This critical stage of development in most infants occurs at the same time they begin to reach out and bring food to their mouths. It is at this stage that many parents begin to use a high chair and not infrequently offer children food from their plates.

When introducing table food at this stage, the selection and size of food is important. The child may choke on small bites of food (e.g., raisins, corn, coconut) or on foods that splinter in their mouths such as graham crackers. Well-cooked vegetables and fruit, cooked cereals, and mashed baked potatoes are excellent transitional foods. Children like soft and ground well-cooked meats. Many accept hamburger in gravy or sauce. They do not like dry, cold, hard pieces of hamburger. Easy to chew pieces of Vienna sausage, frankfurters with the casein removed, tuna fish, and liverwurst are also appropriate transitional foods that provide protein of high biological value for the baby. Size of the food should be considered carefully at this stage. The child picks objects up with a palmar grasp and often has difficulty in securing and mouthing small items. Peeled Vienna sausage, oven-dried toast, and arrowroot biscuits are appropriate finger foods for the child at this point.

As the pincer grasp develops, large curd cottage cheese, dry cereal, or cooked vegetables can appropriately encourage this manual behavior. Use of large amounts of high-carbohydrate food of low-nutrient quality such as cookies, candies, and crackers should be discouraged, since they can interfere with the child's appetite at mealtime or encourage an excessively high-calorie intake.

As the child learns to release, it can be "great fun" to have his parents retrieve what he drops. Parents who do not respond appropriately may encourage this game and create a situation that can cause later conflict around eating. Counseling parents about ignoring this behavior at this stage of development can permit the child to learn the skill without creating a situation which may later lead to problems.

Between 6 and 9 months of age the infant shows an awareness of the cup. When a cup is presented, he frequently comes forward to it. When the mother holds the cup to his mouth, he extracts the milk with a sucking pattern. Milk frequently leaks at the corners of his mouth; this is because the tongue projection reflex is still present. Frequently, part of the milk is expelled during a feeding. At about 1 year of age, since the infant has greater mobility in tongue action, a true drinking pattern develops. He can hold the cup alone but usually willingly accepts help. Not infrequently he bites the cup, blows bubbles in the milk, and spills milk from the cup. It is during this stage of development that many children reduce the volume of milk they consume appreciably. Counseling regarding the use of other calcium-containing dairy products is appropriate. Many children enjoy yogurt and cheese or will accept powdered milk dissolved in other foods they eat.

Between 9 and 12 months of age, infants frequently reach out for the spoon during feeding. Offering the spoon during a feeding gives children an opportunity to begin to learn how to feed themselves. When they are hungry, they prefer to finger feed and on satiety may bang the spoon in the dish or on the tray. During their second year, most children insist on feeding themselves. They experience difficulties at first in scooping food in the spoon and may initially need help. They may be messy and drop food, but if they are permitted to practice, most are skilled self-feeders by 2 years of age. The choice of food is also important. It is much easier for the child to learn to feed himself mashed potato, custard, or yogurt, which sticks to the spoon, than soup, which spills easily, or fruit canned in heavy syrup, which is slippery and often difficult to get on the spoon.

Understanding the developmental stages of eating is important in helping parents to establish realistic expectations for their child in relation to feeding skills and to select appropriate foods for the stages of development.

PRESCHOOLERS' FOOD BEHAVIOR

During the last half of infancy the infant reduces his milk intake and increases his intake of semisolids.[17,18] Preschoolers often show a disinterest in both milk and cooked vegetables. Not infrequently children go on food jags, reject specific foods or groups of food, are disinterested in food at mealtime, and do not consume as much food as their parents think they should. Parents who do not understand that this is

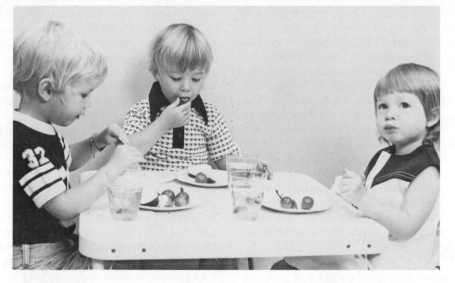

Fig. 9-2. Assessing the nutrients of three young children at snack time.

normal behavior frequently become concerned that their children are not eating enough of the right kinds of food. They may bribe, force, or reprimand their children, and often conflict between the parents and child develops about what and how much should be eaten. These conflicts can become so severe as to influence the child's nutrient intake. Merely telling the parents not to worry, that their child will eat when he is hungry, may only increase their anxiety. Assessing the child's food intake even though it appears that the child is receiving sufficient food can reassure the parents. Frequently, parents focus only on mealtime and are not aware of between-meal food eaten, which, when totaled into the daily nutrient intake, reveals a perfectly adequate intake. On the other hand, frequent snacks of low-nutrient quality can adversely affect the preschooler's nutrient intake.

The Seven-Day Food Record can be an invaluable tool in making the parent aware of both the quantity and quality of food that their child is consuming, as well as the influence and quality of the between-meal fillers. In the process of keeping records, parents often have said, "I simply was not aware of how much Johnny is eating; he's eating a great deal more than I thought." If, however, the parent, child care professional, or both continue to have concerns, calculations of the nutrients consumed give definitive evidence of the adequacy or problems of food intake.

Too often the studies of Davis[19] have been misused by individuals who failed to properly interpret them. Information has been passed along by a number of health care professionals that Davis proved that children left alone would select and consume foods to support an appropriate nutrient intake by themselves. These individuals failed to recognize that in her studies, children were offered in a nonjudgmental manner only the following simply uncombined foods without the addition of salt or seasoning:

1. Meats (muscle cuts): beef, lamb, and chicken
2. Glandular organs: liver, kidney, brains, and sweetbreads (thymus)
3. Sea food: sea fish (haddock)
4. Cereals: whole wheat (unprocessed), oatmeal (Scotch), barley (whole grain), cornmeal (yellow), and rye (Ry-Krisp)
5. Bone products: bone marrow (beef and veal) and bone jelly (soluble bone substances)
6. Eggs
7. Milk: grade A raw milk and grade A whole lactic milk
8. Fruits: apples, oranges, bananas, tomatoes, and peaches or pineapple
9. Vegetables: lettuce, cabbage, spinach, cauliflower, peas, beets, carrots, turnips, and potatoes
10. Incidentals: sea salt

The children in Davis's studies[19] consumed meals that were considered odd by our culturally defined meal standards. She describes a breakfast of apples and liver, a noon meal of raw beef and lactic milk, and a supper of orange juice, bananas, and milk. The children went on food jags that lasted a few days to a few weeks. The quantities of food eaten at meals varied. Large meals were usually followed by small ones.

The children did select an adequate and balanced nutrient and calorie intake from the foods presented to them. It is important in interpreting these studies to recognize that it would be difficult to select and eat foods from those presented and not select a balanced intake. These children had no exposure to children's television programs and had heard no conversations from parents or siblings about food likes and dislikes, nor were foods used as rewards or withheld for punishment.

Davis's studies clearly show that if children are not satiated by an abundance of between-meal snacks and are presented with foods that support an appropriate nutrient intake in a nonjudgmental manner, they will select by choice an appropriate nutrient intake.

Many lessons can be learned from her studies by day-care operators and institutions in which children are cared for, as well as parents, nurses, dietitians, and nutritionists. One must remember, however, that the preschool child is totally dependent on his caretaker for the selection of food offered to him and that he can select an appropriate nutrient intake only if foods providing those nutrients are available to him. It is important also to note that no sweet foods (e.g., candy, cookies) were offered to children in these studies.

Preschoolers sometimes do present problems of inappropriate nutrient or calorie intake. Simply offering foods that provide the nutrients a child needs does not ensure that he will eat them. Satiating the child with frequent between-meal snacks dulls his appetite at mealtimes. The child who eats an abundance of cookies, candy, carbonated beverages, bread items, and other foods between meals will not be hungry or want to eat at mealtime. The child with a brittle appetite who is presented with large portions may be overwhelmed by the task of "cleaning his plate" and not even try to eat.

Presented with utensils (adult-size spoons and forks) that are difficult to manage and parents who have unrealistic expectations about neatness in eating can discourage a child to the point that he does not try. Tension at mealtime discourages the consumption of a balanced food intake. Children need to feel secure of their place in the family. They need to be included in the family conversation. Mealtime should be a pleasant time. It is not the time for family squabbles.

Occasionally preschool children do not eat because they have become so hungry that they have lost their appetite. Most preschoolers need food at intervals of at least every 4 hours. Well-planned snacks of high nutritional quality can be important in planning food for such children.

Other preschoolers may not eat because they know that by not eating the food presented to them, parents concerned about total intake will offer ice cream, cookies, or other "sweets" they would rather have. They may refuse to eat or may dawdle and play with their food because they receive parental attention by doing so. It is important that children receive appropriate social reinforcement and that attention not be focused on not eating.

The consumption of a large meal may make it unnecessary for children to consume large amounts of food at a following meal. Fatigue is another factor that interferes with consumption of appropriate amounts of food. A rest period shortly before a meal may make mealtime more successful.

It is apparent that in assessment of food intake and counseling of the parents, the child care professional must attend not only to the foods offered but also to the manner in which they are presented and to the environment at mealtime.

There is good evidence that preschool children presented with foods that provide the nutrients they need in a setting which promotes acceptance of those foods will select and consume an appropriate nutrient intake. Parents may need counseling not only about which food to offer their children but also about normal food behavior of preschool children.

EVALUATING DIETARY INTAKE INFORMATION

In the preceding discussion, emphasis has been placed on calories, iron, and appropriate vitamin supplementation and on development and behavior because these nutrients and factors have been seen clinically to be the most frequent causes of problems. The other nutrients share equal importance in the child's nutritional needs. Other factors operate in the conflicts children have with and about food.

Infants who consume breast milk or cows' milk-base formulas, receive a utilizable form of iron from fortified food or supplements in amounts sufficient to support normal growth, and are provided appropriate vitamin supplements will receive the other nutrients they need. Assessment of the food intake of infants who are intolerant to milk and/or other foods or who have disease entities that require dietary modification may require quantitation of a greater number of nutrients.

Since the preschool child consumes nutrients from a greater number of foods, assessment of this child's nutrient intake will require more detailed evaluation.

Foods that are primary sources of selected nutrients which may be of concern to many parents are shown in Table 9-2. For a more comprehensive list of foods that are sources of nutrients, one is referred to tables of nutrient composition of foods most commonly used.[20,21] It is important to remember that in calculating nutrients provided by a diet, any vitamin supplements or mineral supplements should be included in the totals. In judging adequacy of intake, an average of nutrients consumed for a 3- or 7-day period should be used. No 1-day record of food intake should be considered sufficient for making judgments about a child's food intake.

Dietary histories and food records do not give definitive information on the nutritional status of the individual. However, they can give clearcut information about what and how much the child is consuming.

Assessment of nutritional status includes biochemical evaluation of nutrients within the body; clinical evaluation including anthropometrical measurements, and dietary intake data.

It is obvious that to have the nutrients needed to provide the tissue reserves for optimum nutrition, the child must consume those foods which provide the necessary nutrients. Dietary intake data can give clues to potential or real problems and are important in anticipatory guidance, prevention, and health promotion.

Recommendations for use of vitamin supplementation should be made only on the basis of an evaluation of the child's food intake. Use of high-potency and expensive vitamin supplements should be discouraged.

COUNSELING

Parents are the decision makers as to the formula, milk, or food fed to the infant or child. If efforts directed toward modifying the child's diet are to be effective, the parents must be included as decision makers in the plan for change. It is important that the mother's and father's attitudes and beliefs about food, the money available for purchase of food, and the family's cultural food habits receive careful consideration in developing a strategy.

In addition, parents need to know why change is important and how their actions and attitudes affect the child's food intake. They may need help and support in dealing with grandparents, relatives, and others who offer food to their children. Counseling efforts should be directed toward nutrition education for the family and creating a relationship with the parents so that they feel free to ask questions and express their concerns.

Fathers often play an important role in the child's food intake not only because of the example he sets but also because mothers most frequently prepare the foods their mates enjoy. Children unfamiliar with new, strange foods are reluctant to eat them.[22] Fathers also play an important role in the child's behavior at mealtime because they often determine the environment at mealtime and establish the limits that will be tolerated in regard to eating behavior. Thus it is important that the father be considered and, if possible, included in the counseling.

Counseling regarding the addition or deletion of foods or the addition of vitamin supplements, mineral supplements or both, based on the nutrient and/or caloric values of foods, should be approached by sharing with the parents the child care professional's concern. The counselor should also give them information about foods that will provide the nutrients and calories which appear to be in short supply or cause concern because they are consumed in excessive amounts. Parents may need help in locating community programs and resources that can help them provide the food their children need. Simply pointing out to the parents that their children receive few sources of iron in their diet and suggesting that they feed their children food that supplies iron may be totally ineffective if the cupboard is bare and cash reserves are nil. The food stamp, supplemental food, and school lunch programs are important resources in helping the family plan for feeding their children.

It may also be important for the child care professional to focus on the food itself rather than the nutrients it provides. Children are good judges of good food. Frequently, they will not eat food that is not well prepared, is difficult to eat, or is not presented in small enough pieces for them to manage. Foods that do not adhere to the spoon such as soups are difficult to handle for the child who is learning to feed himself, and the child with a brittle appetite simply may not try.

The child care professional may believe that it is important to focus entirely on the feeding practices of the parents and the environment at mealtime. Aid in establishing reasonable expectations for children at mealtime both in relation to the quantity of food consumed and the manner in which it is eaten and in appropriate parent-child interactions at mealtime may lead to solution of feeding problems.

Frequently, by showing parents evidence that their children are consuming greater amounts of nutrients than they had thought, anxieties may be relieved, and as a result the focus and attention previously placed on feeding may be redirected to other areas.

Success begets success. In any program for modifying a child's food intake, plans should be made so that the parents and child feel success in their efforts at change. Thus small increments of change should be suggested. Parents need to be reinforced for their efforts at change and should be taught to reinforce their children for their successes in eating. They may need continuing support in their efforts to modify the child's food intake.

Parents do have concerns about what their children should and do eat. Some of the concerns are reasonable, whereas others may seem inappropriate to the health caring professional. It is important that regardless of how insignificant the concern appears, the parents be given a chance to discuss it.

A typical example of parental concerns is shown in the following letter received in a clinical setting:

Thanks for saying I could ask you questions about Susie's diet.

Breakfast
  2-3 times a week—3 oz ground chuck
  Remainder—½ cup oatmeal with raisins and milk
  Now and then—Rice Krispies
  ½ cup Tang in tomato juice
Lunch
  1 cup milk
  Peanut butter and jelly or American cheese sandwich or 3 or 4 fish sticks
  Sometimes canned vegetable soup
Snacks
  American cheese
  ½ cup Tang or milk
    or
  When cold, hot chocolate

Dinner
  6 times a week—cooked ½ cup vegetable
  3 or 4 times a week—½ cup coleslaw
  1 cup milk
  We have a "pure" meat dish once a week (i.e., roast) and the rest of the time we have casseroles—lasagna, bacon and cheese pie (usually ground beef things)
  Twice a month—chicken, etc.
  2 or 3 times a month—pudding
She usually gets a candy bar once a week with her allowance and I give her one pack of sugarless gum each week. Outside of that she doesn't eat much. We rarely have crackers, cookies in the house—once in a blue moon she has a glass of ginger ale.

My questions are:
1. Does this seem like a good/fair/poor diet for a 50-pound 5-year-old?
2. She won't eat eggs. Are cereals really so awful?
3. Is Tang (which Wes and Susie love) an adequate substitute for orange juice?
4. Enough vegetables? She loves vegetables but rarely is interested in eating more than she eats.
5. Enough meat? Protein things?
6. Health food friends tell me that even one drop of chocolate prevents milk from being used by the body. True?

I hate all the fashionable agony about food. I worry so much. Half of my friends are "into" health foods and wouldn't dream of letting their kids near a box of Rice Krispies. The other half give their kids sugar coated cereals every morning of the year plus three bites for lunch, soda and pretzels in the afternoon—all afternoon, dinner without any vegetables, and the kids seem just as healthy. I stand solidly confused. I really would like to do right by everyone. I wish I could return to the days when everyone killed their own turkey and that was that!

Susie's mother expresses well the confusion that many women face in trying to decide what is reasonable to feed their families. The food she presented her family did indeed provide the nutrients they needed, and Susie's nutrient intake was adequate. This mother had been exposed to so much conflicting information from so many people important to her (relatives, friends), from her own reading, and from advertising, that she really did not know who to believe or how to approach planning for her family.

Counseling regarding nutrient intake and nutrition education for the family is one important aspect of the child care professional's role in preventive health care.

REFERENCES

1. Harris, L. E., and Chan, J. C.: Infant feeding practices, Am. J. Dis. Child. **117:**483-492, 1969.
2. Laupus, W. E.: Nutrition and nutritional disorders. In Vaughan, Victor C., and McKay, James,

Nelson, Waldo E., editors: Nelson textbook of pediatrics, Philadelphia, 1975, W. B. Saunders Co.

3. Fomon, S. J., Filer, L. J., Jr., Thomas, L. N., and others: Relationship between formula concentration and rate of growth of normal infants, J. Nutr. **98:**241-254, 1969.

4. Knittle, J. L.: Obesity in childhood: a problem of adipose tissue cellular development, J. Pediatr. **81:**1048-1059, 1972.

5. Asher, P.: Fat babies and fat children: the prognosis of obesity in the very young, Arch. Dis. Child. **41:**672-673, 1966.

6. Heald, F. P., and Hollander, R. J.: The relationship between obesity in adolescence and early growth, J. Pediatr. **67:**35-38, 1965.

7. Owens, G. M., Krum, K. M., Garry, P. J., Lowe, J. E., and Lubin, A. H.: A study of nutritional status of preschool children in the United States, 1968-1970, Pediatrics **53:**597-646, 1974.

8. Martinez-Farres, C., and Layrisse, M.: Interest for the study of dietary absorption and iron fortification, World Rev. Nutr. Diet. **19:**51-70, 1974.

9. Callender, S. T., Marney, S. R., Jr., and Warner, G. T.: Eggs and iron absorption, Br. J. Haematol. **19:**657-665, 1970.

10. Andelman, M. B., and Sered, B. R.: Utilization of dietary iron by term infants, Am. J. Dis. Child. **111:**45-55, 1966.

11. Cook, J. D., Minnich, V., Moore, C. V., and others: Absorption of fortification iron in bread, Am. J. Clin. Nutr. **26:**861-872, 1973.

12. Ministry of Health: Iron in flour, Reports on Public Health and Medical Subjects, no. 117, London, 1968, H. M. Stationery Office.

13. Committee on Nutrition, American Academy of Pediatrics: Iron-fortified formulas, Pediatrics **47:** 786, 1971.

14. Ziegler, E. E., and Fomon, S. J.: Fluid intake, renal solute load, and water balance in infancy, J. Pediatr. **78:**561-568, 1971.

15. Gesell, A., and Ilg. F. L.: Feeding behavior of infants, Philadelphia, 1937, J. B. Lippincott Co.

16. Illingworth, R. S.: The development of the infant and young child, normal and abnormal, Edinburgh, 1974, Churchill Livingstone.

17. Beal, V. A.: Nutritional intake of children, J. Nutr. **50:**223-234, 1953.

18. Eppright, E. S., and others: Eating behavior of preschool children, J. Nutr. Educ. **1:**16-19, 1969.

19. Davis, Clara M.: Self-selection of diet experiment; its significance for feeding in the home, Ohio State Med. J. **34:**862-868, 1938.

20. Church, C. F., and Church, H. N.: Food values of portions commonly used, ed. 12, Philadelphia, 1075, J. B. Lippincott Co.

21. Watt, B. K., and Merrill, A. L.: Composition of foods—raw, processed, prepared, U.S.D.A. Agriculture Handbook no. 8, Washington D.C., 1963, U.S. Government Printing Office.

22. Lowenberg, M. E.: The development of food patterns, J. Am. Diet. Assoc. **65:**263-268, 1974.

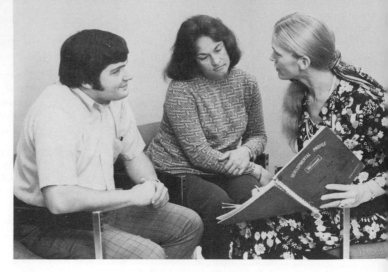

10

MEETING THE
NEEDS OF PARENTS AND
CHILDREN IN WELL-CHILD SETTINGS

If health care professionals are to meet contemporary family needs in highly effective ways, it is essential that they establish meaningful communication patterns with parents and their children. Parents are becoming increasingly aware of potential emotional and physical health hazards and are becoming oriented to health promotion measures. As a result, parents are seeking and expecting different and broader responsibilities from health care professionals. Parents and consumers in general are becoming more aggressive and conspicuous in stating their dissatisfaction with traditional approaches to health care and the failure of health care professionals to provide guidance and counseling in specific areas of concern. According to Hansen and Aradine,[1] parents expect to receive assistance in the following areas:

1. Child growth and development and the parents' role in fostering positive development
2. Common child-rearing issues and the rationale for proposed approaches
3. Child behavior and management, discipline, social and school behavior, and learning
4. Measures for home care and the rationale for management

5. Family issues and balancing the needs, care, and problems of all family members
6. Utilizing and relating to health care professionals and community resources effectively
7. Identifying and managing needs and problems of the parents themselves
8. Family relationships associated with personal and interpersonal crises, single-parent families, and extended family issues

GAPS IN COMMUNICATION
BETWEEN PARENTS AND HEALTH
CARE PROFESSIONALS

The majority of parental needs and concerns are both valid and reasonable and should be expected by health care professionals. However, observational studies by researchers in various care settings suggest that parents are justified in their dissatisfaction with health care delivery and that some health care professionals are neither prepared nor motivated to provide guidance and counseling appropriate for contemporary family needs. One study showed that many parents did not think that well-child settings were designed to meet the psychosocial needs of their families, nor did they view well-child care settings or the health care professionals associated with them appropriate for discussing well-child care or growth and development.[2] Findings of several researchers regarding the degree of health care professionals' attention to or awareness of parents' behavioral and physical concerns clearly indicate factors contributing to the dissatisfaction of parents with care delivery and the continuing gap in communication and interaction between parents and health care professionals. Following is a summary of these findings:

1. Little or no time was ostensibly used for discussing children's behaviors and development during well-child visits.[3]

2. Generally, health care professionals' awareness of somatic complaints was far greater than their awareness and recognition of behavioral complaints.[4]

3. Less than half of parental concerns were addressed by health care professionals unless they were somatic concerns.[4]

4. Some health care professionals did not know their clients nor did they take opportunities to know them as individuals.[5]

5. Some health care professionals believed that they were experts in fields other than those in which they were educated.[5]

6. Some health care professionals believed that they knew what was best for their clients because they were the "experts" and viewed the client as unschooled or unprepared to make such decisions.[5]

7. Some health care professionals did not give parents opportunities to ask questions. If questions were asked, they were often ignored, given vague answers, or the subject of conversation was changed.[6]

FACILITATING EFFECTIVE COMMUNICATION AND INTERACTION

The most often cited critical variable affecting the degree of parental satisfaction with well-

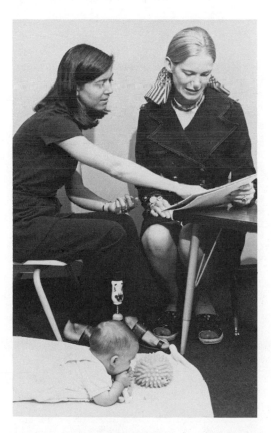

Fig. 10-1. Encouraging a mother to ask questions after the completion of a developmental assessment of her infant.

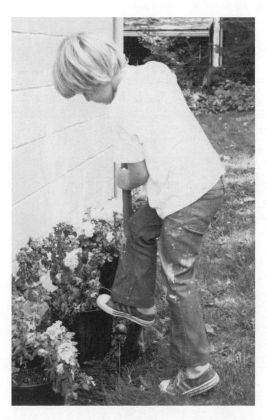

Fig. 10-2. Assessing a child's gross motor skills with digging.

child visits is the attitude of interest, concern, and friendliness conveyed by the health care professional.[6,7] Another consistent obstacle to parental satisfaction with communication and interaction is the health care professional's use of technical anatomical and physiological terminology in describing or explaining health problems.[6] These factors along with the health care professional's existing attitude that parents lack the capability or knowledge to determine their own needs undoubtedly suggest that traditional approaches to health care delivery are no longer adequate to meet the needs they were intended to serve. Epstein[5] suggests that if health care agencies and professionals are to serve their clients in more effective ways, provisions must be made for the client to become involved and participate in the decision-making process. Epstein also suggests that health care professionals' knowledge is only partial and that they need the information clients have to approach contemporary needs and concerns in a professional way. Including

family members in decision-making and problem-solving processes presents new challenges and responsibilities to both consumers and health care professionals. Both groups must learn to develop mutual trust and to appreciate and acknowledge each other's areas of competence. They must also develop new skills, expanded knowledge, and, most importantly, experience meaningful communication transactions that are mutually perceived and validated.

Mutual participation model

Utilization of the mutual participation model described by Szasz and Hollander[8] can greatly contribute to alleviating parental dissatisfactions with health care in general and at the same time help health care professionals realize that parents are indeed capable of determining goals and priorities that are best for themselves and their children. The success of the mutual participation model relies on objective data based on mutual identification, validation, and reevaluation by both parents and health care

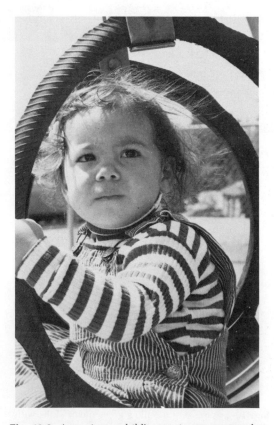

Fig. 10-3. Assessing a child's reaction to a new play activity on a swing.

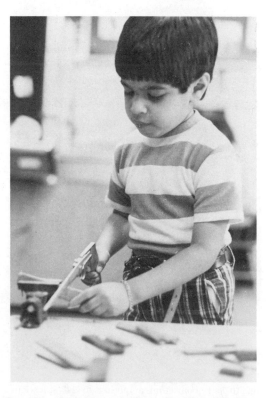

Fig. 10-4. Assessing a child's eye-hand coordination.

professionals. To attain this objective, parents are expected to willingly assume new roles and responsibilities in facilitating successful well-child care as follows:

1. Parents must be willing to actively participate in mutually identifying and validating their concerns and problems openly with health care professionals.

2. Parents must be willing to participate as partners with health care professionals in the management and maintenance of their own health status, as well as that of their children.

3. Parents must assume greater responsibility for interacting with their children and for developing observation skills to detect clues that children present as indicators of their health and developmental status.

4. Parents must be willing to keep records and compile data to facilitate identification of specific problems based on valid information and observations.

DEVELOPING SKILLS IN OBSERVATION AND COMMUNICATION

Health care professionals must also assume greater responsibility for expanding their knowledge, particularly in areas pertaining to human behavior patterns, child growth and development, and patterns of family living and development. More importantly they must develop expertise in communication and interviewing. Health care professionals must also give greater attention to the teaching roles of parents, assist parents in carrying out their own responsibilities, and help parents view themselves as effective facilitators of change now and in the future. It is essential that health care professionals discontinue utilizing stereotyped models and assuming that all families have the same needs and concerns.

Also significant to remember is that just because the mother, father, and child appear together as a physical unit, this in no way implies

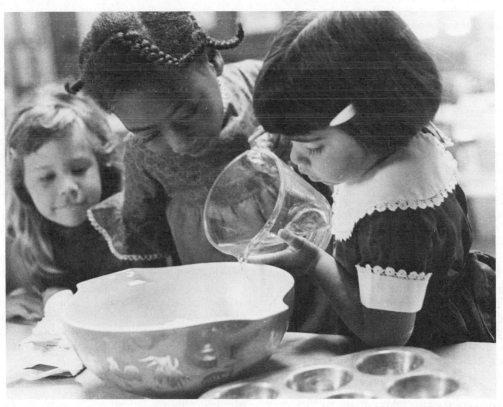

Los Niños Head Start

Fig. 10-5. Assessing the social interactions of children at play. (From Hendrick, Joanne: The whole child: new trends in early education, St. Louis, 1975, The C. V. Mosby Co.)

that their individual concerns, needs, or difficulties are the same. The physical appearance of togetherness can be misleading and may result in an attempt to use the same care planning to meet the individual needs of all family members simultaneously. Each parent and child is a separate individual with vastly and distinctly different needs that require individualized approaches to ensure effective delivery of health care.

It is increasingly recognized that most parents are committed to do what is in the best interests of their children. However, they may experience varying degrees of uncertainty about the approaches and methods they utilize in attempting to solve family problems. In addition, occasionally the needs of parents will be greater than those of their children and will appropriately require greater attention.[9] Therefore it is important to realize that parents are challenged with the responsibility of meeting their children's needs while simultaneously meeting their own needs, which deserve equal attention, care, and planning. The challenge of perceiving the mother, father, and child as individuals and meeting their needs differently is a complex, yet attainable goal. However, the degree of satisfaction experienced by *all* involved is directly related to the extent of meaningful communication, interaction, and mutual systematic planning between parents and health care professionals in identifying and meeting family needs.

THE INTERVIEW

Professional expertise and knowledge of normal growth and development, family dynamics, behavioral sciences, and human development do not guarantee success in effectively meeting family needs. However, broad knowledge combined with expertise in interviewing techniques and family teaching greatly enhances success potential if used skillfully. One method of promoting open communication at the beginning of the interview is to encourage parents to talk freely about their favorite subject—their children. The person who begins the interview in this manner also conveys to the parents a sense of genuine concern for them as individuals and for their concerns for their children's well-being. At the same time, the interviewer has also taken a positive first step in meeting the parents' expectations. From this point, the conversation can be directed toward encouraging the parents to identify and describe what needs and concerns are important to them.[10]

Frequently, parents are immediately advised what to do, with this advice based on potential problems that are identified by someone else. This results in approaches and plans based on what the health care professional has identified as being needed rather than what the parents have identified. The needs as defined by another person have little motivational significance to the parents nor are they likely to have any direct bearing on parental actions.[10]

Ideally parents should be encouraged in a nonthreatening and empathetic manner to identify their primary concerns and the specific changes they want to make. It is important to realize that when parents recognize or feel the lack of a ready-made feedback system, they begin to seek help from health care professionals.[2,4,11] Essentially they are asking whether they are doing the right things or if there is a better or different way or are seeking some indication as to whether what they are doing to meet family needs and concerns is even normal. Mutual identification of objective data is helpful in reducing inconsistencies in how parents may view a situation, what they may be attempting to alleviate particular concerns, and what they think they should be doing to reach solutions. Generally, most parents have a history of successes and failures with certain goals they have formulated for child-rearing, and most have had successful experiences and reasonable gratification with the techniques and approaches they have tried. Some parents, however, may have experienced repeated failures at just about everything or at least describe their failures as chronic parental inadequacy.[11]

The manner in which a health care professional responds can be perceived as reassuring and conveying a sense of genuine concern, or it can precipitate expressions of extreme parental dissatisfaction and verbal confrontation with the health care professional when a parent, particularly the mother, feels compelled to admit defeat or is threatened by the manner of questioning. One study by Korsch[12] indicates that mothers are sensitive to the nature and manner of questioning and feel an extreme sense of threat when asked direct questions such as "What is your problem?" Korsch singles out the following two questions as highly useful in obtaining pertinent information regarding the child's overall health status: "What worried you the most?" and "Why did that worry you?"[6]

REDUCING BARRIERS TO EFFECTIVE COMMUNICATION

Findings from a number of studies suggest additional ways of reducing barriers to communication while helping to convey interest in identifying parental concerns. No single approach can be universally applied in all situations, since different individuals will view similar conditions or circumstances differently. However, the following suggestions to the child care professional can serve as an indication of the kinds of responses that can reduce obstacles to communication and ultimately foster improved health care:

1. Asking broad general questions is one less threatening way of helping parents identify and take the initiative in expressing those aspects of the parent-child relationship that cause them particular concern.[11]

2. An attitude of supportive inquiry must be actively manifested and conveyed.[11]

3. A nonjudgmental attitude should be conveyed toward parents, the parents' behavior, and modes of living.[11]

4. The child care professional should assume a position of helping parents help themselves rather than solving problems for them or giving the impression that "it is not my problem." Problems can be resolved together.[11]

5. If parents present themselves in a helpless way or actively attempt to shift the responsibility for parenting to the health care professional, this behavior should not be accepted or reinforced. If such behavior is condoned, the parents may become convinced that they are indeed helpless, resulting in unhealthy dependency on the health care professional.

6. The child care professional should avoid giving advice or guidance before finding out what the parents have identified as being their concerns or needs and their ideas regarding how they can be corrected.[13]

7. History-taking techniques should not be limited to identifying only physical problems but should also allow parents an opportunity to discuss or identify any psychosocial problems or needs of particular concern.[13]

8. An attempt should be made to explore and reduce any feelings of guilt and/or blame that parents may experience. This is particularly necessary when mothers do not respond and give clues of dissatisfaction after lengthy explanations of the etiology of the child's illness, behavior, or disability.[6]

9. Parents should be allowed an opportunity to ask questions at the beginning of the interview, during, and after well-child discussions. One opportunity alone is not always enough.

10. Parents' questions should be answered as they arise. If the child care professional does not have the answer immediately, the parents should be informed that perhaps the question requires further attention such as additional observations of the child's typical responses and determining how often the behavior occurs. If this is the case, the parents should be allowed to participate in finding the answer to the question.

11. The child care professional should answer the questions that the parents initiate before asking his questions.

12. The child care professional should refrain from responding "don't worry." This answer avoids addressing the parents' concern and does not ensure that they will not worry.

13. One should be sensitive about asking parents a series of questions and expecting them to give answers. The child care professional should ask the parents one question at a time until both the parents and the interviewer are satisfied.

14. Parents should be asked to keep records on child behaviors such as eating, sleeping, growth and development, and others. These records provide useful data and facilitate mutual communication and interaction.

15. Parents should always be asked if the discussion was useful. Regardless of whether their response is favorable or critical, one should try to determine the significance of the discussion and its real implications for the parents.

Indirect questioning gives parents the opportunity to enter into general discussions that reveal broad and specific aspects of their concerns. The inclusive nature of parental responses also gives the interviewer a data base for further exploration and inquiry. At the same time, parents perceive that their views and observations are important and that they are being included in the problem-solving and decision-making processes. Most importantly, the parents sense and feel reassured that they are being listened to and that genuine efforts are being made to understand and meet their needs and those of their children.

SUMMARY

Greater effectiveness in interviewing provides the basis for establishing a supportive framework that helps parents solve their problems through knowledge and mutual understanding. By helping parents communicate their concerns clearly, by providing objective input, and by not taking sides in family issues, the health care professional can act as consultant and teacher. This atmosphere is maintained by encouraging parents to be responsible for their own choices, decision making, and evaluation of successes or consequences. This role requires that health care professionals become more knowledgeable in the areas of growth and development, human behavior, and family development to provide parents with new knowledge and tools for mutual participation and decision making. Even though change is slow in coming, parents and health care professionals can ultimately become partners in health care by accepting the challenge and responsibility for adopting new attitudes toward each other through the development of mutual trust, respect, and greater understanding.

REFERENCES

1. Hansen, M. F., and Aradine, Carolyn R.: The changing face of primary pediatrics, Pediatr. Clin. North Am. **21:**245-256, 1974.
2. Korsch, Barbara, Negrete, Vida Francis, Mercer, Ann S., and Freeman, Barbara: How comprehensive are well child visits? Am. J. Dis. Child. **122:**483-488, 1971.
3. Stine, Oscar C.: Content and method of health supervision by physicians in child health conferences in Baltimore, 1969, Am. J. Public Health **52:**1858-1865, 1962.
4. Starfield, Barbara, and Borkowf, Shirley: Physicians' recognition of complaints made by parents about their children's health, Pediatrics **43:**168-172, 1969.
5. Epstein, Charlotte: Effective interaction in contemporary nursing, Englewood Cliffs, N.J., 1974, Prentice-Hall, Inc.
6. Korsch, Barbara M., Gozzi, E. K., and Francis, V.: Gaps in doctor-patient communication: doctor-patient interaction and patient satisfaction, Pediatrics **42:**855-871, 1968.
7. Deisher, Robert W., Engel, W. L., Spielholz, R., and others: Mothers' opinions and their pediatric care, Pediatrics **35:**82-90, 1965.
8. Szasz, Thomas S., and Hollander, Marc H.: A contribution to the philosophy of medicine, Arch. Intern. Med. **97:**585-592, 1956.
9. Mechanic, David: The concept of illness behavior, J. Chronic Dis. **15:**189-192, 1962.
10. Knutson, Andie L.: The individual, society, and health behavior, New York, 1965, Russell Sage Foundation.
11. Coppolillo, Henry P.: The questioning and doubting parent, J. Pediatr. **67:**371-380, 1965.
12. Korsch, Barbara: Practical techniques of observing, interviewing, and advising parents in pediatric practice as demonstrated in an attitude study project, Pediatrics **18:**467-490, 1956.
13. Balint, Michael: The doctor, his patient, and his illness, New York, 1957, International Universities Press, Inc.

ADDITIONAL READINGS

Auerbach, Aline B.: Parents learn through discussion: principles and practices of parent group education, New York, 1966, John Wiley & Sons, Inc.
Bell, Robert R.: The impact of illness on family roles. In Folta, Jeanette R., and Deck, Edith S., editors: A sociological framework for patient care, New York, 1966, John Wiley & Sons, Inc.
Benedek, Theresa: Parenthood during the life cycle. In Anthony, E. James, and Benedek, Theresa, editors: Parenthood: its psychology and psychopathology, Boston, 1970, Little, Brown & Co.
Clyne, Max G.: Night calls: a study in general practice. In Mind and Medicine Monographs, vol. 2 London, 1961, Tavistock Publication.
Goldfarb, William, Sibulkin, Lillian, Behrens, Marjorie L., and Jahoda, Hedwig: The concept of maternal perplexity. In Anthony, E. James, and Benedek, Theresa, editors: Parenthood: its psychology and psychopathology, Boston, 1970, Little, Brown & Co.

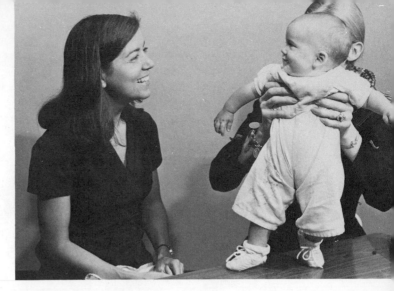

11

CONSIDERATION OF PARENTAL NEEDS DURING THE DEVELOPMENTAL SCREENING PROCESS WITH CHILDREN

Parents may require assistance in being assured that they are capable of meeting their children's needs during stress, crisis, critical periods, and transition periods of developmental change. Parents can learn that they are capable of coping with uneven growth patterns and accelerated or delayed developmental achievements. They can also develop greater tolerance and coping mechanisms for dealing with deviations from the normal, once these are adequately defined. That is, parents can learn that they are capable of coping with both regularities and irregularities in a child's developmental patterns (e.g., a child who is verbally advanced and slow in motor achievements).

In our culture, parents are sensitive to the normal and can become tense at any deviation from the ideal. Some parents need permission to relax their continuous efforts at parenting and assistance in helping their children relax also. They may need help in developing more tolerance to deviations from the ideal or "better-than-average" concept. In addition, they may need help forming realistic expectations, identifying strengths, and learning to respond to assets instead of weaknesses of the child and themselves.

Not only are nurses, physicians, and other health care professionals in immediate and intimate contact with parents in the newborn nursery setting, but they also have access to natural home environments of children and their families. They see the child and his mother or other care providers during routine home visits, which are scheduled on a preventive basis, rather than having the mother bring the child to a health care facility when he becomes ill. Home visits serve many purposes, are often seen as less threatening by mothers, and provide health care personnel with a unique approach to preventive care. The home visit can serve the purpose of monitoring a child's responses in his own environment during well periods. The child care professional can use the home visit for teaching mothers to become more sensitive to their child's needs on a well-care basis rather than a sick-care orientation.

An additional value attached to home visits is that the child care professional not only teaches the mother, gives her feedback concerning her effectiveness in teaching, and gives her encouragement for the child's progress in attaining certain developmental tasks but the child care professional may serve as a role model during the home visit. As a role model in this

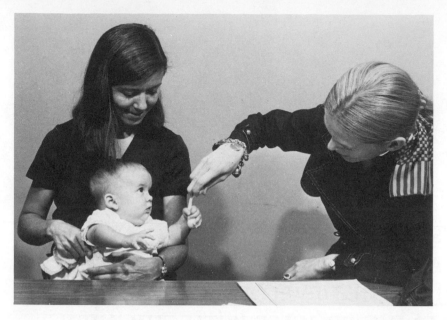

Fig. 11-1. Developmental screening for personal-social abilities. The examiner gives the infant a toy and while the infant plays with it, gently tries to pull the toy away. The infant passes the item if she pulls back on the toy. The examiner observes if the infant actually resists having the toy taken away.

sense, the mother receives approval and reassurance.

Nurses, social workers, educators, physical therapists, and others can become more comfortable, feel more secure, and use more creative approaches to reassure parents about their children's growth and development because of the screening tools that have become increasingly available. It is not necessary to memorize rates and levels of development or to know for sure that a developmental task is supposed to be performed exactly at 3 months of age. Nurses, physicians, and other health care professionals should not feel responsible for trying to make a diagnosis when using screening tools. They should be more conscious of a child's adaptive behaviors, strengths, and independent behaviors but also be alert to the need for continued observations. Health care professionals should be able to recognize the need for testing with more sophisticated equipment if actual delays are seen and be prepared for referral. They should be ready to help prepare the mother if there is a need for comprehensive or extensive evaluations of the child by specialists in a child development setting.

With the availability of numerous tools that have been designed for quick screening, health care professionals find it easier to carry out developmental screening and to a greater extent

are more secure in reporting what they observe within a framework of variations of normal growth and development. The criteria for passing or failing a developmental item must be present for child care professionals to refer to. When using screening tools, child care professionals should not feel compelled to assign a developmental age, since this corresponds to making a diagnosis. They can make recommendations for further screening and observations.

Child care professionals are more sensitive in regard to cues from the mother and child that a delay in a task is possible. Health care professionals have gotten away from one-shot interpretations of behavior and can say with equanimity, "No, I can't say that he is doing as well on this task as others; however, we will continue to observe, or I'll reexamine his performance on this item again soon." They also feel more comfortable in asking and preparing parents to obtain accurate observations in the interim between visits. Child care professionals have more confidence saying, "Yes, I can see that you are concerned that she isn't talking yet," instead of, "Don't worry, some children just aren't talkers." Those in the field of child care are also able to admit more readily that they do not have all the answers.

As a result of gaining more knowledge about

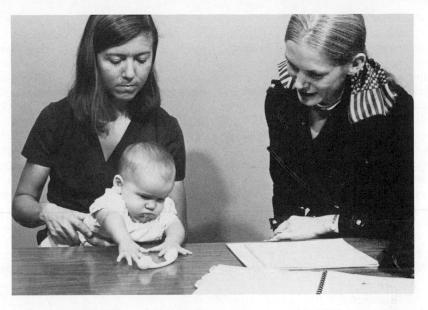

Fig. 11-2. The examiner places a toy that the infant enjoys on a table a little out of her reach. The child passes the developmental screening item if she actually tries to get the toy. The infant is stretching arms, head, shoulder, and trunk in purposeful movements to reach the rattle.

developmental screening tools, child care professionals can say, "I don't know" and go one step further with "but I'll find out," or "To answer that question in a way that won't continue to frustrate you, I need to make some further observations and together we can work this out."

This approach can be applied when answering parental questions about motor development, language, play, and social skills. For example, if a mother asks when a child will be able to talk, the health care professional must help her focus on the preliminary efforts that the child has already made, using such methods as counting consonant and vowel sounds that are heard and possibly having the mother keep track for a week of how many times the child articulates a sound or word clearly. The same approach applies with motor development. If parents want to know what a child will do in the future, child care professionals should help them concentrate their observations on present behaviors. For example, if parents ask how soon the child will be walking, the child care professional should ask the parents what they have already observed about the child's crawling movements forward. Do his legs alternate? Does he get from one place to another? Is he pulling himself up to an upright position? Is he hanging on and moving his feet from one place to another? Does he walk between two pieces of furniture? What have the parents observed about his balance? Can the child keep himself upright when he does get to a standing position? Does the child tend to catch himself when he falls by extending arms and fingers as if to break the fall? If he is not walking and the parents expect this to occur soon or think the child should be walking already, the child care professional should focus on assets of behavior already present that are preliminary to walking. The parents should be asked what they judge as necessary for walking.

The mother of a 2-year-old child may be concerned that he does not play cooperatively. This may be an undue concern and beyond the child's age level anyway. The mother should be assured that play patterns emerge sequentially like other behaviors and that solitary precedes parallel play and cooperative precedes collaborative play.

If a mother reports that her child is a "loner," the child care professional should listen to her descriptions first. It is possible that in-depth observations of the child's play will be required in different environmental settings such as at home and at nursery school.

It is helpful to have the mother describe precisely what she means by "loner." When does her child play alone? For how long? Most of the time? Does she ever see him playing with other children? When? Are they the same age as her child? These descriptions serve as a preliminary basis for judgments about the need for increased attention to the child or to the structure of the environment for play with other children.

In addition, it is important to find out from the mother when this behavior began to concern her, what brought it to her attention, and what she thinks should be done about it.

For purposes of clarity and judgment about the need for further observations, the mother should be asked if she has noticed whether her child looks at other children, has eye contact with them, and maintains it; whether the child goes near another child, how close he gets, and how often this occurs; whether her child initiates an action such as touching the other

child, taking another child's toy, or offering a toy; whether her child says a word or makes some attempt at communicating; and how often the child goes near another child but does not touch him or goes near the other child, touches, and leaves. These observations would indicate the presence or absence of beginning socialization skills and would point to the need for further observation or the need for intervention.

If these observations are gathered, certain behaviors can be shared and pointed out, thus relieving anxiety of an all-or-none variety. Parents may need help in getting accustomed to looking at parts of their child's developmental tasks rather than the entire task in one finished performance. Children learn and master certain behaviors and skills before they perfect the entire task that is sometimes expected of them.

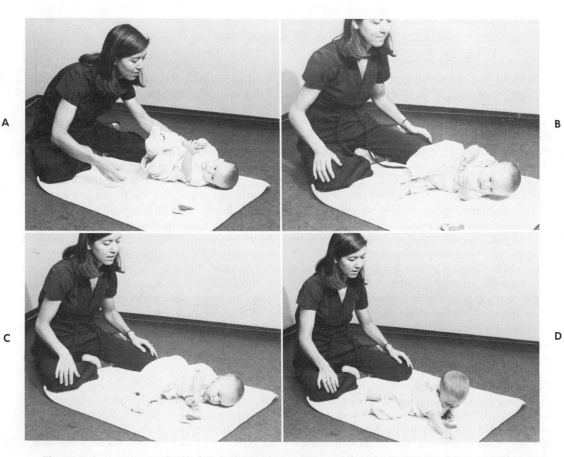

Fig. 11-3. Assessing an infant's ability to roll over from back to stomach. **A,** The infant is on her back and sees toys. **B,** The infant goes through a sequence of head righting, shoulder righting, and rotation of trunk. Her hands are in the midline. **C,** The infant moves head, shoulders, and trunk and rotates hips. **D,** The infant rolls over purposefully to stomach to reach toys.

Parents occasionally must be informed that certain preliminary skills are being mastered in preparation for the developmental task that they expect now.

Levels of parental frustration can be reduced through a systematic approach, and this is occasionally helpful to the child who is receiving disproportionate amounts of pressure. Parents can learn to relax and see positive behaviors that are already unfolding.

It is noteworthy to mention the importance of helping parents observe their infants or children in a routine developmental screening procedure. One mother of a 2½-month-old child was present as the Denver Developmental Screening Test (DDST) was being administered. It appeared that the infant did not follow briefly, lock on, or track visually a red pompom. The infant did not lock on to the examiner's face or make eye movements to the left or right or up and down. This lack of behaviors was expressed as a concern to the mother. She was asked if she had noted the infant looking at her in the face, and she could not recall any instance that the infant did look at her. This mother was asked if she would be willing to jot down during the next week any obvious visual locking on or following of the mother's face, even for brief periods of time. The mother was not alarmed and agreed to carry out this observational task.

When the infant was retested a month later on the DDST, she was looking at faces and parts of a face, locked on, and followed vertically and horizontally, and the mother was pleased. This mother was not originally told that her child had a visual delay; she was simply asked if she had noticed the child's visual attending behaviors and if she would keep records. The mother, with this minimal amount of support and guidance, was able to follow through, make observations of her infant, and supply the needed visual stimulation that so obviously was lacking. The mother even reported that the child was smiling now and was pleased with this behavior, which she had not noticed before. The mother's efforts were acknowledged, she felt pleased, and it seemed that the infant had a better opportunity to enhance her capabilities for seeing objects, interacting more visually with her mother, and perhaps processing more information than otherwise would have been forthcoming if the problem had not been brought to the mother's attention in a positive way.

Traditionally child care professionals have told mothers what to do, but a mother's need to feel adequate, to be able to act on her own, and to act creatively and competently at that is increasingly being recognized.

With their increase in knowledge about variations in growth and development, child care professionals can be more reassuring to mothers when they ask about an uneven development rate. In addition, when they are administering developmental screening tests such as the DDST or Developmental Profile, child care professionals are advised to reinforce appropriate actions of mothers with comments such as "that's nice, the way you're talking with him" at the time they occur, or at the end of the procedure.

Developmental screening is repeated for a child because of changes that he undergoes or that may occur in the environment which either negate or promote growth and development on a longitudinal basis. As children change, the responses of others to their changes are altered. Just as one measurement of head circumference is valueless, so is one developmental screening. Repeated screening of a child is necessary at any period of his development to find out if his behavior is on time, delayed, or even ahead according to a comparison with established norms or according to a comparison of his present behavior with his behavior at an earlier period of time. This can be useful for reassurance about the range, sequence, and timing of experiences, activities, and expectations that are appropriate for the child's current needs and abilities, as well as for consideration of ways of attaining the next levels of development.

A determination of the parents' current expectations, their plans to promote development, and their investment of efforts in one or more different aspects of development can be useful in defining the type of support or guidance they may require.

Child care professionals have tended to underestimate the danger of casually and quickly reassuring parents about children's development regardless of whether they are well children or those with developmental delays. It is important to remember that just because parents are told not to worry, they do not cease. As pointed out in Chapter 10, health care professionals may cut them off and also convey unwittingly that they are silly to worry anyway. This practice must be changed, and health care professionals must convey by means of verbal responses, body language, and, most particularly, facial expression that parents are indeed expressing a concern.

Occasionally child care professionals do a disservice to parents by trying to predict the child's future or what he will be like without the benefit of sophisticated assessment tools. It is necessary to check with parents about what they think or expect from their child or how they view the child's behavior. Before one assesses the future,

it is advisable to assess the present. One inventory such as the Developmental Profile (Chapter 13) can be useful in determining how accurate the parents' judgments are about their child or how well they think the child is doing in five different categories. Parents are key participants in the assessment process. In addition to the appraisal and estimation of the child's performance by his parents, the Developmental Profile serves to facilitate communication between

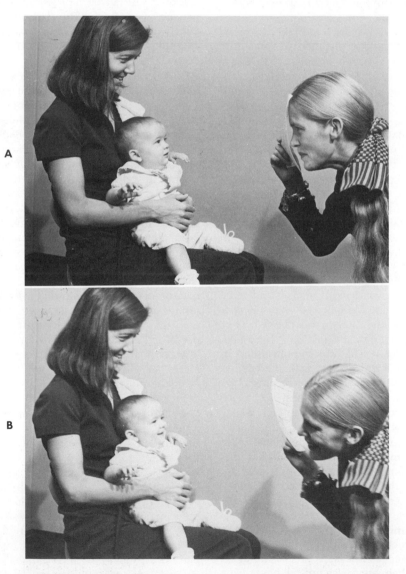

Fig. 11-4. A, The examiner elicits the infant's response to playing peek-a-boo by making a small hole in the middle of the test form. When the infant is looking at the examiner, the examiner hides her face with the test form. **B,** The examiner looks around the test form twice and says "peek-a-boo." The infant passes this developmental item by looking in the direction where the examiner's face appeared before.

parents who may never have systematically discussed their assessment of their child.

Parents also report that reviewing items is useful, with the results being that for the first time they are thinking about what their child should be doing and are leaving the assessment procedure with definitive ideas about what they will plan with and for their child.

It is not by chance or an accident or a mystery that a child passes developmental items for his age on the DDST (Chapter 12) or the Developmental Profile. A combination of vital factors contributes to the progress a child makes in developmental achievements. Helping a child attain maximum development and even rates in progress requires that parents be sensitive and respond to his needs most of the time, provide him with challenging and new tasks, and acknowledge mastery of old tasks. It requires ignoring some of the child's behaviors, selecting appropriate play toys, approving of interactions with playmates, talking to him and not talking for him, helping him initiate tasks, assisting or not assisting him with completion of tasks, and giving him positive feedback and encouragement during success and failure. These and many other variables exert a potent influence on a child's mastery of skills and determine the proportion of successes and failures he experiences, the progress he makes, and, more notably, the abilities he displays in the future.

THE VALUE OF DEVELOPMENTAL SCREENING TOOLS IN MEETING NEEDS OF PARENTS

Most parents find it helpful to know that children vary in their patterns of individual developmental rates, the times at which they will master a task vary, and their rates for mastery of some developmental tasks are different at different age periods. Whether it is during the newborn period, infancy, or preschool period, most parents need varying degrees of reassurance about the progress of their children's development. In general, parents need to know that there is a continuum of sequences toward achievement of developmental tasks. That is, developmental tasks emerge in a sequential or step-by-step process for most children.

Children show individual differences in their rates of growth and development, and there is a tendency for individual differences to be apparent early in their lives. They also show differences in their temperaments, personality, and readiness for change in development. They master developmental tasks at different time periods. One child's timetable for beginning or ending a task may be different from that of another child, but mastery of any developmental task occurs within an established time period. Some children develop a skill sooner than other children, and some accomplish the same task but at a later time. However, their behavior may still be acceptable and considered within normal

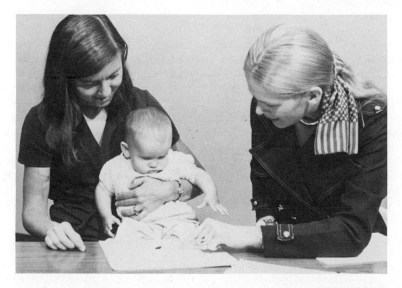

Fig. 11-5. Screening the infant's ability to visually focus on a dropped raisin.

limits. There is an approximate range of time during which parents can anticipate new achievements in developmental tasks. Children give numerous cues in their behavior and parents can learn to pay more attention to periods of readiness. Parents can also be helped to reduce pressures or to minimize demands on children when readiness for taking on new tasks or becoming more independent is an unrealistic expectation.

Progress in development may be marked by unevenness, irregularities, and starts and stops. Children may begin learning a new skill while discarding or showing disinterest in a previously acquired skill. New behaviors that are adopted and mastered may temporarily disappear and reappear at a later time. Some children may need permission to not perform at the same consistent rate that has characterized their behavior previously, if they are acquiring new skills.

Children require different amounts of stimulation at different periods in their development. Their needs vary from one time period to the next. Sometimes they show advances when these are least expected. Occasionally children do not meet with parental expectations of their performance. Different experiences and stimuli should be provided according to each child's progress in gross and fine motor skills, cognition, and social needs at a given time.

Children are considered more vulnerable at certain times than others. Their development in a particular direction or achievement of certain skills can be affected by stress, change, or differences in others' expectations. A child's developmental pattern or status is a direct result of the interplay among learning, growth, and maturation rates; genetic makeup; and environmental conditions.

It is recognized that there is an orderly, predictable sequence that characterizes the progressive maturation, integration, and organization of the central nervous system. Valuable clues about the progress and indices to central nervous system maturation are present from the newborn period on. Observations that are carefully planned and systematically and objectively carried out are valuable adjuncts in gaining evidence and reliable data that developmental progress is being made. The use of standardized developmental assessment tools can indicate individual levels of development, the sequence of tasks that a child is passing through, and individual rates of development from the newborn period through childhood.

The use of developmental tools and observa-

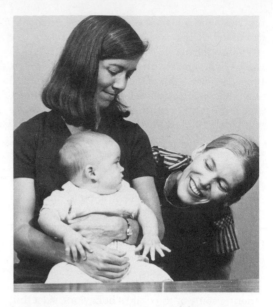

Fig. 11-6. Screening an infant's ability to turn to a voice. While the infant is seated on the parent's lap or on the table facing the parent, the examiner approaches the child from within 20 cm (8 inches) of either ear. The infant's name is whispered several times. The child receives a pass if she turns to the direction of the voice.

tions can indicate to or alert parents about what to anticipate in regard to their child's readiness to master new tasks or put aside old ones. A child may not master a developmental task at the exact time that one of his peers does, even though both children started showing signs of readiness to advance in a particular skill such as language at the same time.

Although one child may perfect a task or skill earlier or later, there is a sequential pattern to achieving a goal. Mastery of one task contributes to the ease or accomplishment of another skill that will unfold next.

There are definite time periods or ranges in which children exhibit various clues of their readiness to attempt a new task. There are also peaks of readiness for new behaviors, and these periods can be critical for either enhancing and nurturing or interfering with the mastery or success that is possible for the child at that unique period of time.

A child may also be learning more advanced skills, trying out new behavior, exploring more of his environment, and having success with more than one developmental task.

Parents in general need support in view of these developmental principles. If some irregu-

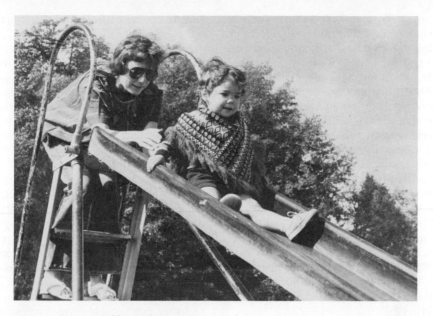

Fig. 11-7. Determining a child's readiness to coordinate arm and leg movements to go down a slide independently, as well as the child's readiness to go down the slide without the parent's assistance.

larities appear in a child's growth pattern, as they are expected to, such as a child having difficulties in motor coordination or balance but showing advances in expressive skills, his parents may need help and support in exploring what it means to them that the child is not meeting their expectations for being equally advanced in both areas. Perhaps they can reduce their high expectations for their child in all areas. Perhaps they can be helped to view the verbal skills in a positive way and also appreciate the child's attempts, beginnings, or starting efforts to achieve more coordination in walking. Occasionally parents need help in viewing parts of behaviors that add up to mastery of an entire task.

Instead of ignoring the parents' orientation to "failure," "weakness," or "slowness" of the child in motor development, the child care professional might point out sequences of behaviors, and maybe it will be easier for parents to gain a new perspective on the child's advancing skills. Parents can explore and think of ways that they can help promote skills in motor development. If a delay in fact is evident, they can also begin thinking of a variety of ways to support and promote the child's efforts to master the skills of motor development. Again the strengths of the child should be carefully and thoroughly made apparent to the parents, and their reactions to the child's progress should be explored.

Children need periods of freedom from excessive pressure for performance, and parents need permission and support to reduce pressure. It may be helpful for parents to experience relief from feeling the need to identify gains immediately. Occasionally parents need help in taking it easier on themselves and in reviewing the sometimes inordinate expectations they have of themselves. Their principal worries about the child's differences in one skill as compared to another skill should be explored, and reassurance should be provided based on objective evidence.

When children are learning new tasks, they need opportunities to practice, to have success, and to experience the ability to cope and master certain amounts of frustration and difficulty. If tasks are too unrealistic, children experience unnecessary failure, and a negative cycle can emerge. Parents need help in learning how to give positive feedback to children for their attempts at certain tasks, imitation of certain behaviors, and beginning mastery of tasks instead of holding back their approval until the completion of entire tasks. Parents should explore the best times for a child to attempt a particular task, how long the child should try, when help is needed, and the criteria for determining if a task is too difficult during a particular developmental period. Just because a child has not yet mastered a task does not imply he never will. Perhaps parental attention in the form of approval will make a difference in success rates or will influence the period in which he can complete a task.

Since growth and developmental patterns are established according to a sequential order, during developmental assessment, emphasis can be placed on what is anticipated next in the child's developmental achievements. The individuality of the child's rates of growth should be stressed with a positive orientation, and his own unique rate of growth within a sequential framework can be emphasized. The emphasis should be on the uniqueness of the child's rates of growth rather than on stereotyped progress in development. This is a time also to inform parents about the wide variations in reaching various levels of development. A variation does not imply "bad" for a child; rather it might signal the unique, individual pattern that is right for this child.

As the child passes through successive changes, which are generally indicators of progress for him, attention to the parents' responses to these changes may be beneficial to them.

Because growth and development are viewed as continuous, it is important that parents know that what has occurred at one stage may carry over and affect later and subsequent stages in development. What kinds of observations have they made about one period so that they will know what to anticipate in the next and not be taken by surprise?

Although most children pass through the sequences that are established as normal, some may omit steps and move ahead. These omissions may be a source of concern for parents. For example, if a child does not finger-feed but learns to independently feed himself with a spoon, the mother's primary concerns must be expressed and reassurance given that coordination is present. The mother may need approval for going ahead and giving table or finger foods. What does she want to give to the child? What does it mean to her?

The unique aspects of a child's behavior, growth, and maturation rates must be stressed to parents if he is also to gain confidence in his mastery of developmental tasks. Parents must be reminded that not all children are cut from the same mold, that yes, variations are expected, and that this child is unique even though he is not putting on weight, talking at the same time as the neighbor child, learning to take turns

exactly like his cousin, or learning to toilet train when his older sister did.

Parents can sometimes create unnecessary problems in feeding, produce unnecessary stress, and maintain unrealistic expectations. They may try to force change, force development, or apply so much pressure that serious interferences in the parent-child relationship occur, learning is interrupted, and both parent and child end up experiencing the negative effects of frustration.

Results from a developmental screening can be used to stress the child's strengths and can be a reference for acknowledging the parents' unique approaches to assisting the child. Both parents can discuss their views of the child's development and can state their expectations and desires for the child, what their developmental goals are, and, most importantly, how they wish to meet these goals in the most realistic, comfortable, and successful way in view of the child's developmental capabilities, his readiness, and their readiness. What will make it easier for them as parents and easier for the child for whom they are trying to promote success in learning and living?

Once pressure is removed by the parents and goals are realistic, both parents and child have a better chance of reaching objectives in a mutually satisfying way. Frequently, readjustments can be made based on a developmental assessment. If a child is assessed in a systematic way and the child's functional levels, adaptive behaviors, and skills are shared with the parents, goals are more easily reached.

If a child is making strides in one area such as accomplishing fine motor tasks, this may signal the need to provide him with activities that will promote this advancement. If changes occur in verbal output, the parents may need assistance and reinforcement for their efforts at responding to his communicative efforts. If it is evident that the child has difficulty controlling or coordinating gross motor activities, the parents may benefit from a discussion of suggested measures that will allow him to make progress and that will provide him with appropriate activities to enhance the mastery of these skills.

HELPING PARENTS UNDERSTAND THE BENEFITS OF DEVELOPMENTAL ASSESSMENTS

Assessment tools have been developed to determine the progress or lack of progress an infant or child is making in developmental achievements. Assessment and screening tools help to objectify, quantify, and aid in determining how well or poorly children are doing generally in self-care skills, personal-social abilities, receptive and expressive communication skills, fine and gross motor achievements, and preacademic behaviors.

Criteria for passing or failing individual children are carefully defined and are present in most standardized developmental screening tools. Scoring procedures are clearly outlined, and a format is present for recording the degree of success or failure. Less attention has been given to clearly describing, instructing, suggesting, or encouraging how to present the results, negative and positive, to the parents, who usually are participating as informants about the child's abilities.

Health care professionals clearly do not follow any uniform pattern of input or feedback to parents. Some clinicians do not even share partial results of assessments with parents. Others share pieces of information. Some child care professionals neglect comment, whereas others give complete, useful information. After developmental screening is completed, it is not always clearly established if the child's performance was typical under the circumstances, if the child would perform the same in a similar environment, and whether interactions with an unknown person who administered the items made a difference in the child's performance.

There are inconsistent approaches in determining whether the developmental screening was understood by the child's parents, whether the results aided them in a clearer understanding of the child's developmental needs, whether the parents were supported in their efforts to promote the child's development, or how they thought they could best carry out a plan to meet the changing needs of their child according to the findings of the developmental assessment.

The learning needs of parents are deserving of more attention than they generally receive before, during, and after a developmental assessment of their child. The personal needs of parents for support for the activities they plan, the environment they provide, and their response to the child's ever-changing needs clearly require more professional acknowledgment.

Unequivocally parents are entitled to the following:

1. Increased understanding of the purpose of developmental assessment and screening tools
2. Increased understanding of the value of developmental screening for their child on a periodic, regular basis
3. A comprehensive definition of what each assessment tool is intended to assess and how well or poorly their child performed
4. Opportunities to ask questions before, during, or after a developmental screening procedure
5. Opportunities to express concern or relief
6. Opportunities to ask for assistance in planning ways to promote change
7. Encouragement for appropriate stimuli they have provided

Parents are entitled to a comprehensive introduction to the purpose of developmental screening tools, as well as to a comprehensive presentation of the results of the developmental screening procedure. Results should be presented in a clear, systematic, understandable way whether the child's development was being assessed or the child's environment was being evaluated. Parents have the right to know whether the environment that is being observed meets the child's changing developmental needs. In addition, parents are entitled to know about the environment's strengths, as well as its deficiencies that could be adjusted in accordance with established norms.

Parents should receive answers to their questions that are accurate. It is permissible to advise them that further observations, more data, or increased information is desirable to answer their question in the fairest, most accurate, and comprehensive way possible. Parents can be advised that complete answers to their concerns and questions might best be attained at a future time after pertinent information is obtained. At the same time they can be recognized for their appropriate questions.

RESPONDING TO NEEDS OF PARENTS BEFORE, DURING, AND AFTER DEVELOPMENTAL ASSESSMENTS OF CHILDREN

Child care professionals in a wide variety of settings have increasingly paid attention to the available developmental screening tools and have refined skills and techniques in using them appropriately for assessment and screening.

It is acknowledged, widely recognized, and not disputed that emphasis has been correctly placed on the proper ways to administer, score, and record results obtained from assessment tools. However, it is also recognized that too little emphasis has been placed on the ways that assessment results are to be shared with parents.

Basically child care professionals should be more sensitive and more responsive to the needs of parents before, during, and after assessments of newborns, infants, and children. Their approaches to parents must be modified if they are to meet the needs of parents and children in more comprehensive ways.

Most parents need support and encouragement for the efforts they make, ideas they have, and methods they have thought of to promote the growth and development of their children. Child care professionals should verbalize the strengths that parents present, validate the observations that parents share about their children, and concur and encourage those measures that are obviously appropriate for the age and developmental abilities of a child. More effort should be invested in periodically and regularly expressing sensitivity to the need that parents have to know if they are doing what is right for their children at a given point in their development.

Most parents demonstrate the capacity to respond appropriately to the full range of their children's behavioral cues. At the same time, they show the capacity to provide appropriate stimulation, activities, and interactions that enhance their children's development.

Generally, parents express satisfaction in doing what is right for their children. Most parents are oriented to a norm-sensitive culture. It is important that their children perform as well as, if not better than, other children of the same age.

Most mothers view their children's developmental progress and status as a reflection of mothering capabilities and adequacy as a parent. Generally, a mother will do what is right or best for her child to ensure his being average if not better than another child.

The paramount question for which mothers want a comprehensive answer in a typical assessment procedure asks, "Is my child doing all right in his growth and development?" This is an appropriate question, deserving a fuller answer than child care professionals have been able to give. This question must be answered with consideration of the parameters of parental needs, values, and expectations.

Parents may not receive complete answers to their questions, let alone positive ones, with regard to their strengths, values they identify, and approaches that indeed have influenced the developmental status of their child.

The type of informative feedback parents receive can be equally beneficial to them and their child. For example, a mother can be encouraged by the feedback she has received concerning her approaches to promote the child's well-being, the decisions and judgments she has made about what is best and what is right, and whether she is doing everything that is appropriate to promote her child's development. The child may then continue to receive and benefit from appropriate stimuli, positive experiences, and successful interactions, which are governed and regulated by the mother who is attempting to create a growth-fostering environment.

The question "Is my child all right?" generally reflects the mother's concern that she has provided appropriate experiences, has timed the readiness of her child to learn or respond to new events, has selected toys and activities appropriately, paced stimuli, has governed and regulated stimuli coming in, and in general has monitored and overseen the quality and organization of his learning environment. Most parents have influenced their children's mastery of developmental tasks and do not receive the credit they unequivocally deserve. Most parents want to hear that their children's growth and development are satisfactory and that the methods they have selected for enhancing and promoting their children's development are adequate.

Child care professionals must make a greater effort to let parents know that they are accurate and sensitive about the changing needs of their child and that they have the capacity and ability to respond appropriately to the child's needs in developing language, fine motor skills, gross motor skills, and personal-social achievement, if indeed they are observed to show appropriate behaviors toward their child. If child care professionals are to rely on the mother's capabilities to be a maximally effective agent of change by providing appropriate interactions, activities, and experiences, they must "tune in" and be more sensitive about giving encouragement, support, reassurance, and advice when it appears appropriate.

Before anticipatory guidance can be planned with a mother, child care professionals rely on a comprehensive assessment of a child's developmental status. It is necessary to explore the mother's perceptions of how the child is doing. It is important to use this opportunity to evaluate whether her perceptions are influencing the expectations she has for the child. Is the child doing what the mother expects or wishes the child to do? Anticipatory guidance rests on a foundation of assessment.

MAJOR POINTS TO CONSIDER IN GIVING REASSURANCE ABOUT A CHILD'S DEVELOPMENT

Parents may expect infants and children to accomplish a number of tasks or skills simultaneously. Parental concern about "unevenness" in their child's development could be explored during a routine screening of the child, using either the DDST, the Developmental Profile, or any other appropriate developmental screening tool.

For example, the child might be making gains in motor development but not progressing in language skills, although not falling behind either. By using screening tools at regular and periodic intervals, the mother can not only receive reassurance about what the child has already mastered but also be helped to identify the beginnings of new accomplishments.

Anticipatory guidance is an important facet of assessment. It can be considered a learning process in which the child's present skills and abilities are observed, defined, and acknowledged. Since some abilities and skills are preliminary to or precede the next level of skills that a child acquires, anticipatory guidance is a process of identifying what behaviors, skills, or abilities the mother can realistically expect next, plan for, and perhaps begin encouraging.

If parents can be encouraged to watch for, be alert to, notice certain aspects of the child's behavior, or relate what they think the child will do next now that he has successfully and progressively made gains in one task, they are better prepared to respond appropriately and positively to the child's gains, to experience increased certainty about the validity of their expectations, and to feel more comfortable in the approaches they have selected to help the child change. Developmental screening may give parents more objectivity in planning appropriate activities for the child and increases their feelings of adequacy in helping their child, not hindering him, or placing too much pressure on him at an inappropriate time.

It is significant that parents are encouraged to seek assessments of their child, and developmental assessments are planned when parents admit discomfort, fear, apprehension, or anxiety about their child being behind, being slow, or not keeping up with children of his own age. Parents need a response to the signals they are receiving from their child, alerting them to possible developmental delays, and may need assistance in defining exactly what they are concerned about.

Increased sensitivity and a willingness to listen to parents giving accurate descriptions of their child's behavior are critical. A parent's report or statement that a child is behind, slow, or unusual always merits consideration for developmental assessment and observations.

Child care professionals should remember that some parents may unrealistically expect their child to acquire a skill swiftly and should be given information about a more realistic timetable for the child to have total mastery of a skill. It helps parents to know their child is beginning a developmental task, showing interest in it, getting better at it, and increasing in his abilities, although not yet totally accomplishing the task. Parents may be relieved to know that the child need not successfully achieve a developmental task right away, and they can be satisfied with objective data about partial rather than complete gains toward mastery of a developmental task. Parents often experience relief and are helped to reduce their worries and levels of unnecessary anxiety by the appropriate timing and administration of developmental screening tools.

VALUES AND ADVANTAGES OF SCREENING TOOLS

Screening tools have been increasingly useful in finding children with early developmental delays, in detecting potential difficulties that might arise for some children, and in planning approaches to meet developmental needs of children.

One aspect of developmental screening tools that is receiving considerable recognition is their potential value and usefulness in teaching parents, reassuring them, offering them anticipatory guidance, and supporting them in their decision making about ways to respond to the changing developmental needs of their children.

During a screening procedure, many questions, concerns, and future uncertainties can be explored with the parents by the child care professional when discussing the observations obtained from a standardized tool. Parents can learn if the child is progressing as expected, whether there are clues indicating his readiness to acquire new skills, and whether the child is accomplishing developmental tasks at a similar or different rate of speed as compared to his rate at a different age. More importantly, the opportunity may be available to reassure the parents that indeed the child is succeeding and that they are responding appropriately to the child's changing developmental needs. Child care professionals need to give parents appropriate feedback when they have been resourceful in promoting the child's independence, greater mastery, and steady movement and progress.

A developmental screening procedure can be used as a time to explain the significance of stacking blocks, why it is important to assess a child's progress in gross and fine motor skills, and, most significantly, the interrelationships among the following variables: the child's readiness for new skills; the appropriateness of practice he is receiving; the degree or lack of success being experienced; the regularity or irregularity of his patterns or rates of achievement; the support and responsiveness of his learning environment to his needs whether he is 3 days, 3 months, 2½ years, or 5 years old; and whether expectations for his performance are realistically based on his level of ability to perform tasks expected of children of his same age.

A developmental screening procedure offers an appropriate occasion to encourage the mother to express concerns, doubts, and anxieties. It offers the opportunity to reassure her about the child's abilities or lack of them and to discuss whether he is being asked to do more than is appropriate for his abilities or not enough and whether opportunities are available for continued learning. A developmental screening procedure offers an opportunity to assess the child's reactions to failure and success, how well he attends, how hard he attempts to succeed, his understanding, his cooperativeness, his unique needs, whether his environment is responsive to his needs, whether the parents are accepting of his abilities, and whether expectations are appropriate. In addition, the child care profes-

sional can use this opportunity to give comprehensive input to parents about decision making, alternatives, their resourcefulness, strengths, ability to make accurate observations, capability of evaluating progress, capacity to change in response to the child's continuous changes, and ability to discuss concerns that are experienced by most parents.

When results from the developmental assessment procedure are shared with parents, attention is not only focused on the child but is equally focused on identifying parental needs, strengths, capabilities, and capacities. The opportunity of screening a child for his strengths and weaknesses also serves as an occasion to explore other ways of solving old problems. Most importantly, parents can be supported for the appropriate judgments they have made, the decisions they have made, and the alternatives they have examined.

SUGGESTED READINGS

Bee, Helen: The developing child, New York, 1975, Harper & Row, Publishers.

Berlin, Irving N.: Advocacy for child mental health, New York, 1975, Brunner/Mazel, Inc.

Chinn, Peggy L.: Child health maintenance: concepts in family-centered care, ed. 2, St. Louis, 1979, The C. V. Mosby Co.

Ginott, Haim G.: Between parent and child: new solutions to old problems, New York, 1969, Avon Books.

Hendrick, Joanne: The whole child: new trends in early education, ed. 2., St. Louis, 1980, The C. V. Mosby Co.

Hobbs, Nicholas: The future of children, San Francisco, 1975, Jossey-Bass, Inc., Publishers.

Illingworth, R. S.: The normal child: some problems of the first five years and their treatment, Boston, 1964, Little, Brown & Co.

Jenson, G. D.: The well child's problems: management in the first six years, Chicago, 1962, Year Book Medical Publishers, Inc.

Maier, John: Screening and assessment of young children at developmental risk, Washington, D.C., 1973, U.S. Department of Health, Education, and Welfare.

Thorpe, Helene S., and Werner, Emmy E.: Developmental screening of preschool children: a critical review of inventories used in health and educational programs, Pediatrics **53:**362-370, 1974.

Whipple, Dorothy V.: Dynamics of development: euthenic pediatrics, New York, 1966, McGraw-Hill Book Co.

12

THE DENVER DEVELOPMENTAL SCREENING TEST

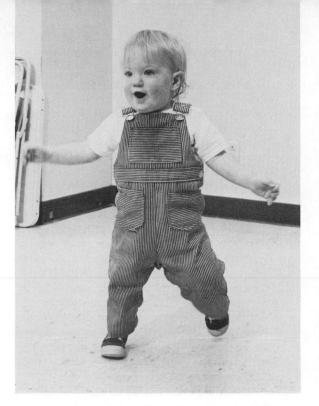

It has become increasingly clear to child care professionals that screening tests can be used effectively to find and prevent handicapping conditions in early childhood. The Commission on Chronic Illness[1] in 1951 defined screening as "the presumptive identification of unrecognized disease or defect by the application of tests, examinations, or other procedures which can be applied rapidly. Screening tests sort out apparently well persons who probably have a disease from those who probably do not. A screening test is not intended to be diagnostic. Persons with positive or suspicious findings must be referred to their physicians for diagnosis and necessary treatment."* As pointed out by the Commission on Chronic Illness, screening affords early detection of handicapping conditions for large groups of the population. Screening should serve the purpose of detecting handicapping conditions in their incipient stages so that child care professionals can do something about them.

The need for designing a screening tool that

*From Commission on Chronic Illness: Chronic illness in the United States: prevention of chronic illness, vol. 1, Cambridge, Mass., 1957, Harvard University Press, p. 45.

would aid in the early detection of delayed development in children was discussed in 1967 by Frankenburg and Dodds.[2] These investigators pointed out that a large number of young infants and children were not receiving routine developmental examinations after the period of infancy, nor were they the recipients of standardized and objective evaluations even if they were seen. It was also suggested that parents as well as child and health care professionals might deny the possibility of developmental delays in young children. Frankenburg and Dodds also reported that the incidence of diagnosed cases of developmental delays became strikingly higher at the age of school entrance. All these findings suggested that there were unnecessary delays in the detection of abnormal development in young children. These same major findings pointed to the critical need for a simple method of screening for evidence of delayed development in infants and preschool children. Frankenburg and Dodds[2] responded to this identified need by developing a test format that would "be simple to administer, easy to score and interpret, and useful for repeat examinations of the same child." Thus the Denver Developmental Screening Test (DDST) was devised to provide a simple method of screening for developmental delays during infancy and the preschool years. The DDST yields a developmental profile of an infant or child in four areas. These four areas include gross motor, language, fine motor-adaptive, and personal-social skills. The DDST is designed to help alert professionals and others to do a more in-depth evaluation of a child once it is discovered that development in any of the four areas is questionable or abnormal when comparing it to normal standards.

The DDST is not an IQ test; instead it simply helps to give a rough approximation of a child's current developmental status. It therefore serves as a screening tool.[3] Because the test is standardized, it serves as a valuable frame of reference aiding child care professionals in observing what children can do at different ages, assessing the progress a given child makes in all four categories from one time period to another, and comparing a child's abilities with those of other children of the same age.

Researchers developed the DDST by testing more than 1,000 infants and children under identical conditions.[3] Each child was asked to perform an item in the same way, using the same test materials; each was given the same number of chances to successfully complete the task; and each was scored according to predetermined indicators. Some of the children had no previous opportunities to perform certain test items, and occasionally children simply refused to comply. These occurrences were taken into consideration, and the children were scored accordingly.

The actual test form correlates each test item with the ages at which 25%, 50%, 75%, and 90% of the standardization population could perform a particular item.[1] Each item is designated by a bar, which is so located under an age line to show the age at which 25%, 50%, 75%, and 90% of the normal children were able to perform a developmental task. It is important to remember that each bar represents a time continuum.

RELIABILITY AND VALIDITY

The DDST has been subjected to a number of reliability and validity studies. As Frankenburg and associates[4] reported:

Tester-observer agreement and test-retest stability of the Denver Developmental Screening Test (DDST) were evaluated with 76 and 186 subjects, respectively. The correlation coefficients for mental ages obtained at a 1-week interval were calculated for 13 age groups between 1.5 months and 49 months. Co-

efficients ranged between .66 and .93 with no age trend displayed.[*]

With regard to the validity of the DDST, Frankenburg and associates[5] reported the following:

A study was undertaken to evaluate the validity of the DDST. 236 subjects were evaluated with the DDST and the following criterion tests: Stanford-Binet, Revised Yale Developmental Schedule, Cattell, and the Revised Bayley Infant Scale. Correlations of mental ages obtained with the DDST and the criterion tests varied between .86 and .97. Scoring for DDST as normal, questionable, and abnormal agreed very highly with IQs or DQs obtained on the criterion tests.[†]

The results of the validity study led Frankenburg and associates[5] to the following conclusion:

The over-all impact of data . . . is to lend strong support to the use of the DDST as a screening test for identifying developmental deviations. The consistency with which children with low IQs are identified without grossly calling "deviant" children who actually are normal is especially encouraging at the upper ages.[‡]

The majority of studies done with the DDST support the instrument in regard to face and concurrent validity.

There is concern that child care professionals and others recognize its limitations in terms of its predictive validity, particularly with minority ethnic groups.[6] Child care professionals and others who use the DDST must keep in mind that the DDST "is not a definite predictor of current or future adaptive or intellectual ability."[7]

UNIQUE FEATURES OF THE DDST

Frankenburg[8] has identified six criteria for evaluation of screening tests and screening programs: acceptability, simplicity, reliability, validity, appropriateness for the population being screened, and cost.

The DDST has received extensive support of child care professionals; it is recognized for being a simple test to administer, score, and

---

*From Frankenburg, William K., Camp, Bonnie W., Van Natta, Pearl A., and Demersseman, John A.: Reliability and stability of the Denver Developmental Screening Test, Child Dev. **42:**1315, 1971.

†From Frankenburg, William K., Camp, Bonnie W., and Van Natta, Pearl A.: Validity of the Denver Developmental Screening Test, Child Dev. **42:**475, 1971.

‡Ibid., p. 484.

interpret. It has been subjected to rigorous reliability and validity testing and meets criteria for both.

Stedman[7] states that "the number of children involved in the standardization, the matching of community characteristics, the spread of age range, and the careful item selection make this one of the better standardized survey instruments available." Stedman[7] points out, however, that one weakness of the test is the "difference in characteristics of the Denver population and other major urban areas in the United States."

There is evidence that it meets criteria for cost. According to Stedman,[7] "it provides a reliable, economical, and useful device for the early identification of developmental disability."

Frankenburg and associates[9] emphasize that the best screening test for screening individuals for asymptomatic disease is one that is economical in regard to professional manpower, accuracy of screening (as revealed by overreferrals and underreferrals), and cost of screening one child.

Accumulated evidence from many sources suggests that the DDST meets the six criteria of an efficient screening device as outlined by Frankenburg.

EDUCATION OF THE EXAMINER

Both professionals and paraprofessionals can learn to administer the DDST with a high degree of accuracy. The degree of accuracy in testing a subject will depend on both a proper training program and a proficiency evaluation. Self-instructional units are available to ensure that each individual uses a standardized method of test administration. An instructional unit is available for a classroom session using the manual, workbook, and a film combination; a practice testing session; and a proficiency evaluation.

Importance of proficiency training and periodic retraining

There is increased sensitivity to the need for periodic checks of screening results. It has been found that proficiency of test administration and observation skills decline when the examiner using the DDST no longer thinks his screening is being checked.[9] To assure the highest level of screening accuracy, examiners must have periodic checks of their screening practices and results.

Hunt[10] cautions that results from the validity studies of the DDST point to the need for exten-sive training for nonprofessional health aides who have had no previous experience or advanced education.

Stedman[7] states that the DDST can be learned and performed by at least high school–level personnel. He also reports that study programs are underway to determine the effectiveness of using sub–high school, indigent, and parent populations for screening. In addition, Stedman asserts that "persons trained in the area of health or allied health professions, education, social sciences, and human development are excellent trainees and screeners."

Hunt[10] suggests that proper training for anyone giving the test should not be too readily assumed because of the specificity of administration and the nature of scoring.

Stedman[7] suggests that training time may range from a few hours to several days, depending on the level of formal education, experience, and availability of children in different age groups for demonstration and practice and trial evaluations.

Frankenburg encourages potential users of the DDST to be properly trained in administration, scoring, and interpretation of items. He recommends that a trainee of the DDST should go through a training period and pass a proficiency test. Persons using the DDST must be properly trained to assure meaningful results with the DDST.

A proficiency evaluation is available for the purpose of measuring the skills of the individual learning to administer the DDST. It helps determine if the learner is meeting minimum testing standards. Each evaluation consists of a written test, a film, and an observed testing session, wherein the learner's skills are observed and assessed. The proficiency test helps ensure that the learner is administering items according to the standardized method for which the developmental items were validated. It is questionable whether test results are accurate if the learner does not pass the proficiency test.

USING THE DDST

The DDST manual sets forth scoring criteria for each item, contains general information on how to score, and presents symbols to be used in scoring.[1] It also offers numerous do's and don'ts regarding the preparation, administration, scoring, and interpretation phases. However, developmental screening of an infant or child requires more than just presenting selected items correctly and in a prescribed manner. It requires more than merely informing a parent that a child passed or failed to achieve a certain score. Using the DDST well requires sensitivity to each child's uniqueness, attention to the child's individual ways of responding, and regard for the strengths as well as the weaknesses that are observed. It also requires attention to the parents' personal needs.

CONSIDERATION OF THE CHILD

Of major importance is the examiner's orientation to each child's optimal performance under the most favorable conditions. To maintain this positive orientation the examiner must be continuously aware of the variety and number of cues a child emits in response to requests being made. The child's attention to a task, interest in participating, and eagerness to please are all equally important to consider. Most children need time to become comfortable with a new person and a new environment. Encouraging the child as he tries to initiate tasks, complete them, or do the best he can promotes maximum feelings of security, certainty, and comfort. The examiner should be clear and affirmative in orienting the child to what is expected through-

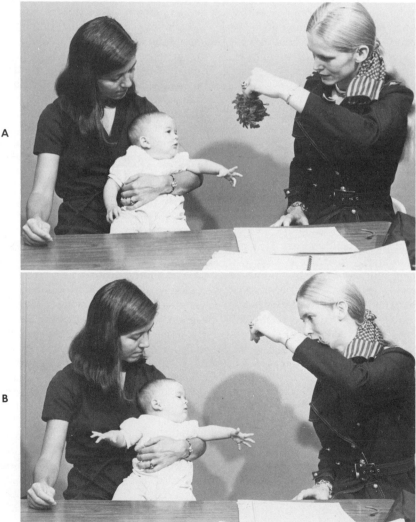

Fig. 12-1. Developmental screening for fine-motor adaptive responses. **A,** The infant's attention is attracted to the red pompom of yarn. As the infant focuses on the yarn, it is dropped out of her vision. **B,** The infant sits and looks to see where the yarn pompom disappeared.

out the session, remembering to do the following:

1. Offer explanations at a child's level of understanding.
2. Obtain the child's visual and listening attention for each task and maintain it.
3. Use consistently a format that the child understands.
4. Repeat instructions if the child does not respond or acts confused or in doubt.

Children are sometimes unpredictable in their behavior and need time to adjust to requests being made of them. Consequently rescheduling the test may give a child a greater chance of success.

CONSIDERATION OF PARENTS' NEEDS

Parental needs during screening should be actively considered by the examiner, who must listen attentively to what parents say about themselves and about their child's abilities. An examiner can acknowledge the objective, important observations parents make during the screening procedure, respond to their concerns, and praise the approaches they selected to help their child make steady developmental gains. Other supportive statements can refer to the parents' perceptiveness about the child's needs at different stages, their judgments regarding the child's readiness to progress further, and their problem-solving and decision-making efforts.

Several phases are inherent in the screening process, and each requires special consideration and appropriate responses by the examiner. The first phase involves preparing both child and parent for screening. The second phase concerns administering individual test items. The third phase, scoring, is extremely important; attention to the scoring criteria in the DDST manual ensures the only correct score for each child. The last phase, interpreting the results, is crucial for meeting the parents' needs and for supporting the child's efforts, as well as for accurately portraying the significance of the child's behavior.

I have used an approach that emphasizes a mutual participation model—one in which the mother participates from the beginning to the end of the screening process. First, the DDST is explained and its purpose clarified. The clinician stresses what the screening test can and cannot do. Its limitations are clearly spelled out. (It is not an IQ test.) It is useful to explain that items are designed for both younger and older children. It is important to explain to the parents that they will not receive a specific age estimate because that is not the intended purpose of the screening test. Some practitioners have given parents age estimates, which is considered to be a dangerous practice. Second, it is productive to find out how the parents think the child will do in all four areas. After completion of the screening, it is useful to ask the parents how well they thought the child performed.

It is extremely helpful to use a positive model in sharing the results with parents. First, present the child's strengths in all areas; second, present the child's weaknesses; and third, ask the parents if they agree with your observations of the child's strengths and weaknesses in performance.

Avoid falling into the trap of making some hasty recommendations of what the child or parents should do if the child has had any seri-

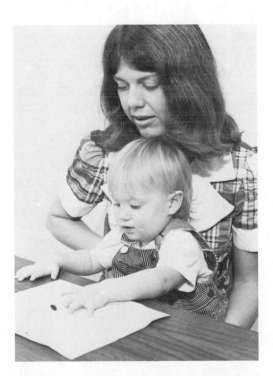

Fig. 12-2. The child is seated on his parent's lap so that he can place his hands on the table. A raisin has been dropped directly in front of him within easy reach. The child is observed to reach for and ready himself for picking up the raisin, using a thumb and finger grasp.

ous deficits in performance. Find out initially what the parents think is a weakness or developmental problem and have them define it in their own terms. Avoid defining their problem or concern. Let the parents state in their own way the goals they have for their child. Comment on whether you think it is appropriate after considering the systematic observations made while the child was being screened. Specifically be attuned to whether the activities that parents are planning are appropriate for the child's development. It is of value to find out what the parents want or have done to correct a developmental delay if one actually exists.

Always consider a rescreening if it seems to be warranted for the child. If the parents ask for instant advice, think instead of ways to collect data on the child's questionable performance. Once appropriately timed and sufficient data are collected on the child, then a program of intervention can be planned in a mutual way with the parents participating in a problem-solving manner.

Generally, parents are basically wondering or actually asking, "Am I a good parent?" Use this time after screening to comment on the parents' appropriate behaviors and interactions with their child.

COMMON ERRORS IN ADMINISTERING THE DDST

Having observed a wide number of child care professionals administering the DDST, it has become clear that a number of errors occur during this vital test. The following list depicts the most commonly made errors in the preparation, administration, scoring, and interpretation of results of developmental assessments. These errors need to be avoided to ensure that the DDST remains valid and reliable as its original designers intended.

1. Failure to place yourself at ease.
2. Failure to use the manual.
3. Failure to place the parents at ease.
4. Failure to ask the parents how they think the child will do in all four areas.
5. Failure to ready the child for the task by getting and maintaining his attention.
6. Forgetting to distinguish for the parents that it is a developmental screening device and not an IQ test.
7. Not informing the parents of the purpose and then clarifying their understanding. Ask directly, "Do you understand? Do you have any questions?"

8. Not informing the parents ahead of the purpose of screening.
9. Forgetting to encourage the parents not to prompt the child on items and advise them that the child is not expected to pass every developmental item.
10. Failure to remind the parents of the intent to go from simple to complex items.
11. Failure to ask if the child's performance is typical or different and to have the parents describe their expectations before the DDST is used.
12. Forgetting to let the parents know once the child is into a more complex task at the time it occurs.
13. Failure to make a supportive statement that it must be difficult for the parents to observe their child when it is obvious they are tense or anxious about the failure of their child to comply.
14. Failure to attend to the parents' anxiety when the child is obviously refusing or failing an item.
15. Forgetting to ask the parents what they thought of the child's performance after the DDST is completed.
16. Failure to share specifically what the child is achieving in each area he passed after the test is administered.
17. Failure to encourage the parents in their efforts and to give credit for their obvious and appropriate contributions to the child's progress.
18. Failure to ask the parents if they have any questions about the tool.
19. Failure to ask the parents if they have thought of ways or approaches to encourage progress in one area or another.
20. Failure to use phrases like, "It wasn't as easy as other items," when a child obviously is not passing selected items.
21. Failure to share positive findings and strengths before discussing weaknesses of the child, that is, the use of a positive approach instead of a deficit model. Find out from the parents their perceptions of the child's strengths.
22. Failure to let the child get comfortable with the examiner and environment first.
23. Failure to allow the child three trials with all items.
24. Failure to present one item or activity at a time, particularly for a younger child or child who may have difficulty attending to tasks that are presented.

25. Failure to familiarize yourself with items of the child's age level before administering the screening test.
26. Forgetting to subtract for prematurity.
27. Forgetting to place P, F, R, or N.O. at the 50% hatch mark.
28. Failure to reassure the parents that children are individuals in their responses to a screening test; that is, some children react in different ways as the examiner brings them under "instructional control."
29. Forgetting to reassure the parents that some tasks are easier for children than other tasks.
30. Acting surprised when a child passes an item.
31. Failure to use a positive tone of voice and facial expression when you intend to be supportive to the child.
32. Failure to capitalize on the parents' resourcefulness and encourage them to try out methods of promoting the child's progress in each of the four areas that they have thought of, if they seem appropriate.
33. Putting words into the parents' mouths when interviewing for items that are to be reported.
34. Dismissing a concern that the parents have by using a ready-made statement such as, "He'll catch up" or "Don't worry."
35. Asking the child if he thinks he can rather than taking a more positive stance and saying, "Show me how you can do this."
36. Not remembering, when interpreting results, to ask the parents if they have questions about the areas you have just reviewed rather than moving on to cover the entire profile.
37. Failure to use reassuring phrases that the child may not be able to do this item because he is not ready for it or not yet capable, but he is showing strengths in getting there, if in fact you observe the prerequisite behaviors.
38. Failure to watch for cues that signal fatigue in younger children.
39. Failure to remember to start with items that automatically give the child and caregivers a feeling of success.
40. Forgetting to get comfortable with not having answers to all of the parents' questions and being able to say, "I need to observe further. It's difficult to make predictions. I'm not certain I can answer your question now, but perhaps I can later after further observations." (Learn to refrain from giving instant advice.)
41. Not attempting to find comfortable ways to discuss questionable developmental delays without threatening the parents.
42. Failure to consistently show social approval and acknowledgment when appropriate for both parents and child.
43. Failure to encourage the child to work harder when he says, "I can't."
44. Failure to remember to change activities to keep pace with an individual child's interest.
45. Failure to remember to secure the child's attention for building with blocks, answering questions, drawing with a pencil, getting ready to catch a ball, and watching you demonstrate activities.
46. Failure to attempt to give the child one instruction at a time rather than a series of instructions.
47. Failure to remember to let the parents know that you are getting into more "advanced" tasks rather than more "difficult" tasks.
48. Failure to be certain that the parents are defining the child's ability to do certain tasks rather than relying on their report that "We think she can."
49. Failure to remember to define each area when interpreting it and allow the parents to know which category you are discussing.
50. If uncertain about the parents' questions or answers, failure to ask for specific examples of behaviors they are discussing.
51. Forgetting to establish eye contact with the parents when interpreting results. Failure to interact with the parents rather than through the child.
52. Not attempting to point out to the parents that "Maybe you have noticed I am moving into a more advanced area now" to give them credit for their observations.
53. Failure to remember to encourage the parents with their appropriate attempts. Try to include the father during screening.
54. Failure to remember to let the parents know when you are moving from one

area to another before administering items to the child.

55. Failure to introduce expectations to a child that are appropriate for his age level and attention span and to let the child know what is expected of him with simple explanations of a positive nature.

56. Giving the specific age level in which a child is functioning. The DDST is not intended for this; it is intended as a screening tool, not a diagnostic test.

IMPORTANCE OF VALID RESULTS

Developmental screening tools are increasingly being used by persons of different educational backgrounds. Ideally these people learn at the outset about ways to avoid making common errors during each phase of the screening procedures. Without such knowledge, they might produce invalid results.

Results of developmental assessments are primarily used to determine whether a child is progressing at expected rates in developmental tasks, to reassure parents regarding their child's progress, and to give parents guidance about what to expect next in the child's development. There is an increasing trend to use screening results to decide whether in-depth neurological and psychological investigations are needed. DDST results influence many decisions made by parents, nurses, physicians, early infant educators, and paraprofessional workers; thus invalid results may jeopardize the welfare of both the child and the parents.

Examiners can avoid common errors by following the DDST manual closely and adhering to the advice given for each phase. Some instructions are highlighted here that appear in the DDST manual. The examiner can refer to the DDST manual for other pertinent points for the entire screening process.

PHASES OF THE DDST PROCEDURE
Preparation phase

The preparation phase of the DDST procedure involves the following steps for the examiner (these steps are outlined in the DDST manual but are emphasized here because of their importance):

1. Become familiar with items at the child's age level before beginning the screening procedure.

2. Place the parents at ease. Make the distinction that the DDST is a developmental screening device, not an IQ test. Inform the parents of the purpose of the DDST and then

clarify their understanding by asking directly, "Do you understand? Do you have any questions?" Have the parents describe their expectations before beginning the screening procedure.

3. Ask if the child's behavior has been typical so far before carrying out the test. Ask whether the child has had his nap and eaten and whether the parents have prepared the child so that he will not be frightened or feel uncomfortable.

4. The parents should be reminded of the examiner's intent to go from simple to complex items.

5. Inform the parents to refrain from prompting. Explain that if it becomes apparent that their assistance might make it easier for the child to succeed, they will be told exactly how to ask the question or how to instruct the child (carefully following the directions specified in the manual).

6. The examiner should allow the child to get comfortable with him and the environment before the screening procedure.

7. Tell the child what is expected of him, using simple explanations of a positive nature such as the following: "Today you and I are going to take turns with some toys, questions and answers, and activities I have selected just for you to do."

Administration phase

Although directions on administration are carefully spelled out in the DDST manual, it is important to emphasize certain points about the administration phase.

The examiner's instructions for the administration phase are as follows:

1. Ready the child for each item by getting and maintaining his attention.

2. Present one item or activity at a time, particularly to a younger child or a child with a short attention span. In addition, give the child one instruction at a time rather than a series, and watch for signs of fatigue in younger children.

3. Allow the child maximum trials for each screening item.

4. Begin with the personal-social area so the child can relax, become accustomed to his new environment, and start looking at some materials he will be using such as the blocks, pencil, and red pompom (depending on age).

5. In making the transition from the personal-social area to the other areas, explain to the child, "I've asked your parents a number of questions and we've spent some time together.

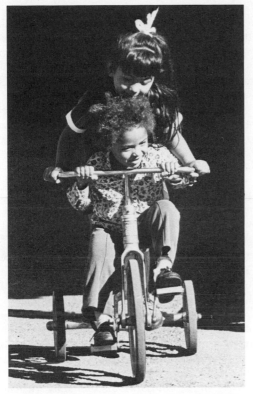

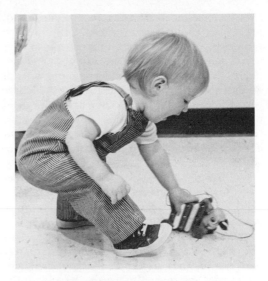

Los Niños Head Start

Fig. 12-3. Screening a child's motor coordination while riding a tricycle. (From Hendrick, Joanne: The whole child: new trends in early education, St. Louis, 1975, The C. V. Mosby Co.)

Fig. 12-4. The child is observed for his gross motor skills of bending over and picking up a toy. The child is observed while standing on the floor away from all support and is told to pick up a small toy in front of him. The child is able to bend over and pick up the toy without holding on or touching the floor. Although the child is not seen returning to stand, he shows the ability to coordinate eye-hand trunk and leg coordination for this task.

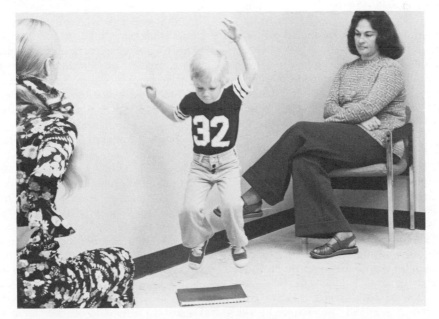

Fig. 12-5. The child is observed for his gross motor skills of doing a standing broad jump across the width of paper (8½ inches).

Now I would like to ask you some questions and have you help me like they did." Or, "Now it's your turn to spend some time doing special things with me. I have some little toys and activities that are planned just for you and we will do these things together. First of all, I will ask you some questions and then it will be your turn to answer them. Some things will be easy for you and later on maybe some won't be so easy, but I know you will try to do what I ask you to do. Are you ready?"

6. Change activities to keep pace with the individual child's interest.

7. Tell the parents when the child is moving from one area to another before administering items to the child.

8. Within each area, first introduce items that are appropriate for a child younger than the child being tested to assure that the child can experience success and positive experiences from the beginning.

9. Let the parents know when the child is moving to a more complex task. Speak of more "advanced" tasks rather than more "difficult" ones if the parent manifests anxiety about the child's test behaviors.

10. Attend to parental anxiety when the child is obviously refusing or failing an item. When the child does not comply immediately with a request, reassure the parents that children are individuals and are not necessarily predictable in their behavior. Reassure them that some tasks are easier for children than other tasks.

11. Refrain from acting surprised when a child passes an item.

12. Consistently show social approval and acknowledgment to both parents and child, even when the child fails an item. Maintain a positive tone of voice and facial expression when you intend to be supportive to the child.

13. Encourage the child to work harder when he says, "I can't."

14. Interact directly with the parents rather than through the child. Refrain from putting words in the parents' mouths when interviewing for items that are to be reported. Ask for examples of behavior if the meaning of the parents' response is unclear.

15. Refrain from making assumptions just because a 4½-year-old child quickly passes social, fine motor, and language areas with almost advanced skills. Do not assume he will pass on gross motor items!

Scoring phase

The DDST manual presents clear and simple directions on how to score items. The item scoring section of the manual presents a discussion on the symbols used and provides examples of scoring when the subject's performance is normal, questionable, or abnormal.

The examiner must be certain that the parents are defining the child's ability to do certain tasks rather than just guessing if he can.

Interpretation phase

The examiner is advised as follows for the interpretation phase of the DDST procedure:

1. Establish eye contact with the parents when interpreting results.

2. Ask the parents what they thought of the child's performance. Validate observations with them, and ask if they have any questions about the screening tool.

3. Convey the attitude that it is appropriate to share, validate, and confirm screening findings with the parents; get away from the mystique that data about a child's growth and development are for professionals only.

4. Even though the test is scored as a whole, it can be helpful to define each area when interpreting it and be sure the parents know which category is being discussed. Ask if the parents have questions about each area as it is being reviewed rather than asking for questions after all the results have been covered.

5. Share positive findings and specific strengths of the child before discussing the child's weaknesses, particularly when presenting information on questionable or abnormal test performance.

6. Find comfortable ways to discuss developmental delays without threatening parents or alarming them unnecessarily.

7. Encourage the parents in their efforts and give credit for their contributions to the child's progress. Ask if they have thought of ways to help their child progress in one area or another. If so, capitalize on their resourcefulness and give them confidence to try the new ideas that seem appropriate.

8. Attend to each concern the parents have. Do not dismiss these concerns with a ready-made statement such as "he'll catch up."

9. Become comfortable about not having answers to all the parents' questions, and be able to say, "I need to observe further. It's difficult to make predictions. I'm not certain I can

answer your question now, but perhaps I can later after further observations" or "I can answer your question about your child's two delays when we retest her in 2 weeks."

10. Include the father at every opportunity and encourage his participation in the screening process.

11. End the session by asking the parents, "Has this been helpful to you?" Their answer will help identify what they gained from the screening procedure, what they heard, and what they saw as the salient part of the screening, as well as whether it reassured them. Their answers will also give clues about their priorities and goals for future visits or assessments.

12. Discourage parents from teaching DDST items to the child. Such a teaching approach may lead to false assurance that the child is progressing normally in his development. The DDST was designed for screening.

SAMPLE DISCUSSIONS WITH PARENTS

Following are five sample discussions between parents of children of various ages and the child care professional who administered the DDST to these children. These discussions are presented as a means of showing the differences in concerns that parents have, as well as different approaches that can be used to interpret the results of the DDST to parents of younger to older children. Three normal test performances, one abnormal test performance, and one questionable test performance are presented. The variations in the following discussions about development are due to the children's age differences. It should be noted that in the last three examples presented, the children were not present during the discussions.

Discussion 1—normal test performance (child's age: 9 months)

During one screening session, a mother commented that her 9-month-old boy was "usually a joy, but sometimes I don't do the right things for him." The infant had passed all the items for his age level and was advanced in motor development, so the mother realized that she was indeed doing appropriate activities with her infant. When asked to clarify and define what she meant by not doing right things, she stated that she did not spend as much time with him as she would like. The examiner pointed out that the child was developing progressively, but for her own sense of comfort,

she could spend 10 to 15 minutes with him three times a day, engaging in activities that she enjoyed. The mother also related that this was her sixth child and that "no one really pays much attention if you've had a number of children." She went on to clarify that people take it for granted that older parents know what they are doing, forgetting that they need attention for rearing their children too. The examiner spontaneously agreed and proceeded to reassure the mother about her excellent nurturing qualities, the way she reinforced her infant's sounds, the number of times she smiled and touched him, and her patience in allowing him to begin and complete a task. During the discussion the mother also said, "He didn't get enough rest, he couldn't you know, with five other children around." The examiner explored this statement and discovered that the mother needed more time for herself and some extra rest. As they talked, the mother thought of ways to make arrangements for getting out by herself and for getting a nap if she needed it and considered the possibility of getting to bed earlier.

Comments. By being sensitive to verbal cues, the examiner focused attention on the mother rather than the infant. The examiner acknowledged the mother's needs and went one step further—problem solving in a mutual way to find alternatives that met the mother's needs, as well as the child's.

Discussion 2—normal test performance (child's age: 9 months 21 days)

Examiner: Now I'd like to review with you how M did today. Before we begin, was his performance typical for him today?

Mother: Yes.

Examiner: Good. This is the score sheet I've marked to show how he achieved the tasks expected for his age level. You can see that the top shows a child's ages in months, and that each of these bars shows the age range at which most children pass a certain item. M is short 10 days of being 10 months, so this is his age line here.

M passed everything in the personal-social area. I noticed that he cried in distress during the short time when you were out of the room. This behavior suggests his awareness of the difference between people and suggests that he's beginning to differentiate that you, for example, are separate, different, and apart from him. You responded well by assuring him that you would indeed return. He needed that assurance, and your return did make a difference in his anxiety and comfort level.

It was *not* as easy for him to patty-cake and I didn't mark it as a pass.

Mother: That's right. We've never even done it with him.

Examiner: Even though he did not imitate me clapping my hands together, he immediately responded to the idea of the action by hitting the table with his hand. He did this in response to my patty-cake at least three times, so he's getting the idea. It's a new item for him.

Going on, he did feed himself a cracker, and we noticed how he got it to his mouth and coordinated tongue, mouth, and teeth to bite, chew, and swallow.

You saw how he resisted when I tried to take his block away.

He could voluntarily grab onto something and purposefully pull it toward him rather than just reacting with a reflex response, which is more characteristic of early infancy. This demonstrates his ability to use his smaller muscles, his developing strength, and his beginning problem-solving abilities.

He played peek-a-boo very well, reached out for a toy, played ball with me; he indicated what he wanted by pointing, and you said he could drink from a cup. These are all tasks we expect him to have achieved. It seems you have done nicely in allowing him independence to do some of these things like feeding himself. He's exhibiting behaviors that indicate learning is taking place in all these tasks, and you are doing some appropriate things with him to help make it possible for him to learn, to develop, and to accomplish increasingly more complex tasks for his age.

In the fine motor area, M is showing good progress. He was able to sit and look for the red pompom when I dropped it out of sight.

He was able to use his finger and thumb to pick up the raisin. It was not as easy for him to pick it up with his index finger and thumb. Most infants develop this skill in a sequence of increasingly complex steps: first, they pick up small objects with a raking motion of the palm of their hand; then with the second or third finger and thumb; and finally, with a purposeful overhand motion using both forefinger and thumb in more precise coordinated movements.

He banged the two cubes together successfully.

In using his small muscles he's doing well. He also transferred one cube to another hand when I handed him a new one to hold.

Mother: What do you think I should do to help him? Give him raisins to help him learn how to develop a pincer grasp? I don't like the idea of giving him raisins. He might choke on them.

Examiner: That's a good question. You have to be careful with the little things you give him that undoubtedly go to his mouth. It might be better to use cheerios.

In fine motor development he's passed all the items for his age level.

Examiner: In the language area, he's doing very well. He turns his head toward a voice when his name is said. He's beginning to say dada for daddy. He is not yet saying mama but is *beginning* to make "m-m" sounds.

Mother: When should he be saying "mama"?

Examiner: In imitating speech sounds, he's making "boo-boo" sounds. He is not expected to name objects or persons or you or pictures yet. That will come later. I've noticed how much attention you give him when he makes a variety of sounds. He makes more sounds when you repeat his sounds.

In the gross motor area—the use of his large muscles—he's showing many skills. He's sitting without support, pulling himself to a standing position, getting to a sitting position, standing momentarily while he's holding onto something, and we observed how well balanced he is when he does stand up. You said he could stoop. So as far as his use of large muscles, he's at his age level for these developmental tasks.

Mother: So he's at his age and above for everything except fine motor?

Examiner: He's within his age range for all the tasks: fine motor, personal-social, gross motor, and language skills.

Mother: This is good for me because I sometimes forget the things he's supposed to be doing. He's on his own a lot. It's reassuring to know he is at his age level.

Examiner: Has this been helpful?

Mother: It's always helpful. As soon as you asked if he ever did patty-cake, I realized we hadn't done that with him, but we did it with his 2½-year-old sister. I can tell by what you mentioned about his use of his large muscles that he really is getting ready for walking.

You're right; he does balance well and is standing, so I guess he probably will be walking soon. I'm definitely going to play patty-cake with him and continue to encourage his sounds, even though he isn't saying mama yet. I think I'll get him some little blocks too. He seemed to like holding them.

This was very helpful for me, to know he's doing what's expected at this age and that we're doing the right things with him. It's also a reminder of what he's going to do next so I can help him get ready to do some things in an easier way. I want him to experience nice feelings about what he's doing, and I'm glad he's not behind in anything.

Comments. Throughout the interpretation of results, the examiner emphasized M's strengths and supported the mother's efforts at responding to his developmental needs. This approach allowed for a discussion of M's purposeful behaviors, such as reaching for toys, and his efforts at combining a number of skills—for example, trying to coordinate standing, hanging on to the table edge, and placing a banana in his mouth all at the same time. The examiner suggested that the child was showing clues of increased skills for standing and balancing and was in a stage of learning to prepare for walking; his primary task was to achieve balance while standing now and to coordinate leg movements with upright posture later.

When discussing the results of the infant's fine motor skills, the examiner answered the mother's questions on promoting fine motor development, encouraged her ideas for helping M achieve a pincer grasp, and told her what to expect even though he was not passing some test items, which is all right for "normal" children. Normal children may be delayed on one or two DDST items and still be well within a normal range of variability. The examiner explained how children go from simple to more complex tasks, and that if he did not pass certain items, these would be tasks to expect him to achieve in the future. Significantly the examiner stressed beginnings of skills and did not emphasize any failure.

The mother learned from the examiner that M had made a variety of both vowel and consonant sounds. She was encouraged because she and M's father were beginning to promote word formation. This was an opportunity for the examiner to reinforce the mother's promptness and appropriate efforts at repeating what M says and to point out that it is important that

she talk with him when he makes a sound rather than later when he was not making sounds.

The examiner paid special attention to reassuring the mother that M was at his age level for the majority of items that had been presented to him. The examiner also attempted to use more open-ended questions in the discussion to encourage the mother to talk about her concerns rather than cutting her off after she had been asked to describe her child's abilities. The examiner was careful not to interrupt the mother. If the mother said "no" in answer to a question, the examiner rephrased it. When the mother declared that she had no concerns, the examiner did not drop the matter but went on to mention other positive interactions she had noted between the mother and the child. By asking the mother questions correctly and in a supportive way, the examiner helped the mother formulate her own decisions.

The examiner also attempted to convey that just because the mother had not encouraged the child to learn patty-cake, the child could still learn it. Sometimes parents might feel guilty for not teaching one particular task to their child.

Discussion 3 normal test performance (child's age: 2 years 19 days)

Examiner: Now that we are finished with all the assessment items, we can discuss the items G did do and those she didn't do. You will probably have some questions that we can discuss together also. First of all, did her behavior look typical and usual for her? Did she seem to respond the way you would have expected her to?

Mother: Yes, she seemed typical.

Examiner: Please look at the scoring sheet where I kept note of how she was doing. This line, from top to bottom, indicates her age line of exactly 2 years and 19 days.

She is able to imitate housework, doing simple things around the house, and she is able to use a spoon without spilling. She is able to wash and dry her hands, which some children her age do, whereas others don't.

As far as dressing herself, she can remove garments, which we expect her to begin doing. Although she's not yet putting on all her clothes, she's beginning to show readiness to cooperate. It is appropriate that you allow her to undress and are helping her with dressing.

Regarding play with other children, you say that she's mostly involved with parallel play? It sounds like she's beginning to get to the point of playing interactively with other children, although most of her play is, like you say, alongside another child. Do you have any questions about this area?

Mother: Yes. How do you teach them how to share?

Examiner: That's a good question.

Mother: It seems that you just keep going over and over it again and you have tears and arguing and I guess it just comes with patience? One child takes a turn, then the next one, and you don't know whether to take a toy from her to show her that it's time to share.

Examiner: Taking turns is learned in a series of steps, and it takes practice to know how, when, and with whom you share. Sharing starts in a simple manner and progresses to more complex kinds of interactions between children. As you say, it requires patience, but children do learn to share like they learn any other task. Usually the way to promote sharing is to praise G when you observe her sharing, whether with a child or an adult. An adult can serve as a model and verbally indicate, "Now I've held the doll. It's your turn." Children learn that sharing is expected of them, and they gradually internalize the concept. At this age we don't expect her to share completely. If she hands you something when you ask her to and thank her, even that helps her learn that something definite is expected of her. In a sense, she shows beginnings of sharing by the fact that she offered you a raisin when she was eating one. That was her idea of sharing.

You asked about play too. Play, like other developmental tasks, is a series of behaviors; a child masters certain simple goals, adds new behaviors, and moves on to more advanced levels of play. Generally, children play with their bodies first; then learn to look at, reach for, hold, grasp, and release toys. They tend to repeat what is pleasurable for them. Through play they learn many things: they act out what perhaps is difficult for them to communicate in language, they master new experiences by acting something out and repeating it; and they learn to coordinate fine and gross motor skills. Through play they learn concepts such as the small or large ball. They also learn about social interactions and cultural expectations. They learn that there

are places where you can play and others where you are not allowed to. They learn simple to complex rules about games. From a very early age they learn to share, to take turns, and this is generally taught through play, so you'll probably notice more sharing as time goes on.

Mother: I agree.

Examiner: On to her fine motor skills. She was able to do some scribbling, to stack a tower of five blocks. It wasn't as easy for her to complete a vertical line, but she tried to imitate it.

Mother: I've never done anything with her with crayons. I have just given her simple coloring books and all she does is scribble all over the pages. Maybe I should concentrate on having her draw certain things like circles and lines on a piece of plain paper. Should I work with her at this age on these things?

Examiner: Well, she seems to show pleasure in holding a pencil and making scribbling marks. She's beginning to show interest in using the pencil and was paying attention while scribbling. She talked about her scribbling and seemed very positive about what she was doing. Copying is something you could encourage if she continues to show interest and likes drawing lines or other forms. She did *try* to copy the line but didn't have it perfectly straight. I didn't expect her to.

She was showing some readiness to draw a circle by drawing round scribbles. She was able to figure out what to do with the bottle with the raisin inside without having someone show her. This kind of behavior indicates that she is attending to what she is doing and is practicing problem-solving skills and is experiencing success with such challenges.

In the language area, she shows the most achievement. She has a wide vocabulary and puts words together in a logical sequence that is perfectly understandable. This is a very strong area for her.

Mother: Yes. I have noticed that she used big words and in the correct context. I'm not sure where she learns this, but when we talk to her, we do not use baby talk. The other day she said she smelled horrible, and indeed she did. She had just soiled her pants, but I was surprised she could come out with such a big word.

Examiner: The way you are talking with her indicates that she's learning how to use words right, and so far it's very appropriate. It doesn't seem that you're expecting too much because she seems so comfortable in her use of words.

She was able to follow directions as to where to put the blocks. You said that she is able to say her first and last name, but she didn't say it to me. It could be that she's shy with me yet.

Mother: Yes, she does use her first and last name together, and I'm surprised she didn't tell you what it was today. We worked and worked on it when she first started walking. We figured that if she could say her first and last name, in case she got lost she could tell people who she was. She's been saying it for a long time.

Examiner: Concerning her gross motor skills, we observed that she is walking well; she can walk both forward and backward and has really developed well in that skill. She's also shown that she can kick a ball forward, although she seems to enjoy throwing it more.

Mother: I haven't allowed her to throw things in the house, but she is allowed to kick a ball when she is outside.

Examiner: You said that although she was not able to put the block in front of or behind the chair today, she is able to do this at home?

Mother: When she's told to pick up something behind her, she'll turn and look behind. I don't recall ever telling her to look in front of her.

Examiner: Many of the skills and abilities she has developed seem to be a direct reflection of the kinds of experiences and activities you have selected for her. Your interactions too indicate many appropriate ways of responding to her past and current abilities and show a consistent sensitivity to her as she changes and progresses from one developmental period to the next and from one experience to others. It sounds like you do spend time with her encouraging her to do things.

Mother: Yes, I spend time in the morning for 2 hours and throughout the day. We will start working on lines and circles though.

Examiner: Was her behavior what you would consider typical?

Mother: She was her usual self, except that she usually spends more time talking. She did less talking today. Usually she's jabbering the whole time.

Examiner: This behavior might be explained by the fact that I was new to her and that she's

in a different place; she needed some time to get used to all the novelty. In addition, I was keeping her pretty busy asking her to do things for me, and she was doing her best to comply and was very eager to please both of us.

Comments. The examiner did not emphasize that the child was failing but instead stressed the child's positive achievements so far and particularly the beginnings of skills. The examiner gave credit for what G was doing and pointed out where she was going in terms of developmental skills, what the mother could anticipate, and that she would be doing more on her own. Thus the examiner helped the mother prepare herself for the probability of her child's increased independence and perhaps even suggested to her that G needed greater opportunities to do more by herself. The mother was glad to hear that G was good at keeping to one activity at a time and that her lengthening attention span was a progressive indicator of her ability to concentrate.

The examiner also explained that although G is mostly involved in parallel play, she is beginning to get to the point at which she is playing with other children in different ways. In response to the mother's question about sharing, the examiner correctly emphasized that G would do more sharing and that the mother was correctly and appropriately encouraging the development of sharing by reinforcing it when she observed it.

The discussion gave the examiner an opportunity to reflect on the mother's excellent efforts in helping G become more independent, in responding to her by showing her how to talk properly, and in spending appropriate amounts of time encouraging specific activities.

Discussion 4—abnormal test performance (child's age: 2 years 9 months)

Examiner: In the personal-social area, she is doing very well. She initiated taking off her pajamas. She's taking off her shoes. You said that you're doing a lot of things to encourage her with dressing, such as putting one shoe on her while she puts on one.

You mentioned that she tries to put away the wash cloths, she watches you do dishes, she doesn't spill much with the spoon, and she is beginning to use her fork. You said she's also showing interest in cutting up her food and is beginning to use a lot of utensils. She can't turn faucets on or off, but she can wash and dry her own hands and you hand her the towel. She dresses with supervision and, as you say, likes to pick out some of her own clothes. Except for taking off tight shirts, she can undress herself. You said she can't unzip or unbutton or lace her shoes. It sounds like she's progressively doing a lot of things herself and that you are helping her learn how to be more independent.

Mother: She will roll a ball back and forth and returns it when you ask, and she takes turns pushing a truck back and forth.

Examiner: She doesn't play games that require taking turns with other children, but there are apparently few children that she really has a chance to play with on a consistent basis. She sees a cousin about once a week, but they don't really play together, according to what you said.

Mother: I wanted to ask what you thought about big puzzles. She loves them. I have bought huge puzzles for her to piece together. She tries really hard to get them together. Just last week she put a big wooden cat together. I helped her with it for 7 days.

Examiner: It must make you feel good to see her put puzzles like that together. As long as puzzles hold her interest, and she responds positively or doesn't show too much frustration and attends to what she's doing, it's appropriate.

Playing with puzzles helps her process information, helps her problem solve, and gives her excellent practice with fine motor movements of her fingers and hands. The puzzle pieces might help her learn that objects have different colors, sizes, shapes, and textures. She's getting practice in learning that a large piece fits into a large hole and that certain shapes fit only in certain places. At the same time, she probably experiences pleasant associations with the comments you make and the fact that you are proud and pleased with what she is accomplishing.

At any rate, in the personal-social area she is doing most of the items. You mention that she still needs some help with dressing but that you're working on that.

Mother: I'm really pleased that she is doing well. I wasn't certain how she was doing in comparison to children of her own age or if I was doing the right things.

Examiner: Screening such as this can be valuable in showing you what is easy for her and what is not so easy for her. In the personal-social area she is doing most of the tasks adequately. She's able to put on her own clothes almost to the point of being able to get dressed without supervision, according to what you said.

Mother: Most of the time I can tell her to go ahead and get dressed, but I must admit she usually needs my supervision and help. She tries to initiate things like taking off her pajamas.

Examiner: She's even putting on her shoes and holding the laces. You're really doing some activities to encourage her and even make a game out of it.

Mother: I've tried to make it a game because I hate to have a hassle every morning. If we don't make dressing a game, she will flatly refuse. Maybe she's just at an age where she's rebellious. One thing really works: she doesn't get to eat until she's dressed.

Examiner: It sounds like you've found some positive, comfortable ways to make it easier for both of you. You are also indicating that you are using a consistent approach every morning, which helps her learn what you expect of her all the time. The hassles that you mentioned sound as if they are disappearing due to the ideas you are trying out. The important thing is that not only did you try out the ideas, they worked for both of you and you found that you do come up with successful ways to cope with challenges such as these.

In the fine motor area, I did not observe her to draw a circle, nor did I see her scribble when I gave her the pencil. She built a tower of five blocks, which shows that she has the beginning skills for the coordination it takes to place one cube on top of another so it won't fall off. Also, she is trying to watch carefully what she sees. She tried to copy my vertical line. It was not as easy for her to get the raisin out of the bottle without coaching and having it demonstrated to her.

In the language area, she is demonstrating that she understands what is being asked of her by placing objects on the floor, in front of her, behind her, and on the table. She also articulates her words, uses a variety of words to express what she wants, and uses three-word sentences.

Mother: I've started noticing more that she is increasing her use of words. She asks me while I'm working what I'm doing.

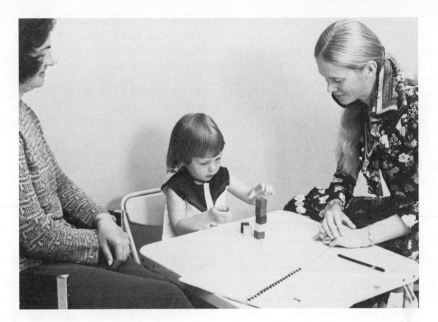

Fig. 12-6. The child is observed for her fine motor adaptive skills at building a tower of cubes. She has successfully balanced five blocks on top of each other and is working on placing three more.

Examiner: Do you find that you talk to her while you're doing your housework?

Mother: I probably could be doing more.

Examiner: It sounds like you must be talking with her and responding to what she says.

Mother: Well, I do ask her to pick up her toys and she puts them away, although it takes most of the afternoon. Also, we spend a great deal of time each day reading stories. She loves simple little stories. I know she's talking more now than she ever was and it's more interesting to talk with her. She seems to understand better what she's saying.

Examiner: Children learn to talk by having others respond to what they are saying or having someone repeat the words they are using in a correct way. All of her accomplishments show that someone has responded very appropriately and creatively to her unique learning needs. She was able to name all the pictures and follow three directions for where to place the blocks. It was not as easy for her to understand in front of, behind, under, and on top of; these are prepositional phrases. She didn't give her first and last name.

Mother: I've never encouraged her to use her own name, although she calls other people by their names.

Examiner: In the area of gross motor skills, I noticed that she stoops and recovers and also walks well. However, I need to check with you on some other observations I made. I also need to know if you observed the same behaviors that I did. First, I did not observe her kicking the ball forward or throwing it overhand. Did you?

Mother: No.

Examiner: I also noticed that jumping in place was not an easy task for her. In fact, she didn't actually do any jumping. I didn't see her balancing on one foot either. Did you?

Mother: No, I didn't see her do any of those things that you mentioned.

Examiner: You mentioned that she doesn't walk up steps or walk backward. I didn't see her walking backward today when I asked her and showed her how. Does she do either of these at home?

Mother: No, I guess I haven't seen her even try. I guess she has been too lazy to learn. She'll catch up though; my sister has a child just like her. Neither one of them is very good at that kind of coordination. It is just something that runs in the family.

Examiner: I'm not certain what you mean by "lazy." Would you share what that means to you?

Mother: She just depends on people to do things for her. We've always babied her.

Examiner: As I have mentioned to you, you have done a variety of activities with her to help her learn and progress. However, since both our observations match and you mentioned that she is not ill, fatigued, or shy today and that nothing is unusual about her behavior, I am concerned about some of the tasks not being as easy for her as the others. She certainly tried very hard, but I did not observe her dump the raisin from the bottle until I actually demonstrated for her. She also acted very perplexed when I gave her the pencil for scribbling. Has she ever scribbled or drawn with a pencil at home? Did you notice that too?

Mother: We have given her boxes of crayons, but she never seemed to get too interested. I just thought she would pick them up and draw when she is good and ready. Yes, I noticed exactly what you are talking about. You're not telling me she's behind, are you? She's okay, isn't she? Is there something wrong? Have I done the wrong things?

Examiner: No, I'm not telling you she's behind; I'm checking to see if you observed what I did today. I'm not telling you there's anything wrong or that she's behind either. I recognize that you are concerned about her. Sometimes it may be upsetting if a child doesn't do as well as her mother expected her to do. I know you are also concerned about not doing the right activities with her. We both observed how well she is performing with her language skills and we both see evidence of her social achievements. I can see that you are as concerned as any parent would be under the circumstances; it can be very difficult if you think something is wrong with your child. Before we jump to any conclusions, let us plan together to observe her again. She needs to be screened on the same items again to give her a chance with the tasks that weren't as easy for her. Does that sound reasonable to you and could you please bring her back within the month?

Mother: Yes. I will be glad to bring her back to this well-child clinic within the month.

Comments. In this case the examiner responded to the mother's needs to be supported in providing S with puzzles by saying that they were appropriate activities for S and that they helped her learn fine motor coordination and the differences between shapes, sizes, and colors. The examiner also praised the mother's creative ways of helping S to become more independent in self-care and stressed the mother's positive approaches and unique capabilities in problem solving to avoid conflict with S. The discussion focused on the beginnings of skills and allowed the examiner to acknowledge the child's vocabulary skills and appropriate parental responses of the mother. In addition, the mother was given support for her efforts to spend time with S while she was doing housework.

According to scoring criteria of the DDST, the child had two definite delays in the fine motor–adaptive section, and she had three delays in the gross motor section. First, the examiner attempted to elicit whether the mother agreed with the observations of her performance. Then the examiner attempted to respond to the mother's natural anxiety and attempted to clarify what the mother meant by the term "lazy." The examiner again acknowledged the mother's concerns as valid ones. The examiner also pointed out the child's strengths before discussing the visible weaknesses. The examiner emphasized the need to "plan together." The examiner did not answer the mother's questions by saying, "Don't worry, she'll catch up," but made appropriate plans for retesting and referral on the second test for a multidisciplinary evaluation. The examiner accentuated that "it's not as easy for her" instead of abruptly saying, "She failed three items."

Plans were made for a follow-up DDST, at which time the child was retested on the items she had not passed. The results 3 weeks later were exactly the same. The mother and father were then encouraged to seek a further diagnostic work up for their child at the local child development center.

Discussion 5—questionable test performance (child's age: 4 years 6 months)

Examiner: Do you have any questions?

Mother: No.

Examiner: She does really nicely in the personal-social area. She is able to put on her clothing, which is quite independent behavior; she is able to button up her dresses when the buttons are in front, and she handles small buttons, as well as the large buttons you mentioned. I agree that it isn't as easy for her to button when the buttons are right under her chin or in back. You also reported that she has reached the point where she picks out her own clothing and doesn't ask for your help with dressing. She washes and dries her hands independently, and she even laces her shoes, which shows fine motor skills and increasing independence in her ability to care for herself.

The interactive games that you described, such as follow the leader, tag, and king of the mountain, are good examples of her learning to be more cooperative in her play patterns with children of her own age. You also mentioned that she separates easily from you and is comfortable when she is left with a babysitter or goes off to preschool. Her behavior with the babysitter indicates feelings of trust and confidence and reflects some appropriate kinds of preparation for being without you and not being distressed about it.

In the fine motor–adaptive area, she does a nice job of copying the cross, circle, and square. Perhaps you've noticed that as she gets older she adds more parts to her picture. I was looking for at least six parts to her picture. Hers had more than that: she added eyebrows, mouth, nose, head, neck, shoulders, and even flowers on the dress.

Mother: Yes, I've noticed the details she's added in the last 3 or 4 months. She's started adding eyes, which is new for her. She's showing more interest too in her drawings. The clothing she added today is much more refined and the best yet and more precise than what it was 6 months ago.

Examiner: You've really done some appropriate things with her. It looks like you've capitalized on her strengths in this particular area.

Mother: She's fun to have around, and she's really responsive to the things I do with her. She likes to do things and we do a lot of things together. Yes, I do try to capitalize on her strengths. I try to find every one of my four children's strengths, and I find the things they do best. She's not as physical as some of the others, so we do the things that really seem to be more interesting to her. Right now we are practicing with hopping and skipping. She hasn't really gotten that coordination down yet. We work at it occasionally. I know it's something that will come with development, but she hasn't gotten it yet.

Examiner: It sounds like you're really trying to help her get there, though.

Mother: Yes, we try and I know it will come with more practice.

Examiner: In the fine motor area she did everything very skillfully. The item she excelled in was drawing the girl, and she is really showing strides in fine motor, purposeful, coordinated use of her fingers and hands. She does have definite strengths, and it seems that she has had appropriate kinds of practice and opportunities to progress with these skills.

In the language area, she is doing a beautiful job of describing and defining what some words, such as ceiling, mean. She is learning more concepts and beginning to define words more completely. She defines some words with greater accuracy than others. She is doing fine and is showing progress in adding to her beginning skills. I noted that she didn't give her first and last name.

Mother: I can see after you asked her again, that she wasn't quite ready for defining all the words, but it makes me happy that she can define some of them.

Yes, I noticed too that she didn't give her first and last name; that really surprised me. I thought she would. I can't figure out why she couldn't tell you what cold, tired, and hungry meant, but she couldn't. You gave her three tries each time.

Examiner: She understands prepositions, colors, analogies, and composition of words.

In the gross motor area, she did everything correctly. Catching the ball wasn't as easy for her as the other gross motor skills. She's getting ready to learn how to catch the bounced ball. She did very well in balancing on one foot and then the other for 15 seconds. She pedals a tricycle forward and backward, she did the broad jump very well, she hops on her left and right foot with excellent balance and timing, and she shows good rhythm in hopping. She didn't lose her balance in the heel-to-toe walk forward and also showed excellent coordination, posture, and movement when doing the heel-to-toe walk backward. She shows motor maturity, balance, posture, and coordination with movements that require spatial judgment, timing, and purposeful, precise movements. Do you agree? Do you have any concerns?

Mother: Yes, I agree, and no, not really. I really don't. I've noticed that she is able to handle herself fine with her own age group, and with children who are older than she is. Socially she is quite good at meeting people and making her own way and holding her own. She's not one that I worry about. I don't feel she is going to be shy or one who can't do things that children of her age group are doing. I have

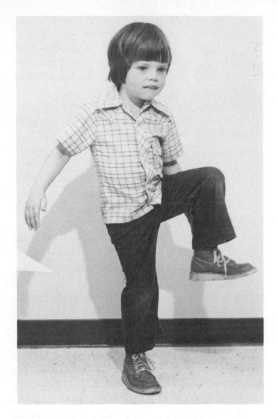

Fig. 12-7. The child is screened for his gross motor skills at balancing on one foot for 10 seconds. He is shown with excellent balance on one foot without any external support or holding on to anything.

confidence in her. I'm proud of her. She's a little quieter when she gets in situations like this. As she says, she's trying her best. She really works hard at doing her best, maybe a little too hard. Maybe she's taking things too seriously and maybe I've caused this.

Examiner: Do you ever see her relaxed and not serious?

Mother: I know I expect quite a bit from her. I expect the best from all my children, but I don't want to overdo it with her. I don't want her to be too serious about working at everything. Not that I'm always evaluating her or judging her, but she seems to feel that she's got to do her best. It doesn't seem to hurt her. I don't want it to harm her.

Examiner: What happens if she's been asked to do something that's too difficult for her?

Mother: I'm not certain if she would quit.

Examiner: What would she do if she got discouraged, or if someone was expecting too much of her?

Mother: I'm just not sure how she would react if I were expecting too much. I have a feeling she would go on trying just to please me. I'm wondering if I push her too much and if she will quit if she gets too discouraged. I'm really concerned that she not be exposed to too many frustrating things in the future. She is 4½ and I'm planning on placing her in kindergarten. I don't want her to experience too much if she is not ready for it.

Examiner: Your concern is a natural one. What kinds of things might frustrate her, or what kinds of things have frustrated her before?*

It appears to me that you have always been observant and sensitive to her needs and to when to present her with new challenges and tasks. You have given thought not only to her present needs, but to her future needs as well.

Mother: Yes, I have even told her kindergarten teacher that I want her to be honest with me about how E does, and I'm confident that she will share her observations with me.

Examiner: It sounds like you are doing some very appropriate planning for your daughter, and you sound as if you feel right about the decision you made. I realize you want to achieve a balance by introducing her to new tasks without causing too much frustration. Is that right?

Mother: Absolutely.

Examiner: It sounds as if you're very much going in the right direction. I have noted that E lets you know when she doesn't want to do something. She has adequate communicative abilities and perhaps will let you know herself if she is bothered, if too much is being asked of her, or if it's too boring. I know you want to provide her with enough and not too much. Do you think she will continue to let you know how she feels?

Mother: Yes. She really does let me know if it's boring or too tough. I think things will be okay. It sounds much easier already.

Examiner: Good.

Mother: She seems to try things. I've never thought of her as a quitter. I'm watching this very carefully to see how she responds to things that frustrate her.

---

*At this point the examiner could have asked the mother the following three questions: "How did you respond to her frustration? Did your response help reduce her frustration? Did you notice a change in her behavior?"

Examiner: I think it's appropriate that you're expressing your concerns and that you're watching for things that might potentially frustrate her. You are aware of her behaviors, and that in itself is appropriate and good. You are showing concern and sensitivity to her needs and so far have shown interest and appropriate responses to her different needs. She responds well to you, and you have elected some appropriate ways of encouraging her in her development. Since we both noticed that she didn't do as well in her language skills as you expected, I'm wondering if you would be willing to bring her back in 1 month for a rescreening.

Mother: Yes, I think that would be a good idea; I simply don't understand why she wouldn't tell you her first and last name. I'm sure she must have said it sometime; after all, she is 4½ years old. I also know she knows when she's tired, cold, or hungry.

Examiner: Has she ever told you when she's tired, cold, or hungry?

Mother: No.

Examiner: How do you know if she is tired, cold, or hungry?

Mother: I'm her mother; I should know. Okay. I'd rather have her tested out than to find out something's wrong before she goes to kindergarten.

Examiner: I recognize your concern about something being wrong. Before we conclude that something is wrong, we really need further observations of her. She needs another chance to try before we reach any conclusions or make any decisions about her.

Comments. This discussion emphasized to the mother her child's increasing skills in adding details to pictures, her greater attention to detail, and her increasing attention span. It also reinforced the mother's astute observations about her child's changing behavior. The examiner pointed out that the mother had indeed capitalized on many of E's strengths.

She could have given more attention to the mother's concern regarding E's physical abilities and carefully clarified the mother's expectations of E. After all, E was passing items for her age level. However, the examiner did point out that although E hadn't learned to skip or hop yet, the mother was helping her attain these skills.

The mother answered her own question about E trying to do her best by stating that it did not seem to be hurting her. She voiced concern about pushing her too far and was carefully observing E for any signs of frustration. The examiner acknowledged this effort, stressing that the mother had thought about E's responses and was aware of expecting too much. She assured that E need not be serious about everything and that the mother's observations would continue to help her judge when to reduce expectations.

The mother's need to discuss her discomfort regarding kindergarten was apparent to the examiner who acknowledged that it was not uncommon for mothers to experience various concerns when their children were going to be separated from them for the first time in a kindergarten setting. The examiner suggested that adjusting to E's new experience in school and increasing independence might be difficult and that another visit could be arranged if the mother wished to discuss E's progress and the mother's reaction at a later time.

Since the child showed two definite delays in the language sector, and one delay in the personal-social sector, the examiner interpreted the test results as a questionable test performance. The examiner attempted to elicit whether the mother agreed with the observations about her performance. The examiner attempted to have the mother give evidence of the child's ability to express her understanding of cold, tired, and hungry. The examiner appropriately requested the mother to bring the child back for a rescreening a month later. At the second retesting period, it was learned that she could express her first and last name with excellent articulation skills. She also expressed her comprehension of cold, tired, and hungry. The mother boasted that she could say these words on her own and reassured the examiner she had not taught her daughter what to say, as she had been instructed earlier. Thus it was concluded that the first test was indicative of a temporary delay, and the child did not require further referral after the rescreening.

SUMMARY

The DDST, which is in widespread use today, is recognized for its unique features: it is simple to administer by professionals and paraprofessionals; it meets test criteria for reliability and validity; it is designed for infants and preschoolers; there is evidence that it requires minimum time to administer and score; and it is a screening device, not a diagnostic instrument. When used by an individual who is well trained in the procedures for administering, scoring, and interpreting results, the DDST can produce valuable information about a child that can be useful in planning for his individual developmental needs.

Information about the time allotment and selection of appropriate materials for training are available from LADOCA.*

---

*Films on the DDST, the proficiency film, test pads, test kits, manual, and the manual/workbook used with the training film can be obtained from LADOCA, Project and Publishing Foundation, Inc., E. 51st St. and Lincoln St., Denver, Colo. 80216.

REFERENCES

1. Commission on Chronic Illness: Chronic illness in the United States: prevention of chronic illness, vol. 1, Cambridge, Mass., 1957, Harvard University Press.
2. Frankenburg, William K., and Dodds, Josiah B.: The Denver Developmental Screening Test, J. Pediatr. **71:**181-191, Aug., 1967.
3. Frankenburg, William K., and Dodds, Josiah B., and Fandal, Alma W.: The Denver Developmental Screening Test, Denver, 1970, University of Colorado Medical Center.
4. Frankenburg, William K., Camp, Bonnie W., Van Natta, Pearl A., and Demersseman, John A.: Reliability and stability of the Denver Developmental Screening Test, Child Dev. **42:**1315-1325, 1971.
5. Frankenburg, William K., Camp, Bonnie W., and Van Natta, Pearl A.: Validity of the Denver Developmental Screening Test, Child Dev. **42:**475-485, 1971.
6. Meier, John H.: Screening, assessment, and intervention for young children at developmental risk. In Hobbs, Nicholas, editor: Issues in the classification of children, vol. 2, San Francisco, 1975, Jossey-Bass, Inc., Publishers.
7. Stedman, Donald: Developmental screening. In Frankenburg, William K., and Camp, Bonnie W., editors: Pediatric screening tests, Springfield, Ill., 1975, Charles C Thomas, Publisher.
8. Frankenburg, William K.: Criteria in screening test selection. In Frankenburg, William K., and Camp, Bonnie W., editors: Pediatric screening tests, Springfield, Ill., 1975, Charles C Thomas, Publisher.
9. Frankenburg, William D., Goldstern, Arnold D., and Camp, Bonnie W.: The revised Denver Developmental Screening Test: its accuracy as a screening instrument, J. Pediatr. **79:**988-995, Dec., 1971.
10. Hunt, Jane V.: Developmental screening. In Frankenburg, William K., and Camp, Bonnie W., editors: Pediatric screening tests, Springfield, Ill., 1975, Charles C Thomas, Publisher.

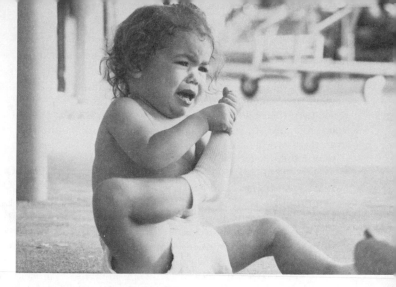

13

USE OF THE
DEVELOPMENTAL PROFILE

For some time, child care professionals have focused attention on constructing assessment tools that are both reliable and valid for estimating the developmental capacities of infants and children; they have also assumed major responsibility for using such tools in the management of developmental changes. However, a new trend is emerging: parental participation in assessment practices is being emphasized, since parents' observations about their child may significantly influence the way they interact with him. Evidence is accumulating that a child's growth and development are influenced by learning experiences and the animate and inanimate stimuli that are offered at appropriate stages in the child's development. Knowledge of growth and development is essential for parents to respond to the developmental needs of their child, to interact appropriately with him, and to encourage intellectual development, social adaptations, and other aspects of development. Such knowledge can be gained by actively taking part in the assessment process.

One optimal and underused time that could be capitalized on for drawing parents into the assessment process is the newborn period. Both mother and father could be included in making early observations so that they would feel that they were collaborating in assessment, as well as in care planning for their infant. The pattern of sharing in assessments during the child's early years could thus be established as a routine expectation for parents.

Parents' capacities for making observations and reaching sound conclusions about planning for developmental change and progress have been underestimated. Parental observations are more uniformly accurate than formerly assumed and deserve far greater and more consistent attention from child care professionals. The majority of studies done on parental assessment abilities have focused on parents of handicapped children, and controls were not uniformly well established. Parents of children of a wide age range were included in those studies, although most were parents of older children. Although some retrospective studies show that parents are incorrect in estimating the developmental levels of their children, some studies showed that parents were generally accurate in estimating their children's abilities; when they were incorrect, they erred in an upward direction, perceiving a child as doing better than he actually did.[1] Mothers were more likely to overestimate children's abilities than fathers,[2] and greater degrees of overestimation were characteristic of parents of more severely handicapped children.[3] However, studies of parents of

205

severely retarded children showed that parents were more accurate in estimating their child's ability if the child exhibited a greater degree of retardation.[4] In light of such findings, examiners are placing increasing reliance on parental abilities to assess children.

One recently developed and standardized tool that assists parents and examiners in objectively determining a child's level of functioning is the Developmental Profile, designed by Alpern and Boll[5] and standardized on 3,008 children from the newborn period through 12 years of age. It responds to the need for a reliable instrument that can supply valid, multidimensional information about a child's developmental status regardless of the child's sex, race, or socioeconomic class. The Developmental Profile is unique compared to other screening tools in that it relies to a large extent on verbal responses from a parent, teacher, older sibling, or other individual acquainted with the child being studied. The inventory provides an individual profile, which can be used to compare a child's developmental skills with normative data obtained for specific ages at which children in the standardized population sample could perform selected items.

COMPOSITION OF THE DEVELOPMENTAL PROFILE

The Developmental Profile consists of 217 items arranged in the following five scales[5]:

1. The physical age scale assesses the child's developmental status by determining his mastery of abilities that require large and small muscle coordination, strength, stamina, and flexibility.

2. The self-help age scale assesses the child's capacities for such tasks as eating, dressing, and carrying out chores at home. It helps determine the extent to which the child is gaining independence in performing daily activities.

3. The social age scale assesses the child's abilities to relate and interact with others. His

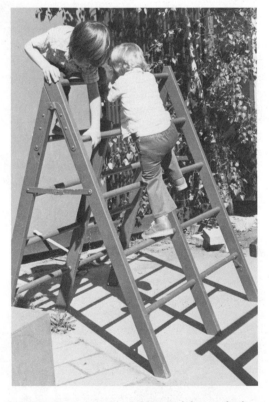

Fig. 13-1. Screening the children's ability to climb up and down on a play ladder and the degree of balance, posture, coordination, and independence exhibited.

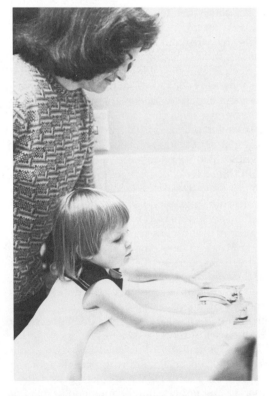

Fig. 13-2. Screening the child's ability to wash her own hands and face acceptably with supervision.

emotional needs for adults and his levels of social interactions with peers, siblings, and adults are measured.

4. The academic age scale assesses the child's intellectual abilities that are required for scholastic functioning.

5. The communication age scale assesses the child's expressive and receptive language skills and determines the age level at which he understands concepts of verbal and nonverbal communication.

Questions in each scale are divided according to age: 6-month intervals are shown from birth to 3½ years of age, then yearly intervals are shown through 10, 11, or 12 years of age, depending on the scale. Representative Developmental Profile questions from each scale category follow. This presentation of partial questions from the Developmental Profile is not intended as a substitute for the Developmental Profile manual.

Physical developmental age scale

Following are sample questions from this scale of the Developmental Profile:

7 to 12 months: When the child picks up something, does he use a thumb and one or two fingers to pick it up? (this is a pass), or does he grasp with his whole hand? (this method is a fail).

2½ to 3 years: Does the child use scissors with one hand to cut paper or cloth? The child must be able to use the scissors to cut rather than merely tear.

6 years: Can the child cut out a magazine picture of an animal or human without being more than a quarter of an inch off anywhere?

9 years: Can the child whistle recognizable tunes?*

Self-help developmental age scale

Sample questions from the self-help developmental scale are as follows:

7 to 12 months: Does the child help with dressing by holding out his arms for his sleeves or his foot for his shoe?

2½ to 3 years: Does the child undo large buttons, snaps, shoe laces, and zippers?

6 years: Does the child use a knife correctly for cutting foods? He may be helped with unground meats such as steaks, roasts, chicken, or chops.

9 years: Has the child prepared at least two of the following foods without help: eggs (any style), popcorn, canned or packaged soup, cake, hot cereal, pudding, or jello?*

Social developmental age scale

Following are sample questions from the social age scale:

7 to 12 months: Does the child wave bye-bye at the right times? This item may also be passed if the child claps his hands (pat-a-cake) copying or playing with someone.

2½ to 3 years: Does the child follow the rules in group games run by an adult? Such rules might

---

*From Alpern, Gerald D., and Boll, Thomas J.: Developmental Profile, Aspen, Colo., 1972, Psychological Development Publications.

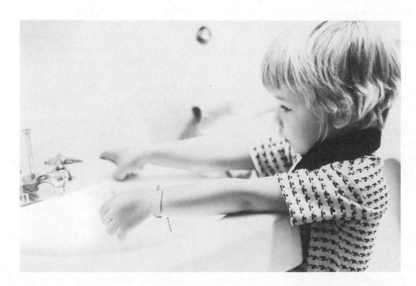

Fig. 13-3. Determining the child's ability to wash his hands acceptably without help.

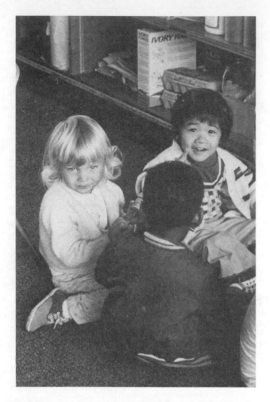

Fig. 13-4. Assessing a child's ability to socially relate to others.

mean being able to sit in a circle and follow directions or imitate a leader, or doing the same thing as the rest of the group.

6 years: Can the child visit and play at a friend's house without needing watching by an adult (except for once-in-awhile checking no more than every hour)? The friend should be no more than one year older than the child.

9 years: Is the child allowed to go anywhere outside his neighborhood (more than four blocks or one mile away) by himself?

11 years: Is the child an active and participating member of a formal group such as scouts, future farmers, band, school athletics, or academic team (football, debate, cheerleaders, etc.)?*

Academic developmental age scale

Sample questions from the academic age scale are as follows:

7 to 12 months: Does the child search in the right place for a thing that has been moved out of his sight? For example, if the child were to see a toy

which was then hidden under a table or a pillow, would he search for it and not just seem to forget it?

2½ to 3 years: Does the child understand the concept of three well enough so that he can hand you three pieces from a bowl of candy?

6 years: Could the child take out 13 objects from a group of 20 objects when asked?

9 years: Can the child multiply through the sixth table with only a few errors? For example, the child will know six times nine, five times eight, four times three, etc.

11 years: Does the child use the newspaper regularly (at least weekly) for new information? Checking the paper for movie listings, radio or TV schedules, or reading comics does not pass at this level. The child must actually read news or sports stories and understand them.*

Communication developmental age scale

Sample questions from the communication age scale are as follows:

7 to 12 months: Does the child sometimes repeat "words" spoken to him such as "da-da" or "ma-ma"? He may not know what these words mean.

2½ to 3 years: Does the child sometimes give his first *and last* name when asked? The child may not do this all or even most of the time, but must have done it when asked.

6 years: Can the child recognize at least five written words and somehow show he understands what they mean? The child must "read" *the words* not just name the things like recognizing a cereal box and naming the cereal.

9 years: Has the child, without help, written and mailed a letter? The letter must be readable; help may be provided with the address and spelling, but not with the message.

11 years: Has the child shown he knows at least three of the following five words by using them correctly in sentences? The words are: fable, microscope, shilling, belfry, and espionage.*

SCORING

Results of the Developmental Profile are recorded on a six-page scoring and report form. Identifying information and a summary of the five scale age scores are placed on the face sheet. A separate sheet for each of the five scales, color matched with the scale inventory sections in the manual, lists each item by number and age level, followed by both a zero and a number. Alpern and Boll[1] recommend that to score items the rater simply circle the zero if

---

*From Alpern, Gerald D., and Boll, Thomas J.: Developmental Profile, Aspen, Colo., 1972, Psychological Development Publications.

---

*From Alpern, Gerald D., and Boll, Thomas J.: Developmental Profile, Aspen, Colo., 1972, Psychological Development Publications.

an item is failed or the number if the item is passed. The number indicates how much credit in months is given for passing a particular item. In determining whether a child passes an item, the rater must be sure the child meets the criteria described for passing, clearly distinguish whether the child "can" do or actually "does" an item, and be sure a child does every item in a series containing the word "and." Each scale is completed when the child has passed all items at two consecutive age levels (referred to as "double basal"), establishing a lower limit, and has failed all items at two consecutive age levels (referred to as "double ceiling"), establishing an upper limit. Scale scores are determined by simply adding up the age credits the child has earned for passing the respective items.

INTERACTING WITH THE PARENTS

When preparing parents to respond to Developmental Profile questions, the examiner should consider the following points:

1. Parents should be reminded that the questions will begin in an area in which the child will most likely be having success and will progress to items that are advanced for his age level. It should be explained that the child is not expected to pass all items. (The examiner should be sure to start one age level below the child's chronological age when asking questions.)

2. The examiner should clarify the purpose of the questions before beginning the inventory. Parents should be told that although it may seem like the same question is being asked more than once, the interviewer is simply getting into more complex questions about a particular set of behaviors.

3. Parents should be assured that they are free to ask for a repeat of questions during the interview, particularly if they are uncertain about what is being asked or about a yes or no answer. They should be told that they are welcome to ask questions and to use all the time they need for answering a question.

4. The examiner should remind parents to wait until the entire question has been asked before they answer.

5. The significance of "can" and "does" should be explained to parents and the examiner should ask them to answer questions with the following in mind: Do they think the child can do a task, or does he actually do it? If in doubt, ask the child to perform the item.

6. The examiner should reassure parents that the results of the questionnaire will be shared with them.

During the inventory, parents should be reminded again that the examiner is moving from

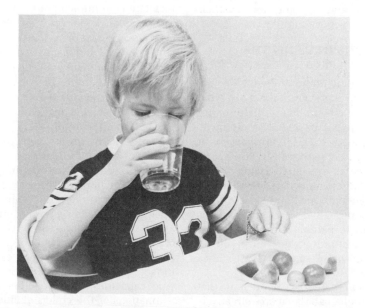

Fig. 13-5. Assessing the child's ability to drink from a glass without spilling.

simple items to more complex ones, which the child is not necessarily expected to be able to perform. They should be assured that their reporting of the child's ability is acceptable, even though they may mention that the child's teacher or someone else might answer the questionnaire in a different way.

INTERPRETING RESULTS

When interpreting the results for parents, it is extremely important to present the findings systematically, indicating the child's strengths (the areas in which he did best) first, then commenting on the areas that were not as easy for him. It is not considered helpful to simply give parents numbers for developmental results. A figure of 5 years, 2 months can be reassuring to a parent but is no substitute for a discussion of concrete and specific developmental information. A figure may indicate that the child is within the expected range for his chronological age but does not begin to clarify or reinforce the strengths he has, his developmental achievements, or the progress he has made from one period to the next. Discussing specific aspects of the child's behavior encourages parents to explore in depth approaches they might use to promote further progress. The examiner should not hesitate to ask them if the questions have been helpful and, if so, in what ways. The interpretative period offers the child care professional an opportunity to be supportive and to discuss what parents are doing, thinking of, and planning next for their child.

CONSIDERATIONS IN USING THE DEVELOPMENTAL PROFILE

The Developmental Profile provides the examiner with a framework for listening to what parents are saying about their children. Administering the inventory requires attentive, purposeful listening because judgments about passing or failing are required. It is of paramount importance to remain oriented to the concept that the way parents perceive the child and his developmental functioning is critical to his development. Child care professionals who are tuned in to parents' perceptions of a child's performance are in the most advantageous position to be of supportive assistance to a child and his family.

Another inherent value of the tool is that mothers and fathers can be more effectively supported in their communicative efforts re-

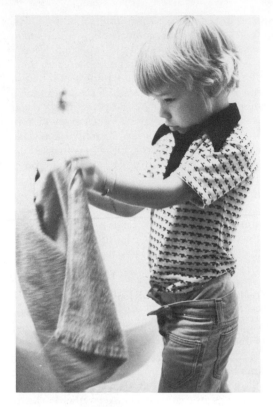

Fig. 13-6. Assessing the child's ability to dry his face and hands after washing without assistance.

garding their child. In addition to assessing a child's developmental status, the tool helps facilitate communication between parents, giving them an opportunity to identify strengths or concerns together. Expressing and coping with concerns and discussing and exploring the child's development may help parents change their expectations to more realistic levels that approximate the child's functional abilities.

Scores that are markedly elevated or depressed merit careful attention because they may reflect the parents' perceptions and expectations of the child. If the child scores high in any scale category, parents might be applying pressure on him to perform at levels that are unrealistic for his current capabilities. In contrast, if parents view a normal child as below his age level in performance, it is important to clarify and obtain more specific examples of the child's behavior. Parental expectations may in fact be low and incompatible with the child's true capacities. On the other hand, parental estimations of the child's abilities may be valid and may indicate the need for further observa-

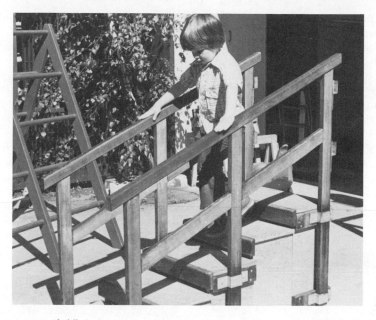

Fig. 13-7. Assessing a child's independent ability to walk up and down stairs without assistance except for holding railing.

tions, in-depth investigations, or planning of approaches to promote the child's levels of performance to more advanced ones. Equally important in the case of either an elevated or a depressed score, the parents may be revealing by their answers how they *wish* the child were functioning, and they may not be accepting and interacting with the child on the levels at which he is actually functioning.

Examiners who use the Developmental Profile do not uniformly calculate the IQ score. If an IQ score is calculated and presented to parents, it is best done by a person highly skilled and knowledgeable in psychometrics and trained in interpreting the meaning, value, and implications of an IQ score. It is recommended that all five scales be used if an IQ equivalency score is obtained.

The Developmental Profile is increasingly in demand because it displays a number of unique characteristics. It has certain advantages over other tools that require direct observations; it can be used with children who are ill and cannot currently perform tasks in their optimal way and with parents of children with acoustical impairments, sensorimotor disorders, emotional disturbances, or intellectual deficits. For example, the Developmental Profile could be highly effective in a pediatric hospital setting.

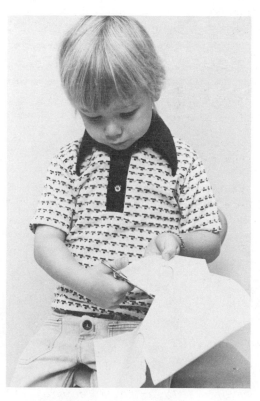

Fig. 13-8. Assessing a child's ability to cut out a printed circle the size of a silver dollar.

Parents could provide important information, which could then be integrated into daily care plans for the child and plans for the child's discharge home. In turn the tool would provide a valid reference for the counseling, advice, and reassurance that most parents need but do not consistently and uniformly receive. Similarly, results of the Developmental Profile can be in-

corporated into planning programs that encourage the advancement of the five skills assessed by the tool in various environments such as schools, homes, day-care centers, hospitals, residential settings, and other educational environments. Direct observations of a child are encouraged whenever possible to supplement information that parents or other care providers give.

Use of the Developmental Profile is increasing.* It offers one more approach to systematically gathering information that can be used to improve health care services to individual children and their parents and is therefore increasingly being integrated into routine developmental assessments of infants and children in a wide range of diagnostic and treatment settings.

The Developmental Profile is increasingly used for the following purposes:

1. *To screen large populations quickly.* Screening technology involving telephone, mail, and sample canvassing, frequently using abbreviated administration, have been developed to identify children in need of early intervention.

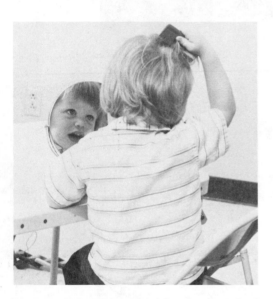

Fig. 13-9. Assessing a child's ability to independently comb his own hair so that adult help is not needed.

---

*Individuals who are interested in individual consultation, direct consultation, or workshops on how to use the Developmental Profile or how to use it for constructing programs and evaluations may direct inquiries to Dr. Gerald Alpern, P.O. Box 3198, Aspen, Colo. 81611.

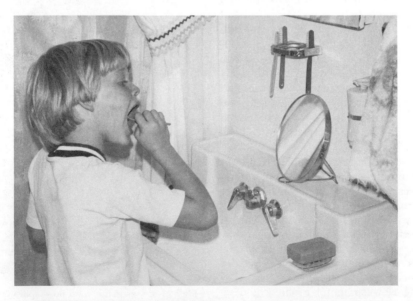

Fig. 13-10. Assessing a child's ability to independently brush his teeth.

2. *To train professionals (e.g., nurses, teachers, teacher aides, field workers) to accomplish developmental evaluations of individual children.* One- and two-day workshops teaching methods are now available, which maximize reliable and effective administration.

3. *To construct individual curriculum prescriptions for children.* Comprehensive manuals on developing and implementing curriculum goals have been published.

4. *To provide before-after form evaluations for various types of programs.* Exemplary agency research reports outlining methodology can be obtained, which then offer guidelines for states to use in developing plans under PL 93-380 as well as other federal and state programs.

5. *To involve parents in parental education–participation programs.* Both home- and center-based parental teaching guides have been prepared in which parents are taught to teach their own children.

REFERENCES

1. Wolfensberger, Wolf, and Kurtz, Richard A.: Measurements of parents' perceptions of their children's development, Genet. Psychol. Monogr. **83:** 3-92, 1971.
2. Copobianco, R. J., and Knox, S.: I.Q. estimates and the index of marital integration, Am. J. Ment. Defic. **68:**718-721, 1964.
3. Barclay, A., and Vaught, G.: Maternal estimates of future achievement in cerebral palsy children, Am. J. Ment. Defic. **68:**62-65, 1964.
4. Kurtz, R. A.: Comparative evaluations of suspected retardates, Am. J. Dis. Child. **109:**58-65, 1965.
5. Alpern, Gerald D., and Boll, Thomas J.: Developmental Profile, Aspen, Colo., 1972, Psychological Development Publications.

ADDITIONAL READINGS

Broussard, Elsie R., and Hartner, Miriam Sergay Sturgeon: Further considerations regarding maternal perceptions of the first-born. In Hellmuth, Jerome, editor: Exceptional infant: studies in abnormalities, vol. 2, New York, 1971, Brunner/Mazel, Inc.

Ehlers, W. H.: The moderately and severely retarded child: maternal perceptions of retardation and subsequent seeking and using services rendered by a community agency, Am. J. Ment. Defic. **68:**660-668, 1964.

Ewert, J. D., and Green, M. W.: Conditions associated with the mother's estimate of the ability of her retarded child, Am. J. Ment. Defic. **62:**521-533, 1957.

Meyerowitz, J. H.: Parental awareness of retardation, Am. J. Ment. Defic. **71:**637-643, 1967.

Worchel, T., and Worchel, P.: The parental concept of the mentally retarded child, Am. J. Ment. Defic. **65:**782-788, 1961.

Zuk, G. H.: Autistic distortion in parents of retarded children, J. Consult. Psychol. **23:**171-176, 1959.

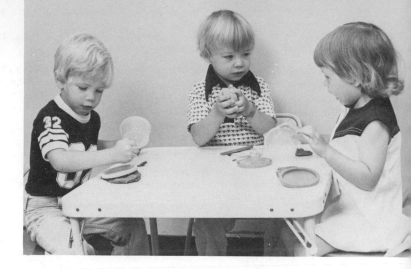

14

BEHAVIOR MANAGEMENT: A FRAMEWORK FOR WORKING WITH PARENTS

It is estimated that 1 of every 20 children experiences behavioral difficulties warranting professional intervention.[1] These figures underscore the need for health care professionals and parents to increase their knowledge about behavior, to know how and when to observe it, to become proficient in analyzing its implications, and to find ways of managing behavior in an effective, constructive fashion. Health care professionals can become more responsive to the needs of parents by expanding their roles in behavior modification techniques, teaching in a preventive model, and offering supportive feedback to the efforts that parents make in response to their children's behavior problems.

Berkowitz and Graziano[2] suggest that child care professionals can direct more emphasis toward examining the powerful potential of parent training in behavior modification as another tool for preventive mental health care. The goal is to assist parents to be future problem solvers, not future service seekers. In the final analysis, parents are responsible for their children's behaviors; thus it becomes imperative that parents be included in a collaborative manner with child care professionals as solutions to behavioral problems are sought. Parents must participate in deciding which of their behaviors and which of their children's behaviors need to

be changed; parents should actively participate in deciding how change can best be implemented, and they need to take an active part in evaluating a child management program.

OVERVIEW OF BEHAVIOR MODIFICATION

A definition of behavior is required before a child management program can be instituted. Behavior can be simply defined as a series of observable responses such as talking, crying, playing, eating, sleeping, or smiling. Behavior modification has one major objective: to strengthen behavior that does not occur often, is weak, or is desired on a more frequent basis or to weaken behavior that is excessive, too strong, or undesirable or inappropriate. Behavior modification accomplishes its goals through the systematic rearrangement of consequences for a child's behaviors. Why does it work? The answer lies in the fact that behavior modification is a flexible approach based on principles drawn from social learning theory.

Learning is defined as a change in behaviors. Reinforcement principles are founded on the premise that behavior is lawful, orderly, and predictable and that the majority of behaviors manifested by individuals are controlled by the immediate consequences of others. For young children, these consequences come in the form of parental attention. Most children's behaviors, if given prompt and consistent acknowledgement or attention by parents either in verbal or nonverbal ways, tend to recur. Behaviors that do not receive reinforcement or attention from parents tend to extinguish or diminish. Parental attention may be demonstrated by social approval, verbal and nonverbal communication, physical contact, restriction, negative responses (punishment), or a combination of these. Parental attentions generally elicit an increase or decrease in a child's behaviors. Consequences of parental attention that lead to an increase, strengthening, or repetition of behaviors are known as "positive reinforcers." Those that lead to a decrease, weakening, or elimination of behaviors are termed "negative reinforcers." "Schedule of reinforcement" refers to the rate at which any response is reinforced. A "continuous schedule of reinforcement" refers to the reinforcement of every observed response. In contrast, if every third response is reinforced, a "ratio schedule of reinforcement" is in effect. Under the ratio schedule, the child must emit a fixed number of responses before he receives any form of reinforcement. When a child is first learning or acquiring certain responses, it is initially necessary to reinforce the desired response on a continuous basis. The pattern can then gradually move to the intermittent reinforcement of the desired behavior. Once parents have selected a behavior of the child that is to be changed, they must not forget to reinforce it.

Many kinds of reinforcers can be used to strengthen or weaken behaviors. Parental manifestations of affection and approval through play, praise, touch, smiles, and talking are effective in strengthening desired behaviors. Food, juice, and water are more concrete kinds of positive reinforcers.

It is important to remember that what is reinforcing to one individual is not necessarily reinforcing to another. For one child the reinforcer might be candy; for another it might be parental attention in the form of positive praise and affection. Frequently, the combination of social reinforcers (smiling, touching, and praising) and concrete reinforcers (candy) is effective.

Some behavioral responses that would not seem to be reinforcing actually are. This explains how parents accidentally teach children problem behaviors. For some children, being scolded or even gently spanked serves as a powerful reinforcing action because it involves attention coming from a parent. Furthermore, any response that is reinforced, not just the responses that the parents desire, tends to be repeated. It is important that parents and child care professionals observe behavior in the most objective way possible to assure that they are not inadvertently reinforcing behavior that is not desirable by inappropriate attention. Parents or others implementing a behavioral modification program must reinforce only the behaviors that they wish repeated now and in the future.

If a child is exhibiting undesirable behaviors and his parents are trying to eliminate them, the objective is to extinguish the child's behaviors *by not reinforcing* them. For example, if a child cries, parents can weaken and eliminate the crying by merely ignoring it on a consistent basis. Since the parents are not trying to talk the child out of crying, are not resorting to spanking, and are not giving other forms of attention, the crying is not reinforced. Parents often believe that their lack of response means that they are ignoring the child. However, they may be making eye contact or even touching the child. Parents should learn to expect a child whose behavior is being ignored for the first time to escalate his attempts to gain parental attention. They must also be advised that ignoring alone is *never* sufficient to effect permanent behavioral changes. A child's desired behaviors must be acknowledged through consistent parental attention—"nice" or "good" behaviors should not be taken for granted.

If a child cannot or will not make a response that is expected or desired, the technique of "fading" is useful. In this approach, the parent holds the child's arms or hands and makes the desired response for the child. The child is thus actively led through a procession of behaviors. As the child begins to master the sequences of responses that make up a task such as bringing a spoon to his mouth, the parent gradually and systematically fades out his assistance.

Another commonly employed technique is known as "shaping." The child is reinforced as he comes closer and closer to making the desired responses. For example, if the desired response is putting away blocks after playing, the child is reinforced as he moves toward his blocks, as he picks each one up, and as he puts them in the proper place.

Consistency, promptness, and appropriate timing of a reinforcer are important in managing desired or nondesired behaviors. The attention to small portions of behavior is as important as the regular rewarding of desired behaviors. Child care professionals can orient parents toward building success instead of perpetuating failure. By adhering to a well-formulated program using natural, potent social reinforcers instead of reacting impulsively to a child, parents can be assured of success in effecting behavioral change.

Most parents give attention to their children. Frequently, they need assistance in administering it in planned, systematic ways which ensure that the desired behavior and not the behavior they are trying to eliminate is reinforced. If parents reinforce a child as soon as he finishes a request, the child is more likely to finish the request when asked again. If parents forget to reinforce the child, he is less likely to carry out the task the next time. Reinforcers strengthen behaviors.

Parents possess an infinite supply of social reinforcers—they should never run out of smiles, thank you's, touches, expressions of praise and approval, or the ability to talk to the child. Behaviors manifested by another person are the most potent and durable reinforcers for either adult or child.

A single reinforcement does not alter changes in behavior. Numerous reinforcements, planned and given abundantly in a spontaneous and natural manner over a period of time and on a consistent basis, produce long-term changes. The process is gradual. Parents should learn to reinforce a desired behavior every time it occurs in the beginning until the child has learned to show it regularly. Once the desired behavior is being emitted regularly, parents can begin to "thin out" their reinforcement (i.e., reinforce the behavior every third or fourth time instead of continuously).

BEHAVIOR MODIFICATION AND CHILD MANAGEMENT

Parents universally seek assistance for a range and variety of behaviors. These can range from self-feeding problems, sleeping problems, sibling rivalry, toilet training, and noncompliance to aggressive actions toward other children. Each problem must be defined according to the degree of concern it presents to the parents, the child, or both and the amount of disruption that is experienced as a result.

Parents need a methodology that can be easily learned and applied systematically to problem behaviors. The approach must not consume too much of the parents' or child's time. Parents

have demonstrated their capacity for learning and applying basic learning principles. The process initially requires time, patience, and practice. However, once success with changing specified behaviors is experienced, the potential for continued success with managing other behaviors of the child is heightened.

A child's behavioral problem does not manifest itself in isolation. The problem usually occurs with a parent, other caregiver, or sibling. The resulting stresses on family interaction patterns can assume burdensome proportions that require a practical, flexible, and successful method of intervention.

The goal of child management is to give parents the means by which they can make decisions and solve their present problems and any that may arise in the future. This means is behavior modification, and appropriate use of it offers parents another resource for problem solving. If parents become aware of themselves and the effects of their behaviors and actions, they will see how they can perpetuate or terminate a child management problem.

Parents can observe clearly and relate a child's behaviors with their own present reinforcement patterns. Parents can learn to help themselves and their children by objectively solving interaction problems in the here and now. Each problem that is solved by the parents makes it easier to discover the solution for the next problem.

Parents can learn that behavior modification possesses the following features:

1. A tenacious attention to observing behaviors systematically
2. Documentation of selected behaviors that can be observed
3. An orientation that environmental contingencies maintain both adaptive and nonadaptive behaviors
4. An orientation to decreasing undesired behaviors or increasing desired behaviors by systematically rearranging environmental contingencies
5. The evaluation of a mutually planned behavior modification program by periodic comparisons of changes in behavior
6. A continuous recognition that contingencies in the child's and parents' environment are related to capacities for change

Child care professionals are becoming increasingly responsible and accountable for teaching parents management methods that are realistic, that reinforce the same approach used by the child care professional, and that are not excessively demanding of the parents' time. For a management program to be realistic, it must contain appropriate goals that simultaneously help the child and meet the needs of the parents. It is therefore important that the child care professional first listen actively to a description of the problem. Observation is the next most important ingredient.

IMPORTANCE OF DOCUMENTATION OF BEHAVIOR PROBLEMS

Under the general rubric of behavior modification, parents have modified specific behaviors of children who have been described as autistic, brain damaged, psychotic, school phobic, and mentally retarded. Parents have had success in modifying specific behaviors such as toilet training, eating, enuresis, tantrums, withdrawal, aggression toward a sibling, crying, and a number of common home problems. How can these problems be sorted out and examined and decisions made about them so that they are solved in the easiest way possible? Finding a solution to a behavioral problem requires the objective description of its occurrence. Parents may underestimate or overestimate the frequency, duration, or intensity of a specific behavior. The picture that parents try to portray of the behavioral problem is often cloudy, mysterious, and confusing—and may be misleading.

Recording and documenting rates of behaviors remove the second-guessing, misperceptions, and confusion that can result from identifying a concern. This recording of information is crucial in determining the success parents can expect to have in solving a child management problem. Data that are obtained on the child's or parents' behaviors ultimately give valuable clues on how to set up a behavioral management program for change. Accurate observations of parent-child interaction patterns give a clearer picture of behaviors needing different kinds of attention.

Behavior modification requires that parents learn how to identify behaviors they wish changed, that they know how to count or even graph the number of times a behavior occurs, and that they are able to apply consequences that will accelerate or decelerate the frequency of a child's behavioral occurrence. Parents are then able to differentiate whether the behavior in question is changing to higher or lower rates.

The documentation of high, excessive, low, or absent rates of behaviors makes it easier to choose specific behaviors that require system-

atic attention. If the documentation or recording of behaviors is not planned, an inaccurate account of the actual behaviors of the child, parents, or both may result. What if behavioral frequencies are inaccurate? What if the events in the environment that tend to maintain a behavior at a high or low rate are inaccurately calculated? In all probability, treatment plans and the behavior modification program are doomed to failure. Parents become disappointed, frustration is high, hope for change diminishes, and the maladaptive behavior originally complained about maintains itself at the usual rate. Opportunities for more adaptive behaviors by both parents and child become simultaneously limited. How can failure be avoided and success a promising reality?

Initially parents can be given a thorough, nonthreatening, supportive introduction to behavior modification and appropriate explanations of how the entire environment as well as how parts of the environment represent the setting for the child's and parents' behaviors. By means of systematic observations carried out in a collaborative fashion, both parents and the child care professionals can find out which events or consequences may be reinforcing and maintaining maladaptive behaviors of the parents and the child. Parents can learn that their own behaviors may limit the opportunity for their children to display more adaptive behaviors. This information may be brought out by discussing problematic behaviors, by collecting records on a planned basis, and by examining patterns of behaviors that emerge as records are kept.

If maladaptive behaviors are to undergo change, it is imperative that the parents and the child care professional are able to identify exactly which behaviors of the parents and child are to be increased or decreased. The identification of one or more behaviors that are to be modified depends on unbiased observations and on the recording of when the behaviors occur, how long they last, if they accelerate, when they decrease or begin to increase in intensity, and what events in the environment follow their occurrence.

OBSERVATION AND RECORDING OF BEHAVIOR

Success with the principle that behaviors are strengthened by their consequences begins and ends with a commitment to observation and recording. Parents and child care professionals can learn the art of observation and recording.

Both observation and recording are important because they free those involved from making judgments or allowing philosophical views to remain barriers to potential behavioral changes. The art of observation and recording also eliminates bias. Child care professionals and parents learn to look at a child in regard to what the child does and says, when he moves, when he interacts, with whom he interacts, how often he interacts, and what and with whom he plays. They learn to observe and document precisely what a child is doing. They become accustomed to observing events, gradually obtaining a picture of the child's overall interactions. Thus it would not be accurate to report that the child played happily with the toy; rather one would more accurately report that the child smiled, laughed or sang while playing with the toy. It is important to concentrate on what the child actually did; otherwise there is the possibility of making a subjective judgment of happiness.

Behaviors can be observed with regard to when they begin or terminate. They can be measured in terms of their duration. Intensity of behaviors can be measured in degrees of escalation or decrease. Events that tend to reinforce a certain behavior can be observed and measured. The consequences that a behavior produces can be observed and subsequently increased or decreased. Behavior is observable, can be measured, and can be changed. Change can occur in greater or lesser amounts. The amount of time involved in changing behaviors varies with the consistency that principles of reinforcement are applied.

Familiarity with objective observation techniques, knowledge of the range of child behaviors for different levels of development, skill at defining behavioral goals, and planning successive steps toward these goals can be useful to parents and child care professionals concerned about behavioral problems.

The initial requirement of observation is the selection of a carefully defined category of behavior to be observed. This process of selection is preceded by a series of observations at different times, since behavior is subject to change under various conditions.

The definition of problem behaviors is often difficult because of the transition that must be made from a perception of attitudes to a behavioral description. In making a total behavioral assessment of a child, one should note carefully the *quantity* of behaviors under consideration. It is easy to describe a child using general terms such as "slow," but this can be avoided by an actual count of behaviors. A mother, for example, may report that her child "always fails" to come to the dinner table, to maintain his bedroom and belongings, to care for his pets, or to wash his hands after toileting. However, what is important here is to determine within a given time limit the precise number of times a child does comply with his parents' expectations.

Behavioral recordings generally begin with a narrative account of the sequences of an individual's behavior. A narrative account is a preliminary procedure to obtain an impression of rates of behaviors. The stage of narrative written accounts should continue until there is satisfaction that the principal problem behaviors can be conceptualized into observable units.

Example of a narrative recording

Observation time: 10 minutes
Setting: Preschool classroom for 12 students (ages 3 to 5 years)
Subject: Chris, age 5 years

C enters classroom with right arm shielding eyes. Moves toward desk. Pulls out chair while observing boy to his left. Rests knee against chair and eases self down across from C. C scoots backward in chair and moves feet forward.

C turns and looks to right; looks at M across from him while wiggling in chair. Moves feet. Hand placed against mouth—scoots forward on chair and leans on desk. Scoots backward in chair; turns head to right, tips chair forward four times, and points with right arm. Places arm down. Moves back in chair; moves feet four times and begins to twist hair with left hand. Wiggles forward on chair and touches counter with left hand. Places fisted right hand to mouth while leaning back in chair. Moves forward, then backward, and turns head to right. Scoots forward. Lowers head down and looks inside desk. Moves left hand five times in searching motions; right hand pulls out booklet. Leans back in chair and turns page, looks at page, turns page, then looks at page. Makes motion of placing booklet inside desk; moves forward and places booklet on desk. Turns around, resting on left elbow with right arm up, wiggling all the time in seat. Sticks tongue out. Twists hair with left hand. (Twenty separate wiggling movements counted in 45-second period.) Teacher approaches after C has had right arm up for 45 seconds. She glances briefly at C's booklet as he holds it up in front of him. C sits closer to desk. C looks at teacher to left as she walks rapidly away. C folds booklet and places against mouth. Teacher returns to C's desk and places paper next to him. C displays booklet; teacher places mark on sheet of paper. C rocks back and forth three times with hand up to mouth. C pulls question booklet from desk. C wiggles in chair. Teacher moves to right, marks on student sheet and moves away. C looks to left as teacher walks away. C moves forward in chair twice. Teacher comes back, makes another mark on C's sheet. C turns pages in booklet, looks at sheet of paper, scoots forward in chair, then moves back in chair. Thumbs through booklet, glances down at page and places right hand to mouth. Scoots forward once. Jiggles feet eight times. (During preceding 2 minutes, C has turned pages in booklet thirty-one times.)

Jiggles feet three times. C looks at booklet while tipping forward in chair (25 seconds) four times. Right elbow rests on desk. Turns pages in booklet and looks at sheet. Turns book. Wiggles in seat and tips chair forward. (Turns pages in booklet a total of twenty-three times in 1 minute. Has tipped forward in chair eighteen times.) Looks at booklet. Elbow rests on desk. Right hand up to mouth. Chews on fingernails. Stares at booklet; takes pencil and makes mark at bottom of answer sheet. Looks back to question booklet and marks another answer. Places hand against mouth, sits back in chair, and raises right hand. (Has moved forward in chair thirty-two times.) Kicks feet forward. Left hand on booklet. Keeps right arm raised. Leans forward in chair; turns booklet eleven times. Right arm up. Right hand used to write in booklet. Marks in booklet. Erases mark on booklet. Turns booklet upside down and makes mark with pencil. Erases and turns booklet to right side up.

METHODS OF RECORDING BEHAVIORAL EVENTS
Use of a table

Some observers prefer the practice of transforming a narrative into a four-column table, which helps gain a more precise picture or impression of the relationships among cues for action, responses, and consequences of selected behaviors. An example is as follows:

Time	Antecedent event	Responses	Consequent social event
9:00	C receives instructions to look at booklet	C picks up booklet	C is praised for holding booklet

Use of a tally

Once a discrete behavior has been observed and records are needed for its occurrence, a tally can be used. When an individual initiates or engages in a specified behavior, the observer marks the incidence of the response and adds the total number to complete a tally. An example

of a tally for recording frequency of behavior follows. Behavior during this observation period is defined as any gross or fine motor behavior, which involves movement of head, eyes, mouth, shoulders, trunk, legs, feet, hands, and fingers.

Observation time: 10 minutes

Record separate actions only to determine how often certain behaviors are occurring.

Nonacademic desk behaviors
Looks to right /
Looks to left /
Hand against mouth //
Scoots forward in chair //// ////
Scoots backward in chair ////
Turns around in chair /
Tips chair forward ////
Moves feet //// //
Twists hair /
Sticks tongue out /
Wiggles in seat //// /
Points with arm /

    Total 41

Academic task behaviors
Raised arm to signal teacher //
Looks at answer sheet //// /
Turns pages in booklet //// ////
Holds booklet //
Looks at question booklet /
Writes on sheet /
Sits close to desk /

    Total 23

From these behavioral accounts, it is important to determine which behaviors are being produced at the highest or lowest rates.

PARENTS AS PRIMARY RESOURCES FOR CHANGING BEHAVIOR

It no longer suffices to give parents the impression that child care professionals are available to "fix up" their child, to remove his behavioral problems, to create more adaptive behaviors, and to eliminate all undesirable or inappropriate behaviors and then return the child to the parents. Increasing emphasis is being directed to helping parents view themselves as more resourceful in the moment-to-moment, hour-to-hour, and day-to-day encounters with and management of their infants and children.

Parents today are viewed as major contributors to parent-child interactions, as well as primary agents for changing these interactions. The orientation that parents are primary resources for change does not mean that child care professionals have abandoned parents or children but that they are encouraging parents to learn, develop, and use parental skills and knowledge in more socially desirable, appropriate ways. Parents can learn to meet the unique needs of their family within a more positive, productive problem-solving framework, using principles from learning theory.

It is generally accepted that parents have the primary and the most potent influence on their child during the early years of his life. Parents are viewed as being responsible for the socialization process of their child and are therefore in a maximal position, in terms of proximity and time, to ensure the child's most favorable adaptations to the environment.

Because of the large number of children presenting behavioral problems, it is possible that the inclusion of parents in training programs cannot even begin to decrease the number of problems for which parents and child caregivers seek help.

Most studies of behavior modification programs with children suggest that individuals whose goals are to effect behavioral change must frequently move into the natural environment of the child to collect data and carry out a program in a consistent manner.[3] A child's environment includes his parents, who usually are present when a problematic behavior occurs and who have control over the contingencies of the child's environment. The retraining of a child's parents is not only desirable in some instances, but it may also be absolutely necessary if certain nonadaptive behaviors in the child are to be eliminated and opportunities are to be created for both a child and his parents for more adaptive behaviors to occur.

EXAMINING PARENTS' BEHAVIOR PATTERNS

In the past, child care professionals have customarily counted how many times a child cries, takes a toy, has a temper tantrum, or refuses to obey. They have not necessarily counted or focused on parental responses. However, there are generally two contributors to a behavior problem: the child and his parents or siblings. In most instances there is a contingency that helps accelerate or decelerate a child's typical response. When records are accurately kept, they often indicate that parents or other family members are major contributors to a child's behavioral response.

Parents can be helped to change their interaction patterns. For example, they can learn to give parental attention to the child at appropriate times, such as when the child is exhibiting socially desirable behaviors that the parents wish repeated, and to reduce parental attention to those behaviors that are disruptive, annoying, or unappealing. It is vital that records be examined for the rewards that the child is receiving when he exhibits undesirable behaviors. Parents can learn how they generally respond to the repeated behavior patterns of a child and can discover new ways to interact.

They can discover what the child's responses gain for him when he whimpers, fusses, cries, or screams. Do the parents give the child any form of verbal or nonverbal attention? Do the parents look at the child, stop what they are doing, ask a question, shout "no!", come closer to the child, or leave the room? What are the behaviors exhibited by the parents in response to an escalated attempt at screaming? Does the child receive a scolding, threats, or pleading from his parents to be good, or is he offered juice, a snack, and a promise for a trip to the zoo or park? If a reinforcement system is operating to increase or decrease a child's behaviors, it is imperative to examine adult behaviors. Generally, child care professionals have been content to say that the child is getting out of his bed fifteen times in an hour. However, what is the parent doing in response during that same time period?

PARENTAL PARTICIPATION IN A BEHAVIOR MODIFICATION PROGRAM

Behavior modification is the most promising technology to date for responding to children's behavior problems in the natural environment. When contrasted with more traditional treatment approaches, behavior modification approaches have been shown to offer certain advantages for training parents to manage children's behaviors. These advantages include the following[3]:

1. Behavior modification techniques are easy to learn. Persons who are unskilled in sophisticated therapy techniques can learn the principles of behavior modification. A college education or professional training is not a prerequisite for successful management of a child's behavioral repertoire.

2. Parents and professionals alike prefer a management model that is not oriented to sick behavior and patterned after the traditional medical model.

3. The majority of children's behavioral re-

sponses possess common features that are amenable to change by the systematic application of behavioral principles.

4. The behavioral principles can be carried out in the natural environment where the behavioral problems are being manifested by the child and responded to by the parents.

Viewed from this perspective, parent training becomes crucial if effective preventive programs are to meet the demand for help with problematic behaviors.

Before change can be planned and success assured in decreasing a behavioral problem, it is necessary to complete a number of preliminary steps. The first step requires a complete description of the behavior problem under consideration. Responses of the health care professional during this beginning stage include proper acknowledgment of the parents' attempts to accurately describe a behavioral problem. Parents can be supported in their accuracy of recall and the difficulty they have experienced in trying to find an appropriate solution to a problem. Both parents and children can benefit from a child care professional's acknowledgment of the frustrations that may have been experienced. Past efforts of parents to change a problematic behavior deserve recognition too. Empathetic comments can be a source of relief to the parents. It is important that emphasis is placed on the prospect for change right from the beginning. Parents need hope and promise for change.

After the stage is set for parents to be involved as the primary resource for changing behavioral interactions, what should be done next? How long and how often should parents observe the child? Should they observe the child every 30 minutes, every 6 hours, all day long, or once every time they think something will occur? Should the parent observe all behaviors, some, or a few? Should parents observe, interpret, or do both? Is it advisable to start praising the child? How soon should parents begin giving attention? How long should it last? How will parents know if their chosen response was correct? Where and when does a person begin? These are typical questions that parents need answered before a behavior modification goal is decided on.

Preparing parents to document behavior

Most child management problems possess common features that are conducive to behavioral programming. Generally, the behaviors emitted by the child occur at a rate that is either too high or too low. Parents can learn to identify behavioral manifestations of children that have reached problematic levels. They can learn to keep accurate records before intervention for changing any behavior is planned. Parents should be reminded that they are *not* to interact differently with their child while they are documenting behavioral occurrences. They should be cautioned about trying out behavioral modification techniques such as ignoring or using positive reinforcement until substantial data are available to plan a management program. Once they have systematically identified a problem that requires intervention, they will be able to apply principles of behavior modification. Parents can both weaken or strengthen behavioral patterns or interactions that they have observed.

Parents can evaluate effectively the success or lack of behavioral changes within the home. As behavioral changes occur in children, parents can keep records of their feelings, reactions, thoughts, and responses to the changes that are occurring. They can learn to reinforce appropriate and desired behaviors in children in a systematic way and to withdraw and decrease parental attention to behaviors they consider inappropriate. Parents can learn the power of ignoring behaviors when they occur instead of inadvertently attending to the behavior they wish eliminated.

The major objective of asking parents to keep records of their children's specific behaviors or their own behaviors is to obtain and identify information as clearly, precisely, and rapidly as possible. It is not feasible for child care professionals to be available at all times in a child's home when misbehavior or noncompliance occurs. They must rely on parents' objective, accurate, and consistent record keeping if they are to be of assistance in solving problems that are unique to the parents. It is possible for child care professionals to make home visits at specified times to observe children eating, dressing, and playing, or to study the parents' limit-setting techniques. Home visits of this type are a regular part of a community health nurse's assessment procedures; pediatricians and other health care professionals make home visits so that they can make in-depth and comprehensive evaluations of children's environments and the behaviors that are occurring within them.

Occasionally parents may not be able to keep records of a child's behaviors. If parents cannot comply with the record keeping request, it may indicate that the problem has reached proportions that are too overwhelming for them to cope with effectively. If this is the case, the goal of intervention should be modified to deemphasize the difficulty of watching or observing the child and should be shifted to meet the needs of parents. This shift in attention allows the parents to verbalize their discomfort, frustration, anger, impatience, or sense of inadequacy. Child care professionals can support parents with the concept that behavior can change and that the current problem is not permanent. Parents can be supported for the strengths they have shown to date and reinforced for verbalizing their need for help. Parents require support for their own needs, their capacities for change, and their willingness to explore new approaches to discouraging experiences and past failures.

Some parents may not be able to follow through with record keeping for other valid reasons. Frequently, parents and children who have no real desire to change are pressured into seeking professional help by neighbors, relatives, or health care professionals.

Parents who are remiss or uncooperative in keeping records can be asked about satisfactory times for record keeping. They can be asked if another time would be more advantageous. Parents should be given permission by the health care professional to not follow through. They can receive support for the difficulty they might be encountering. A lack of record keeping may be a cue to explore the difficulty, frustration, or lack of confidence that parents may be experiencing. Parents may have concluded that a problem either no longer exists or was not of concern enough to pursue further.

THE VALUES AND ADVANTAGES OF RECORD KEEPING

Once recording begins, parents and the health care professional may begin to feel positive about the possibility for change. A primary reason is that they have probably agreed on the definition of the concern. For example, one mother asked for help with "sibling rivalry." Instead of taking a stereotyped approach and telling her to separate the children and give equal attention to both, the health care professional asked her to keep records. As a result of this process it was discovered that the mother was basically more concerned about the younger infant's safety than about giving them equal attention. The mother needed relief from worrying about the young child's safety and found

that she had been giving a disproportionate amount of attention to the older sibling when he acted aggressively toward the infant. The mother planned a program of giving the older child attention according to his specific needs rather than giving him a lot of attention because "you're supposed to."

Also by keeping records, parents profit from the positive experience of finding out that what they thought was happening was indeed occurring at the rate they assumed.

Parents learn that planning positive attention is desirable and can prevent continuing problem occurrences. Eventually they will experience and recall positive experiences with their children instead of complaining about negative interactions. They learn to be more sensitive to the number of times that they respond to positive aspects of the child's behavior.

Some parents have found that keeping records before intervention serves to reassure them of their own independent problem-solving abilities. Keeping records before establishing a plan may help modify parents' behavior because the parents realize for themselves what they should be doing differently. Previously they may not have bothered to observe the relationship between the behavior of the child and their response to the behavior.

Record keeping gives parents immediate and objective feedback that certain behaviors do occur and at individual, different rates. Parents may learn to value their children in more positive ways instead of perpetuating a negative orientation and maintaining expectations that the undesirable behavior will continue. Parents report that once they begin record keeping, their expectations for the child do change. If they are accustomed to only negative, disruptive behaviors, parents relate that this is what they expect to see and tend to look for it to the exclusion of seeing positive activities. Once they begin to note more appealing kinds of behavior, they may express changes in their own attitudes, perceptions, and responses to a child. They also may find that they start reviewing their own individual reactions and patterns of responses.

For example, parents were asked to keep records of their child's language behavior because of an appropriate concern that the child was not talking enough. The child was 3 years old and was not expressing himself or making many verbal attempts to initiate speech. To their surprise and relief the parents found that because he was the third and youngest child in the family, few if any efforts were made to encourage the child to express his wants or needs with words. Most of his behavior was anticipated and his needs fulfilled without his having to ask for anything. The parents learned to modify their responses and reviewed and altered their expectations of the child and themselves. The child began making rapid, progressive, and successful gains in articulating his needs in an age-related and developmentally appropriate way.

According to one parent, one value of record keeping is that "it helps you spend time directly with the child instead of guessing or estimating what he is doing."

As a result of record keeping, parents report that they become more certain about what they like and do not like about their child's behavior. Parents learn to define and express what bothers them most. Fewer feelings of frustration, anger, and guilt are reported by parents as they keep records. Keeping records can serve as a substitute for parental yelling and sometimes prevents physical abuse from parents that causes them confusion and deters them from paying attention to the child's behavior problems. Keeping records helps serve as a structure for parents when they need direction, particularly when they think they must do something in response to a behavior, and at the same time helps parents gain a sense of increased control about themselves.

One mother reported that she was constantly "out of control" with her child. After she began to keep records of her behavioral responses to the child, she learned to be more accepting of her feelings and thoughts about how poorly she was responding, and most significantly, she learned that she was not out of control. Being out of control for a parent, or anyone for that matter, can be a frightening experience. This mother learned that thinking she was out of control did not make it so. Thus record keeping can serve as a way in which the needs of the parents can be recognized and attended to.

Through discussions about records with child care professionals, parents can be supported that it is natural to feel disappointed and angry with frustrating events and unlikable behaviors of children. They can be told that it is healthy to be able to talk about what bothers them most and be encouraged to do so. They can learn that they are not alone in their experiences. Child care professionals can acknowledge parents for

the strengths they have and their willingness to respond in more appropriate ways. Parents can be supported during the difficulties that they experience in finding a solution to a chronic problem. Child care professionals can encourage parents to persevere in trying to discover the right solution for the child and themselves. Parents can learn to set more reasonable goals for their child as well as themselves. Both the mother and father can learn to give themselves more credit for their competence in the approaches they are trying. Parents can learn that it is appropriate to ask for help. After learning the principles involved in one situation, they can expect to apply and generalize these principles to other problematic areas if they arise. Parents can learn to accept approval for their creative efforts, problem solving efforts, and consideration of alternatives for challenging behaviors of their children. They can learn when to increase their attention for behaviors that they wish to see repeated and when to decrease their attention for less desirable, inappropriate behaviors. The process can be done in a systematic, positive way that helps both parents and children experience the process of change in mutually beneficial ways.

Baseline records of a child's problematic behaviors are important for later comparison, particularly when change seems to occur in small increments or gradually. A comparison of a child's initial behavior with his behavior after a behavior modification program can serve as concrete, positive feedback to parents. Changes in a child's and his parents' behaviors can encourage them to continue their diligent efforts at behavior management.

SUPPORT TO PARENTS OF CHILDREN WITH BEHAVIORAL PROBLEMS

Most parents in the United States take it for granted that they can adequately help their children attain such usual developmental tasks as independent eating and toilet training. The majority of parents are confident about their ability to set limits in an effective way so that children learn to conform to expectations of others and to distinguish the difference between what one is allowed and is not allowed to do.

Some problems of children and parents can be eliminated by a concerted approach of anticipatory guidance. An anticipatory approach can reduce fears of dealing with the unknown, teach parents what to expect before it happens, and help parents feel more secure in their abilities to respond to the parental tasks that lie ahead. Parents who are supported from the beginning generally show continued signs of resourcefulness and flexibility.

In addition, more attention can be given to supporting the adequate ways that parents are responding to difficult problems. One helpful approach before a behavior modification program begins is to tell the parents that their strengths are visible. For some parents, there may be guilt and feelings of inadequacy attached to asking for help. Parents who seek advice, reassurance, and guidance from health care professionals about the best way to handle infants' and children's behaviors should not be told not to worry about their concerns.

Sometimes parents receive biased advice. Parents need to know that there are a number of views about the best ways to respond to children's behaviors. Frequently, advice is given without giving the parents any opportunity to participate in creating a solution. Typically the advice given by different health care professionals varies. Often it is given quickly, and there may be inconsistency in the information that is given to a mother or father. Health care professionals feel compelled to offer instant answers to parents. For example, a mother may ask about toilet training; the child care professional may tell her to do something after she has already tried about five different ways of toilet training. If the child care professional responds by giving her some intuitive guidance or advice based on generalizations, the mother may try it only to lose confidence in other approaches available to her. The experience may have a more definite effect on how she values her own capabilities of future problem solving; she may end up needlessly blaming herself for failure. Her child may sense her frustrations, and the person who gave instant advice without either defining the problem, encouraging the mother, or suggesting that data be gathered to determine the best approach to the concern under consideration has made a serious series of errors in responding to the parent. The important point here is that the approach just described is one that lacks sensitivity to this mother's need for an individualized response to her request for help. The mother's problem was not precisely clarified, and a comprehensive approach to assessment was not even started.

Child care professionals can respond to parents' needs by offering advice and reassurance based on scientific principles within a systematic framework. One important aspect of the behavior management process is to find out exactly what is happening in a given situation. For example, if it is a mealtime problem, one should have the mother define what concerns her most and determine what is a reasonable expectation. If she perceives the problem as occurring all through the meal, does she want the behavior to cease completely or could she learn to tolerate its occurrence three times, for example?

Child care professionals need to help parents set reasonable, realistic goals for themselves, as well as for their children. Both parents and children must experience success in decreasing the problems, which are interrelated in a network that is usually negative in nature.

In the case of the mother who says, "I wish he would stop gulping his milk at night, talking with his mouth full, spilling food, and knocking his glass over," what would she be most desirous of seeing stopped first? It is virtually impossible to change a number of behaviors simultaneously; once the mother defines the priority of concern and gathers data to document the severity of the problem, this is a positive start for the process of change to occur.

Parents can learn to begin responding to one set of behaviors in more appropriate ways and gain some practice in setting limits on some behaviors. They can learn how to respond more consistently and systematically and discover some new ways of showing the child how much they approve of what he is doing. An entirely new perspective can begin for both parents and their child. Parents can learn that they do not have to scold and nag, and the child can learn that he does not always have to resort to disruptive behaviors to gain and secure his parents' attention, even though momentarily. Once the problematic behavior has been pinpointed by the parents, they can begin to consistently apply behavior modification principles and either attend to the behavior with greater and appropriate attention or ignore the problem behavior systematically. Once parents begin responding to the child in more appropriate ways, new, positive, and less conflictual interchanges between the parents and child may be possible. The parents simply learn to decrease all attention to a specific behavior at a specific time or to increase attention to a desired behavior at the exact time that it occurs with expressions of praise and approval, touching, smiling, or other ways of showing their child how pleased they are.

SUPPORTING PARENTS THROUGH THE PROCESS OF CHANGE

Most parents require support for the fact that change is difficult and sometimes an uncomfortable process. Parents initially need to know that changing anything can be overwhelming. They can be encouraged that they will have success in changing a few behaviors in the beginning; they should experience positive feedback as incremental change happens, and they need to know that once they have had success in changing a few behaviors, they can add to that success by changing more behaviors if it is desired.

Frequently, parents give information about all the interactions, conflicts, and behaviors that they do not like, cannot tolerate, or will not stand for another day. They must learn that they cannot possibly work with a host of behaviors at one time. They must define priorities and determine precisely what behavior they want to change first. Parents usually ask for help when they are most vulnerable to stress or when their ability to cope with a behavioral problem is decreased. Parents sometimes convey the idea that the behavior must be changed instantly. An individual in a professional capacity cannot respond optimally to these unrealistic requests to change everything at once. Parents and the consulting child care professional must mutually agree on a realistic goal for change. This goal is best determined after records have been completed.

The process of change must be explored with parents. Parents should have opportunities to discuss the time element involved and learn that it is not always easy to create or respond to change. Parents need to know that as children change parents will respond differently. They may experience different reactions to the child's behavior than they had anticipated. They may like what is happening, or they may find that it is not comfortable for them to experience the changes that are occurring. Their reactions may in fact be negative. It will be helpful if they can share their reactions to the changes that are taking place with a child care professional. Children's changes can be explored, depending on signs from the parents that indicate their readiness for discussing or anticipating further change. Parents need to know that their responses are natural and that it is appropriate and ultimately helpful if they can participate in sharing their reactions.

SERIOUS PITFALLS IN PLANNING A BEHAVIOR MANAGEMENT PROGRAM

Success for change is never imminent if there is not sufficient objective information as a source of reference for planning change.

Words such as "poor," "satisfactory," "abnormal," "naughty," "poor attitude," "good," "bad," "quiet," "poor attention span," "hyperactive," "stubborn," "negative," "resistant," "uncooperative," "belligerent," "sad," "unhappy," "depressed," "mad," and "unmotivated" are typically used by parents to describe children and their behaviors. Few of these terms can be interpreted in a uniform way. Parents may be inclined to use hazy terms and to rely on labeling to convey their concerns. Some children are labeled a particular way because of the lack of an objective and appropriate description. Others are labeled because of the confusion that exists about their behavior. It is as if labeling takes care of the concern. Vagueness of the description of a problem is often correlated with vagueness of intervention and lack of success in planning change. Some individuals may think it easier to develop or describe an impression concerning a behavior than to count how often the behavior is occurring. This orientation may result in labeling. The dangerous aspect of labeling is that once one has arrived at a label, it becomes a satisfying end in itself. It can be a disadvantage for the child because people tend to respond to the label first and perceive the child as "unmotivated," "hyperactive," or "uncooperative," instead of looking at his uniqueness. Labeling has a tendency to influence individuals to only negative aspects instead of the assets and positive features that all children have.

Labeling is not a substitute for intervention. Sometimes a child continues to suffer from the stigma of labels that have been attached to him. If he has been labeled in a negative way because of certain behaviors and the same behaviors have been reinforced, his chances for learning and responding in more appropriate and appealing ways are lessened. Children's self-concepts can suffer from images that are a direct result of labeling. Successful intervention cannot be planned on the basis of labeling.

REMINDERS FOR SUCCESS WITH BEHAVIORAL MANAGEMENT

The child care professional should keep the following points in mind when dealing with parents who have expressed concern, asked for help, or sought advice for their child's behavioral problem.

The person responding to requests for parental assistance should not feel obligated to give any particular advice that is designed to solve the parents' problem immediately. It is important to get data first. It is important to have the parents describe their observations that lead them to conclude there is a problem. Both the child care professional and parents must become accustomed to the topography of the child's behavior.

It is vital that child care professionals document data about behavior to avoid dangerous approaches. The more objective they and the parents can be the easier it is to describe the problem, plan intervention, and evaluate change and progress. It is important to tell parents, "Before we work this out together, I need examples of the kinds of behavior you are talking about." As the child care professional begins to express his satisfaction about accurately defining concerns, parents sense it and may experience relief and react in more comfortable ways. If a systematic approach is begun with them, their feelings of confidence about their capabilities of problem solving can be increased. Instead of tackling a problem that has been going on for a long time, child care professionals can help parents reduce their anticipation that elimination of the problem will occur overnight. With this more realistic approach, they are given permission to progress at a reasonable, appropriate rate and may be relieved that they are not expected to come up with an immediate solution, that their goals will take some time, and that their contribution to beginning record keeping is significant. A parent-centered approach is a key to success in management, and parents can receive input immediately for success with record keeping, accurate observations, and their ability to follow through with giving or withholding attention for specific behaviors of the child. This can be extremely important to continued parental efforts, can lessen their guilt feelings, and can lessen or reduce the feeling of child care professionals that they must offer immediate advice. Attention must be directed to the importance of records first, then to problem solving, priorities, planning, and further decision making. Parents at the outset need to know that they have alternatives and that there are consequences to their decision making.

Child care professionals can help parents and children experience more success with the goals they are attempting to achieve. They can help both parents and children experience more positive kinds of interactions together. The success of a behavioral management program relies on the extent to which child care professionals and parents are willing to observe and record behavior before a program of intervention is planned. It is vital that child care professionals become more comfortable listening to what parents are describing. It is also important that parents perceive themselves as powerful, resourceful persons, capable of changing interaction patterns with their children.

Parents need appropriate support for their feelings of frustration, fatigue, and disappointment. Child care professionals should acknowledge the parents' strengths in observing and the fact that they have tried to find better ways to approach and find a solution to the behaviors that are a problem to them. Parents must be reminded that it has probably been difficult for the child as well and that both they and the child have experienced varying degrees of frustration and conflict. Parents need encouragement that change is possible and that it is a process requiring time, effort in planning, and different responses in following through to reach goals that are clearly defined and are judged to be realistic for the developmental level of the child and the parents' current levels of readiness to respond. Parents often need verbal permission to relax their efforts at eliminating a behavioral problem, particularly when they are collecting needed information on behaviors of a child.

Child care professionals should tell parents in advance that the data which are collected by them and the observations made by the helping professional will be mutually shared, discussed, explored, and validated before any new intervention begins. Parents should be reminded that they have been able to tolerate the problem so far and that they have strength remaining to plan more realistic goals for the child and for themselves. They need reassurance that they will be able to plan the best and easiest approach for the child and themselves. They should be taught to avoid planning to change a number of behaviors simultaneously. Parents will be expected to select priorities of problems that are reasonable to change within a reasonable time period, so that parents and children may experience success with the change together. These results are possible with systematic assessments and behavioral observations that are collected in a systematic fashion and examined for patterns that have evolved.

Parents can learn either to decrease or increase their attention to certain behaviors. Parents and others must be cautioned that ignoring a child's behaviors only does not change behaviors or guarantee success. Neither does positive attention alone serve as a remedy for changing difficult parent-child interactions. A carefully blended approach based on planning, systematic efforts, and evaluation of the progress made when appropriate attention is given or withheld for certain behaviors can be relied on to generate success between parents and the child.

Individual consultation with parents and children and direct training of parents are vital for parental success. In addition, parents benefit from ongoing reinforcement of their continual efforts.

Generally, parents benefit from being offered specific verbal advice that they can interpret, assimilate, and externalize into actual behaviors. Some parents find the new training manuals on behavior modification helpful. Parents can benefit from supervised behavioral rehearsals before applying any consequences to a child's behavior. It is also helpful for parents to practice under supervision ignoring behaviors, time outs, and withdrawal or reduction of parental attention. Parents can benefit from the supportive element in the behavioral rehearsal technique.

Most parents benefit from explicit feedback about their successes with behavior contingency management programs. Each phase, from reporting a problem to successfully solving it, requires consideration of explicit positive reinforcement for parents. After the parents' training ends and one problem is solved, parents can generalize principles to new concerns that arise with future child rearing.

Parental clinic visits alone cannot assure the success of a behavior modification program. The use of videotaping, modeling techniques, and direct supervision of parents in their home setting is vital.

Frequently, parents are promised an encouraging outcome with a behavioral program but end up experiencing failure. This can happen without consistent contact and ongoing support by a health care professional. Numerous visits to the home, telephone contacts, and ongoing face-to-face support are important. Adequate support from the data collection phase to the conclusion of a program is imperative for successful results.

Both parents and children ultimately benefit from the involvement of parents in decision making from the starting phase to the completion of a behavior management program. It is important that parental skills in behavior management be instilled and retained long after one behavior modification program is instituted. It is equally important for parents to know that there are fruitful answers to the many questions that arise in the management of everyday behavior problems in young children. The application of learning principles merits continued scrutiny and wider use by parents, day-care personnel, and professionals in early child education.

REFERENCES

1. Pless, I. B.: The changing face of primary pediatrics, Pediatr. Clin. North Am. **21:**223-244, 1974.
2. Berkowitz, B. P., and Graziano, A. M.: Training parents as behavior therapists: a review, Behav. Res. Ther. **10:**297-317, 1971.
3. O'Dell, Stan: Training parents in behavior modification: a review, Psychol. Bull. **81:**418-433, 1974.

ADDITIONAL READINGS

Barnard, Kathryn E., and Erickson, Marcene L.: Teaching children with developmental problems: a family care approach, ed. 2, St. Louis, 1976, The C. V. Mosby Co.

Eisler, R. M., Hersen, M., and Agras, W. Stewart: Videotape: a method for the controlled observation of nonverbal interpersonal behavior, Behav. Ther. **4:**420-425, 1973.

Harris, F. R., Allen K. E., and Johnston, M. S.: Methodology for experimental studies of young children in natural settings, Psychol. Rec. **19:**177-210, 1969.

Herbert, E. W., and Baer, D. M.: Training parents as behavior modifiers: self recording of contingent attention, J. Appl. Behav. Anal. **5:**139-149, 1972.

Johnson, Claudia A., and Katz, Roger C.: Using parents as change agents for their children: a review, J. Child Psychol. Psychiatry **14:**181-200, 1973.

Johnson, S. M.: Using parents as contingency managers, Psychol. Rep. **28:**703-710, 1971.

Karen, Robert L.: An introduction to behavior theory and its applications, New York, 1974, Harper & Row, Publishers.

Krapfl, J. E., Bry, P., and Nawas, N. M.: Uses of bug-in-ear in the modification of parents' behavior. In Rubin, R. D., and Frances, C. M., editors: Advances in behavior therapy, New York, 1969, Academic Press, Inc.

O'Neil, Sally M.: Behavior modification: toward a

human experience, Nurs. Clin. North Am. **10:**373-379, 1975.

Patterson, Gerald R.: Families: applications of social learning to family life, Champaign, Ill., 1973, Research Press Co.

Patterson, Gerald R., and Gullion, M. Elizabeth: Living with children: new models for parents and teachers, Champaign, Ill., 1968, Research Press.

Wahl, G., Johnson, S. M., Johansson, S., and Martin, S.: An operant analysis of child-family interaction, Behav. Ther. **5:**64-78, 1974.

Zeilberger, J., Sampen, S., and Sloane, H.: Modification of a child's problem behaviors in the home with the mother as therapist, J. Appl. Behav. Anal. **1:**47-53, 1968.

15

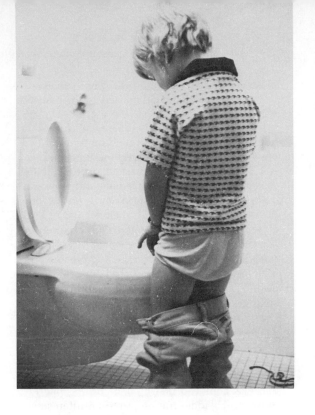

MANAGEMENT OF A TOILET-TRAINING PROGRAM

Toilet training can be a satisfying process only if both the parents and the child are ready to participate. Independent toileting is a major self-help skill that involves a series of complex learning tasks and requires that the child possess a number of physical, physiological, psychological, and motor skills.

Parents' attitudes are major determinants of the child's feelings of comfort about toileting, degree and rate of success, and presence or lack of problems. Typically parents are concerned about expecting too much too soon from the child, are sensitive about starting too late, or will admit to worrying about how much pressure they should exert. Frequently, parents describe their concerns about long-term effects of toilet training on their child's personality and express concerns about the consequences of their methods, approaches, attitudes, and decisions.

TOILET-TRAINING STUDIES

Stehbens and Silber[1] studied parental expectations about toilet training, focusing primarily on sources of advice for parents, time advised for training, and time of beginning attempts at toilet training. Seventy-one mothers whose first children ranged in age from 6 to 10 months participated in the study. Results of the questionnaire showed that 75% of the mothers had

read or were reading about toilet training already, and 77% had discussed it with someone (their husbands, mothers, physician, friends, or others). Two of the mothers had already initiated toilet-training programs to teach independence. Mothers said they would turn for advice to (in decreasing order of preference) a physician; the book *Baby and Child Care* by Dr. Benjamin Spock; friends with children of the same age; their husband, mother, or mother-in-law; friends with older children; a book other than Spock's; and a psychologist or psychiatrist. In this study, 50% of the mothers planned to start toilet training before their child was 15 months old. Of these mothers, 55% expected their child to be trained for daytime control by the age of 24 months. Mothers seemed more realistic about nighttime dryness; most expected it by the age of 4 years. Most mothers expected girls to be trained earlier than boys.

These findings definitely suggest the need to help parents become more realistic about the early goals and expectations that they have for their children as well as for themselves. Stehbens and Silber[1] emphasized the importance of minimizing the aggressive toilet-training methods sanctioned during the 1930s. They described most literature on toilet training as inconsistent and confusing and stated that the most appropriate literature advises a more re-laxed, less hurried method and more realistic expectations.

Brazelton[2] conducted a ten-year survey of toilet-training practices among mothers of 672 boys and 491 girls and found the following:

1. Mothers with their first children exhibited more anxiety about toilet training and more sur-prise and relief when toilet training was accom-plished than mothers with their second or later children. Mothers of second or later children re-ported giving their children more freedom to train themselves at their own rate. Not surpris-ingly, social pressure for these later children to become toilet trained came partially from older siblings.

2. Night training took 1 to 7 months longer for mothers who were training first children than for those training second or later children.

3. Bowel training was achieved first by 12.3% or 144 children, and training for urina-tion was achieved first by 8.2% or 96 children. Bowel and bladder training were simultaneously achieved by 79.5% or 930 children.

4. Of 930 children, 90.3% were between 24 and 30 months of age when success in both bowel and bladder training was achieved. The average age for completion of both bowel and bladder training was 33.3 months.

5. Completion of daytime training was ac-complished by 80.7% of the children when they were between the ages of 2 and 2½ years. The average completion for daytime training was 28.5 months.

6. A total of 80.3% or 940 children were com-pletely trained by the age of 3 years. In the en-tire sample of 1,170 children, 150 did not com-plete training until 3½ years of age.

7. Girls were completely trained an average of 2.46 months earlier than boys.

Brazelton considered the child's psychological readiness for toilet training to be extremely im-portant. The major components of psychological readiness include the feelings of security and gratification a child associates with parent-child interactions, the child's desire to please his par-ents, and the child's wish to control his impulses to eliminate or urinate.

The toilet-training approach that Brazelton[2] advocates is child-oriented. Basing a teaching program on the child's needs and personal time-table rather than on cultural pressures or pa-rental needs for cleanliness can lessen the sense of responsibility that parents have for the child's lack of accomplishment. Discussions about parents' future plans for toilet training should be initiated at least by the ninth well-child visit.[2] Such discussions can help parents withstand external pressures for instituting early, inappro-priate training attempts; help them understand the advantages and importance of a relaxed, unpressured approach; and prepare them to accept the mistakes the child will make during the training program.

Kennell and Boaz[3] also emphasize the value of such early discussions. They suggest inform-ing parents that a child becomes aware of elimi-nation some time between 12 and 18 months of age and advising them not to overrespond but to casually make a verbal connection with the child's act of elimination so that the child even-tually learns to associate a particular word with elimination. (They also emphasize the impor-tance of not training the child at the same time that a new puppy is being housebroken; train-ing methods for a dog confuse and upset a child.)

Brazelton[2] suggests introducing the child's potty chair as a regular chair after the child is 18 months of age; the child can be placed on the potty chair with all his clothes on, talked to, read to, and given food. Thus the child does not initially experience being placed on a cold seat. About a week later, the child can be placed on the potty chair without diapers, but no attempt should be made to catch stool or urine because such an attempt might frighten the child and result in his "holding back" for a longer period of time. The next stage consists of changing the child's soiled diapers on the potty chair and dropping them in front of him into the toilet so that he can see the action of diapers falling down under the potty chair. Then par-ents should gradually begin placing the child on the potty chair several times a day to catch stool or urine. As the child begins to show interest in the toilet-training process, his underclothing can be removed, and he can be given freedom to go by himself to his potty chair when he desires.

Sears and associates[4] documented the impor-tance of timing for success in a toilet-training program. Mothers in their study who started toilet training their children after the children were 20 months of age reached their goal sooner and with greater ease than those who began earlier. Most toilet-training studies suggest em-phatically the need to determine a child's indi-vidual physical, physiological, and psychological readiness. Kagan[5] suggests that toilet training be delayed until the child is conceptually and physically prepared for learning. He believes a child is psychologically ready when the following criteria are met:

1. The child is accustomed to a nurturing relationship with a caregiver so that anticipated loss of nurturance can be an effective reinforcer for learning.
2. The child can understand verbal instructions about bodily control.
3. The child exhibits satisfactory symbolic maturity and can respond appropriately to behavior requirements.

ASSESSING READINESS OF CHILD

Certain specific observations of the child facilitate choosing the best time to implement a toilet-training program.

Physical and physiological signs

Following are questions that help to determine the child's physical and physiological readiness for toilet training:

Is the child able to reach a standard-size toilet, or will a potty chair be more suitable? Can the child sit comfortably by himself? Can he stand alone? Does he balance well, walk forward and backward, and climb onto a chair, his bed, or the couch? Can he undress or remove his trousers or underclothing? Does he ride a tricycle? All these skills require coordinated movement, posture, and balance and suggest that physical and neurological signs of readiness are present. In particular, standing and walking alone indicate that the child's spinal track is myelinated to a level for bowel and bladder control and that he is physiologically capable of sphincter control.

Do records kept by the parents for at least 7 days indicate that the child can retain urine for at least 2 hours? If the child is constantly having to urinate, medical consultation may be in order. Frequency of urination is not conducive to initial success and may indicate immature bowel and bladder control.

Behavioral signs

Certain behavioral observations help assess a child's readiness for toilet training as follows:

Can the parents describe differences in the child's behaviors that signal his need to urinate or defecate or the fact that he has wet or soiled his clothing? Does he become quieter or verbally seek attention? Does he shift his weight? Does the color of his face change? Does he cry, fuss, or become more dependent and clinging? Has the child developed a word, gesture, or symbol

indicating that he needs to eliminate? Does he associate the bathroom with eliminating?

ASSESSING READINESS OF PARENTS

Interviews with parents should focus on their readiness to pursue a toilet-training program that is characterized by a positive, consistent, individualized, nonpunitive, nonpressured style of teaching. It is wise to explore the parents' willingness to participate, the time they have to invest in the program, the advantages they see, the inconveniences that toilet training may cause them, and the reason they wish to start, as well as whether this is the best time for both parents and child to begin a program.

The child care professional should elicit from the parents any past history associated with attempts at toilet training the child. When did the parents start training? Was training their idea, or were they pressured by others? What methods did they use? Did they experience feelings of frustration, indifference, or discomfort? How long did they attempt training and what were their reasons for discontinuing training efforts? Looking back, how do they view the experience for themselves and the child? Were their efforts consistent? Help them define what they did most consistently. If the parents were not successful in the past, do they think that it is important to try again?

Are the parents presently attempting to train? Do they feel comfortable about their decision to continue? Do they regret having started? Do they judge this to be the best time in terms of their needs? Are they rested or are there extra demands on their time now? Are they going through any excessive stress? Have there been any serious crises that have demanded their extra attention recently?

How do the parents react when the child is wet or soiled? Are they so eager for him to succeed that they display anxiety or tenseness when he fails (even by way of facial expressions, which children are sensitive to)? Do they experience negative or angry feelings? If they admit to using punishment in any form (spankings, scoldings, withholding privileges, using suppositories, withholding fluid, getting the child up in the middle of the night, or making the child wash his sheets or clothes), appeal to them to discontinue these unnecessary, ineffective methods.

If the parents are in the process of toilet training, do they stay with the child in the bathroom? Can they describe his behaviors? Is it a pleasant time for both? Do they talk with, look at, smile at, touch, or play special games with the child? Does the child indicate restlessness or boredom, cry, or attempt to get off the toilet? Does the child stay in the bathroom longer than 10 minutes? How often has the child gone successfully in the last 3 days? How did the parents know the child went to the bathroom? How did they respond? How soon? What specifically did they do to show disapproval, disappointment, or approval?

What is the longest the child has ever had to sit or stand at the toilet? Where do the parents teach the child to eliminate? (Encourage them to keep the potty chair in the bathroom, not in the kitchen, bedroom, or living room.) How is the child dressed most of the time? Is he dressed in simple clothes that he could remove if he needed to go to the bathroom and no one was available to help? Does he have imitative models to copy in the bathroom? Are the parents relying on their own verbal cues alone to teach him? If so, what are their usual comments? Do they consistently use the same words for potty, defecation, and urination? Do they use a system of concrete rewards?

If the present method is not progressively successful, what else have the parents thought of? What would they like to try next? If the child is not complying, what worries them or bothers them the most? What is the least of their worries?

Can the parents accept the concept that if the child is not ready, he will learn according to his own individual readiness? Do they expect him to master the entire goal of independent toileting behavior within a short period of time? Can they relax and take it easier on themselves? Can they reduce some of their own expectations to succeed immediately and be satisfied with learning how to systematically observe the child first?

RECORD KEEPING

As part of the procedure for determining the readiness of both parents and child to become involved in a successful toilet-training program, parents should keep detailed records for a period of 7 days. They should be cautioned to discontinue record keeping if the child becomes ill or if fluid intake needs to be changed.

Parents are expected to record exact times that the following events occurred:

- The child ate or drank, no matter how little the child consumed

- The child's behavior was suddenly distinctly different (for example, when the child was noticeably quieter or louder, started fussing or tugging at his clothes, pointed toward the bathroom, cried, or squirmed)
- Parents gave the child attention related to toileting behaviors only: specifically, if the child told the parent he needed to eliminate, maintained dry underclothing, or even indicated that he had just eliminated and the parent responded with praise, concrete rewards, affectionate behavior, or showed approval
- Parents gave attention in the form of scolding, threatening, or spanking if the child had wet or soiled underclothes or did not tell them before eliminating
- The child indicated his need to go to the toilet either by gestures or words
- The child gestured, pointed, or told parents after he was wet or had had a bowel movement
- Parents ignored the child's pretoileting behaviors or activities
- The child was noted to have dry underclothes
- The child was noted to have wet underclothes
- The child's and parents' moods were noted each time they recorded an activity (parents should draw a small happy face ☺ or sad face ☹ to indicate the child's mood and a larger happy or sad face to the right of it to indicate their mood)

Parents should comment if anything unusual happened to them or to the child on any day that the record was being kept.

Parents are most likely to keep accurate records if they keep the record in a convenient place for recording information.

It is crucial to refrain from beginning any toilet-training program until the records are completed because they show how parents are responding to the child's behaviors and what times the child is most likely to eliminate. After the records are completed to the parents' expressed satisfaction, the child care professional should acknowledge their efforts to keep accurate records, their diligence in making observations, and their ability to follow through. The child care professional should ask them whether they learned anything new about the child and themselves, whether they have examined the data for patterns, and whether they judge this to be an optimal time to teach the child.

If parents have not been able to follow through with beginning record keeping, the child care professional should discuss why it was difficult for them, whether the instructions were clear, if there were outside interfering variables, and whether they want to try record

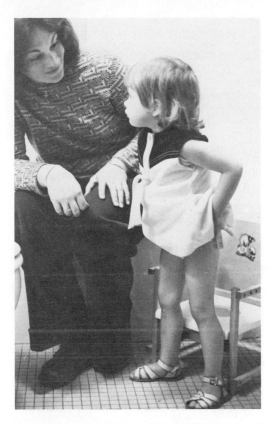

Fig. 15-1. Assessing the parent's readiness to teach and the child's readiness to be involved in toilet training. The teaching environment is assessed for success of both the child and parent.

keeping again. In spite of their verbally expressed wishes, there may be a better time for them to initiate a learning program.

BEGINNING A PROGRAM

The goal of a toilet-training program is to help the child achieve small goals and experience comfort and success and to help the parents simultaneously experience feelings of adequacy, minimal tension, and relief. Parents should understand that they will be capitalizing on the times the child is most likely to eliminate and that they should respond immediately to his behavioral clues indicating his need to eliminate. They must be cautioned to ignore accidents.

A task analysis of toileting reveals a number of discrete steps. Parents must observe and systematically reinforce each step in positive, natural, spontaneous ways. The child is accomplishing one of the discrete steps when he does one of the following:

- Sits on the toilet or potty seat when placed there, without fussing, crying, or attempting to get off
- Eliminates into the toilet on a regular basis when sitting on the toilet
- Waits to eliminate before being placed on the potty
- Indicates his need to eliminate before going into the bathroom
- Asks to go to the toilet or goes by himself
- Remains dry for longer periods of time
- Climbs onto the toilet independently
- Helps undress himself before getting onto the toilet
- Independently undresses himself before getting onto the toilet
- Wipes himself independently
- Flushes the toilet
- Dresses himself
- Washes his hands with soap in a correct manner
- Dries his hands with a towel

Probably the best approach to toilet training is to maintain a positive and relaxed attitude. Parents should begin by leading the child gently into the bathroom, staying with him, and showing approval for each aspect of his cooperative behavior: helping him pull down his pants, accepting being placed on the toilet seat or potty chair, urinating or defecating into the toilet, getting off the potty seat, dressing again, and washing his hands. (If the child has not had any success after 5 minutes, he should be wiped, praised for sitting quietly and appropriately, and asked to get off the potty seat.) Social reinforcers are potent, powerful, and durable in reinforcing desirable behaviors. Some parents may choose to offer concrete rewards such as food or toys. Such additional rewards may be extremely useful but are not necessary. Parents should totally ignore any undesirable behaviors, calmly accepting the child's errors.

Parents should place the child on the potty for voiding when he first gets up in the morning, just before breakfast, midmorning, after snacks, after lunch, midafternoon, before and after dinner, and again before bedtime. They cannot expect the child to have a regular pattern of elimination unless they feed him at approximately the same times each day. The child care professional should specifically caution parents not to use enemas, suppositories, or soap sticks without consulting a physician and not to withhold fluids.

It is important that parents not underestimate their child's ability to learn the task of independent toileting, but it is equally important that they not overrate the child. They should set goals that can be achieved within a reasonable period of time. They should also remember to help the child only when he needs it; it may take longer to accomplish the task, but it is the best way for a child to really learn. Parents should not overprotect the child or give excuses for inappropriate behaviors, and they should learn to feel comfortable setting reasonable limits.

Parents should consistently refrain from feeling and displaying anger, slapping, scolding, spanking, threatening, bribing, and sending the child to his bedroom. A child responds best to a positive, loving, nurturing attitude and should not be told that his parents do not love him if he makes a mistake or does something wrong. For limit setting to be effective, parents must convey an attitude of friendly and positive firmness rather than an orientation to punishment.

Parents should also be encouraged to refrain from using lengthy reasoning and frequent explanations with a younger child unless the child consistently indicates that he understands what is being discussed. Drawn out explanations and reasoning may confuse a child, whereas an immediate behavioral response by the parent serves as explicit positive or negative feedback. Simply talking to a child does not assure his understanding of parental teaching objectives.

In their verbal communication with the child, parents should emphasize what the child *is* to do rather than what he *is not* to do (e.g., "go into the bathroom" instead of "don't wet in your pants"). Parents should act as if they expect the child to behave correctly and should give one simple direction at a time and wait for the child to respond at his own rate. Keeping directions at a simple level will enhance greatly the chances a child has for learning. If these concepts can be carried out in a consistent and spontaneous way while the child is learning a new skill or task or changing an undesirable repertoire of behaviors, both parents and child have a greater opportunity for experiencing successful and more pleasurable interactions at any stage of the teaching-learning process.

If parents follow these general principles, giving special consideration to immediately, consistently, and positively acknowledging elimination into the potty or toilet and, in contrast, devotedly ignoring those toileting behaviors that definitely are not to be repeated, they will have a greater probability of success with the child.

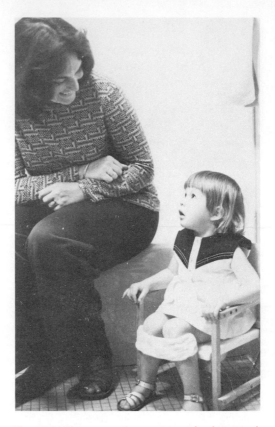

Fig. 15-2. The parent is spontaneously showing the child how much she approves of the child's cooperation and success in learning independent toileting habits.

In summary, when beginning an assessment of both the parents' and child's readiness to be involved in a successful, nonpressured approach to toilet training, it is important to determine the following:

1. Are the parents emotionally prepared to be involved in a teaching process with the child?
2. Are the parents feeding the child at regular times each day?
3. Do the parents know the social and concrete rewards that the child favors?
4. Are the parents prepared to reward toileting behavior as soon as it occurs?
5. Have the parents involved significant others in the assessment and planning stage for toilet training?
6. Are the parents willing to invest some of their time at least four to six times a day in the beginning?
7. Is the child willing to sit on the toilet

without crying, fussing, or trying to get off?

8. Have the parents completed a record of the times that the child seems to eliminate each morning, afternoon, and evening?

9. Have the parents obtained a toilet seat or potty chair that the child will sit on?

10. Are the parents prepared to dress the child in easy-to-remove clothing?

11. Are the parents willing to have the child in training pants once a program begins?

CASE HISTORY

A mother of a 4½-year-old child expressed an urgent desire for help with toilet training. Her reason for seeking help now was that even though the child was 4½ years of age, he could not be entered into a day-care center unless he was fully trained. O was trained to urinate in the toilet and had since he was 2½ years old. Since 1½ or 2 years of age he had bowel movements anywhere he desired in the home. He refused to sit on the toilet seat to eliminate.

The assessment process of the mother's concerns was commenced. Her first request was "I want you to tell me everything I'm doing wrong." The child care professional's response to her request for criticism was, "There are probably a number of things you are doing just right for both you and O." Her young boy passed all the items on the DDST, was above average for his age on the Developmental Profile, and the HOME revealed an environment that met his developmental needs adequately, both currently and from a historical point of view. The mother was reassured that she was in fact doing a number of appropriate things with and for O because he was doing so well developmentally for tasks associated with his age level.

It was learned during an initial parental interview that the mother was avoiding, lacking, and not attempting to set firm limits with O. For example, it was learned initially that O was staying up as late as 12:30 AM every night. (Questions about sleep are helpful and are considered routine child-rearing questions.) When the mother answered this question, she did ask if she was doing all right in letting O stay up so late.

The mother was asked how much sleep he was getting for his age, which when calculated was compatible with his age and needs. The mother related that she simply found it easier to let him stay up late at night with both parents.

When the discussion focused on a more appropriate hour for getting O to go to bed, the emphasis on toilet training was reduced. The child care professional commented to the mother that getting O to bed at an earlier hour seemed like a concern of hers and was appropriate. Had she thought of beginning to change this habit? She agreed that it was a concern but related that she did not know if she could, since the habit was so routine and had gone on so long. Encouragement was spontaneously offered.

A week later she was absolutely thrilled with the results of her efforts to *begin* to set limits with O. She related how difficult it was initially and that she did not want to hurt his feelings, but she was relieved to find out she could do something with him so well.

It was obvious that she needed to learn that just because she started to set limits with O, she was not rejecting him and it would not jeopardize their relationship; in fact, it would help it. It was decided that since she could and was willing to try limit setting with a realistic goal, and one that most parents take for granted, it was not too soon to again explore her concern about O's unusual, undesirable toilet problems. She agreed to collect data and said she would do her best to observe and write down what regularly happened in regard to this behavior. She was not certain that she could keep really accurate records but was encouraged to try.

A record of toileting behaviors, shown on pp. 236 and 237 indicated a definite pattern with O's bowel movements. She recorded times of his bowel movements, where he deposited them, when he ate, what she did in response to his behavior, and how he reacted when she would find him crouching and going to the bathroom.

It is significant to point out that when this mother found it difficult to begin discussing plans for changes, she was given support to progress according to her own needs and feelings of comfort. At one point it was obvious and essential that discussion about O's toileting behavior be dropped. Further attention was focused on how she viewed his behavior, what she thought about it, and the distress she experienced. Alternatives for which she could end up feeling more adequate with her own resourcefulness, abilities, strengths, and decision-making behaviors were explored.

The mother traced historically how she had inconsistently interacted with her child, failed to set goals, limits for him, and limits for her-

RECORD OF BOWEL MOVEMENTS OF 4½-YEAR-OLD BOY

Time for snacks or meals	Time	Place noticed	Child's response	Parent's response
Friday				
9:00— breakfast	9:30 AM	Kitchen	Said "I don't want to be changed," but cooperated	Took to bed-room to change into clean clothes
10:45— snack	11:00 AM	Hiding in kit-chen corner trying to have a BM	Fussed; refused to get on bed to have pants changed	Tried to explain what he was supposed to do
Refused lunch	12:15 PM	Hiding behind couch trying to have a BM	Refused to sit on toilet; made knees go limp; resisted mother when she tried to undress to put on toilet	Took into bath-room
Mother gave lunch (2:45)				
7:30— dinner	7:55 PM		Asked to be changed in bed-room; asked that mother not take him to bathroom	Changed in bedroom
Saturday				
	10:00 AM	Hiding in bedroom	Asked to be changed	Changed in bedroom
10:05— breakfast				
	2:00 PM	Hiding in bedroom	Talked about comic strips as mother changed him	Changed in bedroom
2:05— lunch				
7:00— dinner	7:10 PM	Tried having BM after dinner in kitchen	Told mother he wanted to be left alone in living room to have BM	Explained he had to go into bathroom
	8:15 PM	Living room		Changed in bedroom
	8:45 PM	Living room		Changed in bedroom
Sunday				
	10:30 AM	At kitchen table	Said he liked being changed in bed-room	Parents both just started saying come on and get changed
11:00— breakfast	12:15 PM	Living room	Said he would not go into bedroom	

RECORD OF BOWEL MOVEMENTS OF 4½-YEAR-OLD BOY—cont'd

Time for snacks or meals	Time	Place noticed	Child's response	Parent's response
Sunday—cont'd				
Refused lunch (3:00)	5:00 PM	Yard	Said he liked being changed in bedroom	
5:20—dinner	7:15 PM	Living room		
8:00—snack at bedtime				
Monday				
	10:00 AM	Closet	Resisted being changed in bedroom	Encouraged to come into room to be changed
10:30—breakfast				
11:30—lunch	1:00 PM	Living room		Changed in bedroom
5:00—dinner	6:00 PM	Kitchen	Mother insisted he be changed in bedroom when he said he didn't want to be changed	
7:30—snack				
Tuesday				
9:50—breakfast	12:15 PM	Yard	As mother changed in bedroom he told her not to scold him	Agreed not to scold him
4:00—lunch	7:00 PM	Hiding in closet	Changed subject when mother suggested he be a big boy and stop going to the bathroom in pants	Insisted he go to bathroom from now on
8:00—dinner	11:00 PM	Bedroom	Resisted being changed in living room	
Wednesday				
10:30—breakfast	11:00 AM	Living room	Told mother he wanted to be changed	Said OK and complied with changing in bedroom
12:45—lunch	1:30 PM	Living room	He tried to postpone being changed	Insisted he be changed
4:45—snack	7:00 PM	Yard	No fuss about being changed in bedroom	
7:30—dinner				

self and expressed how she needed experience in interacting consistently. It was decided that working with a complex goal such as toilet training in the beginning would not have been easy for this mother because it required setting definite goals, having realistic expectations, and the ability to follow through on a consistent basis. She first needed the experience of having success with getting him to bed at 8 to 8:30 PM most evenings.

After she was acknowledged and her efforts reinforced for observing him and her excellent efforts in record keeping were reviewed, the possibility of systematically ignoring some of O's behaviors was presented. When she was questioned if she had thought of any new ways to eliminate his inappropriate toileting, she said she could not possibly come up with anything. She said she had begged, pleaded, cried in front of him, and tried everything. There were never any signs of hostility or negative interactions observed between mother and child in regard to toileting.

The child care professional asked her if it might be possible that O was gaining extra attention from this unusual behavior of eliminating all over the house. She agreed, but when it was suggested that she ignore him while changing his pants, she said that this was something she could not do and cried. At this point she was again acknowledged for all her efforts, the fact that she was trying, and how difficult it was for her but was told that it was one alternative and part of the solution to the concern she originally expressed. She was not pressured further. She was left with her records, and it was agreed that further discussion would take place when she was more comfortable in exploring different ways to respond to inappropriate behaviors of O.

The next discussion focused on whether she would be willing to ignore O while changing his pants such as by simply looking at the bed, at the wall, at his shoes, anyplace but his face. She was also asked to refrain from talking or socially interacting during the changing procedure. Generally, after she found him, she took him by the hand, gently telling him about how badly she wanted him to stop having bowel movements all over the house, and took him into the bedroom where he lay on the bed. Then she washed his bottom and put new pants on him, talking to him all the while. It was pointed out that the child was receiving eye-to-eye contact, verbal communication, gentle scolding,

touch by being cleaned, and at least 10 minutes of her undivided attention each time this event occurred at a minimum of twice a day. The mother agreed that it looked like he was indeed getting attention but that it was painful for her to ignore him while changing him, so painful that she simply would make every effort to be firm about making him eliminate in the toilet. She expressed that if she ignored him, O would interpret it as her way of rejecting him.

She was reminded that her attention for this behavior in the form of eye-to-eye contact, touching, and sweet scolding could be given just as exclusively for more acceptable kinds of behavior. She eventually agreed to the plan of completely ignoring the boy while changing him and to implement her plan of making him sit on the toilet for bowel movements according to his individual physiological patterns as indicated by the records. She was enthusiastic also about trying her plan of giving him special rewards in the bathroom. She decided that since he loved lemons, she would try giving him one if he had a successful bowel movement in the toilet. She began to have progressive successes each day in the bathroom within a period of a week and decided that this was "less rejecting" of him than ignoring him while changing him. Within a period of 3 weeks, she had him going to bed at 8 PM every night, going to the bathroom and eliminating in the toilet instead of behind the couch, in the front closet, under the kitchen table, in the bedroom, under the stairs, or in the dining room. The mother was so assured of continued success that she enrolled him in the day-care center that she had wanted to, the one that had originally refused him admittance 6 months earlier. Although she initially missed him during the day, he began to improve in language skills too. This development seemed to be related to being around children on a constant basis for the first time in his life.

His mother related that she had never experienced such gratification in all her years with O, knowing now that she was finally capable of doing what was right for him whenever action was required in the future. She admitted that it was the first time she ever felt genuine success with a goal for her child and herself.

REFERENCES

1. Stehbens, James A., and Silber, David L.: Parental expectations in toilet training, Pediatrics **48**:451-454, 1971.

2. Brazelton, T. Berry: A child-oriented approach to toilet training, Pediatrics **29:**121-128, 1962.
3. Kennell, John H., and Boaz, Willard D.: Infancy and early childhood. In Green, Morris, and Haggerty, Robert, editors: Ambulatory pediatrics, Philadelphia, 1968, W. B. Saunders Co.
4. Sears, Robert R., Maccoby, Eleanor E., and Levine, Harry: Patterns of child rearing, New York, 1957, Row, Peterson, & Co.
5. Kagan, Jerome: Psychological development of the child, In Faulkner, Frank, editor: Human development, Philadelphia, 1966, W. B. Saunders Co.

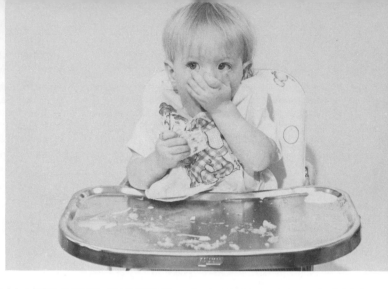

16

PROMOTING
INDEPENDENCE
IN SELF-FEEDING

Adequate assessment of a child's feeding abilities significantly helps determine the type of approach and method of management most appropriate for fostering self-feeding. Independently taking a spoon, filling it with food, bringing it to the mouth, chewing the food, and swallowing it is one of the first major self-help behavioral sequences that children master. It is the first significant developmental step in independently caring for oneself, and the first self-care skill that parents anticipate teaching.

PARENTAL ATTITUDES

Most parents take it for granted that their child will learn how to use a spoon. However, spoon-feeding is not always easy for children to learn. It involves integration of fine motor skills, vision, perception, and gross motor skills such as sitting up and holding the head up. In this culture, parents are expected to successfully teach self-feeding within an acceptable period of time; if they cannot, society judges them to be inadequate. Failing to meet society's expectations naturally influences parents' self-images. Furthermore, in this culture, which places emphasis on industry, getting ahead, and being successful on one's own, asking for outside help with child rearing may be a painful process for parents. An important part of helping parents

teach self-feeding is making them feel comfortable, secure, and adequate.

If parents are skillfully supported during the teaching-learning process, by the time the child is self-feeding, they should be able to give themselves credit for creative ideas, for thinking of new ways to solve old problems, and for making a major contribution to promoting the child's success. Child care professionals can praise parents for efforts at consistency, appropriate reinforcement when it is most crucial to the child's learning, vigilance in watching for the child's readiness to learn more, and the ability to judge when they are expecting too much or too little. Parents should ideally look back at the self-feeding program as a positive experience and a time for learning new ways to interact with their child, discovering new attributes about themselves, and gaining some new perspectives on principles of teaching. They should finish the program with positive views about their child's behavior and progress and feel more confident of their judgment and ability to evaluate progress and make decisions.

Child care professionals have traditionally focused on the readiness of the child for learning a task; however, that approach alone does not guarantee success. It is imperative to also consider the parents' psychological, emotional, and social readiness to be involved in the teaching process. Parents must be willing to accept the fact that the child will make mistakes when first learning a new set of skills. If they anticipate small failures, they can be relaxed and free from tension when teaching. Parents' reactions to a child's increasing independence are also vital. Parents may not actually desire change but may be responding to external pressures. Child care professionals can explore the sources of such pressure with the parents and can be supportive about the stress parents may be feeling in response to the pressure. Parental readiness to talk about concerns, to make observations and record information, to try something new, to plan a specific approach, and to follow through with the approach are major determinants of success in developmental change.

Acknowledging parental feelings should be the first step in any feeding program. Ignoring such feelings and telling parents many different things to do right away simply confirms their worst fears and makes them think that they are failures after all. This disastrous approach can be avoided by finding out what the parents think is not right for their child and what they would like to see change. Each parent's concerns are unique, and each child has unique learning needs; so parents and children must be responded to as individuals. A parent who says "I really did expect things, but I finally came to the conclusion that I couldn't do it now; it wasn't the best time for my child or me" should receive support for making such a good judgment and be told that it was appropriate to stop and to consider other alternatives.

Frequently, parents have not been given helpful advice. For example, they may have been falsely reassured and told, "Don't worry, everything will be OK when he gets older." Allowing parents to express frustration and anger at the pseudoreassurance and misinformation they have received in the past is valuable. The child care professional should explore when the parents became concerned about a feeding problem, what they were told, what helped them the most, what worried them the most, what they tried, what method worked (if any), and what concerns them now.

ASSESSMENT OF THE CHILD

At the outset of any self-feeding program, the child should be assessed with standardized tools. Past and present height and weight measurements should be obtained, growth trends should be analyzed, and the child's current height and weight percentiles should be explained to the parents. If such developmental assessment indicates lags in areas other than feeding, then perhaps the focus of intervention

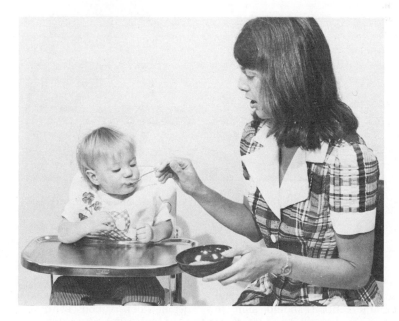

Fig. 16-1. Assessing mother-child interactions before planning a program to teach independent spoon-feeding skills.

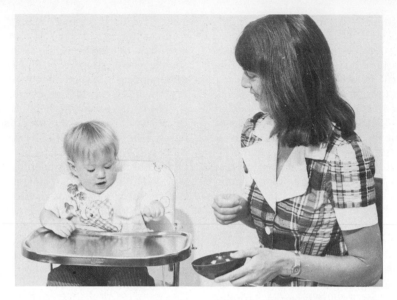

Fig. 16-2. Observing both the mother's and child's reactions when the child is first given a spoon to feed himself.

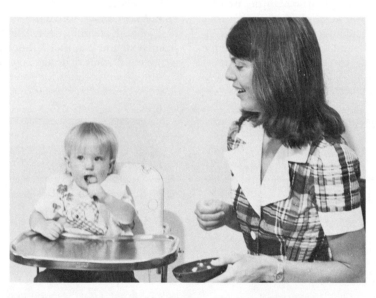

Fig. 16-3. Assessing the child's mastery of feeding himself with a spoon.

should not be on promoting self-feeding. For example, if the child is 19 months old and cannot sit up without support, then in all likelihood a more thorough investigation is necessary, and the priority of intervention should shift to promoting head, neck, chest, and trunk control along with righting responses. However, if a feeding program is in order, a 7-day dietary history should be obtained so that any dietary deficiencies can be corrected.

The child care professional should make detailed observations of the child before planning a program of teaching self-feeding skills. Optimal times for such observations are when

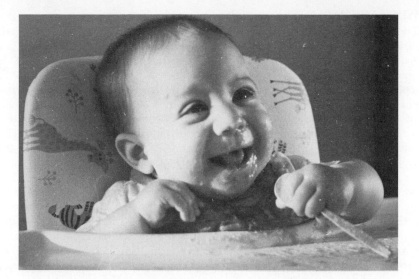

Fig. 16-4. Assessing the infant's readiness to sit without support, to maintain head control, and to coordinate hand, mouth, and eye movements in learning to spoon-feed independently.

the child is alert and is not distracted, is hungry, or is not fatigued and at eating time.

When observing the child's mouth, the child care professional should examine the interior of the mouth, note the shape of the palate, note the presence or absence of teeth, note whether the jaws come together in a symmetrical manner, determine whether the tongue moves laterally or forward and backward in a symmetrical way, determine whether the lips seal around the spoon, and look for evidence of precise lip control.

When observing the child's fine and gross motor abilities, the child care professional should determine whether the child has stable head control; sits without support; focuses visually on the food or spoon; reaches purposely, grasps, hangs onto, and voluntarily releases an object such as a spoon; has stable trunk support; has a fine pincer grasp; finger-feeds; and opens his mouth when food reaches it.

Self-feeding includes many discrete skills that are mastered sequentially. The presence of each skill is related to the maturation, organization, and integration of the central nervous system. The following steps are essential to independent self-feeding[1]:

1. Orienting to food by looking at it
2. Looking at the spoon
3. Reaching for the spoon
4. Touching the spoon
5. Grasping the spoon
6. Lifting the spoon
7. Delivering the spoon to the bowl
8. Lowering the spoon into the food
9. Scooping food onto the spoon
10. Lifting the spoon
11. Delivering the spoon to the mouth
12. Opening the mouth
13. Inserting the spoon into the mouth
14. Moving the tongue and mouth to receive food
15. Closing the lips
16. Swallowing the food
17. Returning the spoon to the bowl

If any steps are missing, helping the child master them must become a part of the feeding program.

Child care professionals must emphasize that parental observations are a vital, integral part of any self-feeding program. Parents can be present (whereas child care professionals cannot) whenever the child is being fed or being taught self-help skills, so they must be encouraged to make and share accurate observations of the child's abilities. Such observations should strongly influence the design and regular modification of a self-feeding program. Continued, open communication between parents and child care professionals is crucial; if their expectations do not coincide, the success of a program may be jeopardized.

INTERVIEWING THE PARENTS

By interviewing parents, the child care professional can find out much valuable information such as whether there is a consistent feeding approach. A child may be fed by several different people (sibling, mother, father, babysitter), each of whom may perceive and interact with the child differently and have different expectations, goals, and teaching approaches. One may wait for the child to chew the food; another may be in a hurry. One may praise the child for appropriate behaviors; another may ignore vital clues of independent progress. One may always smile at the child and make feeding a social occasion, whereas another may be punitive and make feeding an unpleasant experience. An important facet of a feeding program is to explore these factors with the parents and encourage consistency.

Feeding patterns

Following are some important questions that can be answered during the interview: Is the child fed at regularly scheduled times or irregularly? How often is he fed? Is the child fed when he seems to be hungry or at times that fit conveniently in the household schedule? Does the child have the opportunity to experience hunger or is he always satiated? (Some children may be fed continuously, generally in accord with a parent's need to give food, rather than with the child's appetite patterns.)

Does the child have imitative models? A child has greater opportunities for learning if he does. Children learn what socially acceptable behaviors are expected during eating by watching others and by having appropriate eating behaviors constantly praised, acknowledged, and reinforced.

Expectations

During the interview with parents concerning their child's self-feeding, the child care professional can obtain the answers to the following questions:

Are the parents' expectations for the child's behavior compatible with his current capabilities? Are they aware of the child's progress? Is their approach to teaching relaxed? Are the parents of a child who is not ready for some aspects of self-feeding able to identify and accentuate his other skills?

If parental expectations are too high, the child care professional should emphasize the appropriate observations parents have made and activities they have selected for their child to enhance his opportunities for gaining eating skills. The professional should stress small segments of behavior that precede total mastery so that parents perceive success in learning. There is no need to focus exclusively on a child's weaknesses; they are usually obvious to parents.

If parental expectations are too low, it is important to examine the reasons. Parents may have never systematically looked at the child's signs of readiness. Or they may have been told that it is not important for a child to feed himself until he is 19 months old. On the other hand, feeding the child may represent such a source of emotional gratification for the parents that they are not yet willing to give up the pleasure of offering him food. In that case, the parents' psychological adjustment to their child's self-feeding may be painful, and the issue must be skillfully explored as the parents offer verbal or behavioral clues that they are ready to talk about what self-feeding will mean to them.

The significant aspect of discussing expectations with the parents is to help them pick out an objective that can be realistically reached within a reasonable period of time.

OBSERVING FEEDING WITH PARENTS

Observing with the parents as they feed the child makes them feel included and supported. An added significance of joint observation is that the behavior being discussed is happening as it is being viewed and recorded. Such a close working relationship between parents and child care professionals provides an ideal opportunity for recognizing the parents' part in helping their child advance to new levels of attainment.

The best time to observe is when the child is hungry and is being offered food he likes. Even under optimal conditions, children may refuse to eat, turn their heads, whine, cry, spit food out, or make a mess by playing with the food. Most parents find these behaviors unacceptable and difficult to observe; they need reassurance that these unattractive displays are transitory. The child care professional should capitalize on the parents' resourcefulness and competence and point out that such displays are normal and do not reflect on the parents.

Determining how long feeding takes is important. If it requires an inordinate amount of time, the child care professional should be supportive in discussing the effects of such a time demand on the parents. Their feelings of fatigue, insufficient time for themselves, and resentfulness can be acknowledged as appropriate responses. Possible reasons for feeding taking a long time should be considered. Does it take time to find the most comfortable position for the child? Is the time that feeding takes related to the fact that the child cannot see the food, chokes, spits up, coughs, or cannot open his mouth when the food comes near? Are the parents feeding the child appropriate textures, right-size bites, and foods of a consistency that the child can move about in his mouth, chew, and swallow without difficulty? Do the parents admit that the child takes longer with foods he does not like? Are the parents feeding him too often? Are they feeding foods that are too hot or too cold? Is the child ill? What other reasons might the parents suggest for the length of time feeding takes?

Observing in the home allows the child care professional to examine the teaching environment not only for the teaching principles that are being used and the degree of consistency that is present but also for the amount of structure that exists and the parents' sensitivity to reducing extraneous stimuli that distract the child. Parents sometimes need to be reminded that learning a task is more difficult for a child if other children are playing nearby, pets are coming into the room, neighbors are visiting, telephones are ringing, the washing machine is going, and the child's favorite toys are available.

Direct observation provides valuable information. For example, one mother asked for help in feeding her 15-month-old boy. He had all the prerequisites for learning to eat by himself: he finger-fed, was able to get to a sitting position by himself, walked easily, brought toys to his mouth, and was eating some forms of table foods in addition to junior foods. He was in the seventy-fifth percentile for height and the fiftieth percentile for weight, had been in the fiftieth percentile for head circumference since birth, and passed all items on the DDST for his age level. Initial observations of the teaching environment showed that the child was seated comfortably and upright in his chair. His tray was divided into four sections that contained meat, vegetables, fruit, and water; a toy clown about 7 inches high was suctioned to each side of the tray.

As feeding began the mother handed the child an infant spoon, and he slapped it against his vegetable dish. She fed him from a separate spoon, after which he threw his own spoon on the floor. As she dashed to retrieve his spoon, he hit one of the toy clowns and happily watched it bob back and forth. The mother rinsed his spoon, then began a new sequence of offering food from a separate spoon. The mother and child did not establish eye contact during feeding, nor did the mother smile at the child.

After the observation period ended, the mother was surprised to hear that she had picked up and rinsed the child's spoon forty-two times; however, she denied that picking up the spoon was fatiguing for her, said it was not a problem, and stated that she felt it was unreasonable to set limits on a child his age. This mother, although ostensibly asking for help, was not ready for outside advice or input. Apparently she was pressured by relatives to initiate change at a time incompatible with her need to change and incongruous with her readiness level. The child care professional did not want to convey the message that the woman was a bad mother for not being ready to change matters. Instead the child care professional offered positive reinforcement about the mother's request for help and emphasized that if and when she wished to talk again about promoting self-feeding, a professional person would be readily available to her.

BEGINNING A PROGRAM

Success with self-feeding is most likely if the program is begun at an optimal time. The child care professional must explore the family's daily routine and general circumstances with the parents and encourage them to choose the best time for themselves and the child, not necessarily for the professional. The actual time of day is not important; parents should select a time when they are free and feel comfortable and unpressured, even if that means 9 PM. Parents should be cautioned not to begin a teaching program when there are minor or major differences in the family routine. Beginning a program should be postponed if family members are on vacation, relatives or friends are visiting, interpersonal relationships are under stress, marital difficulty or separation is occurring, a family member is ill, the family has moved, a family crisis is being resolved, or anything else out of the ordinary is happening. Other times to avoid are when the child is ill, showing a difference in appetite patterns, on a medication regimen, or receiving extra amounts of fluid.

One indicator of parents' readiness and enthusiasm to get started is careful record keeping. If parents do not keep a 7-day dietary

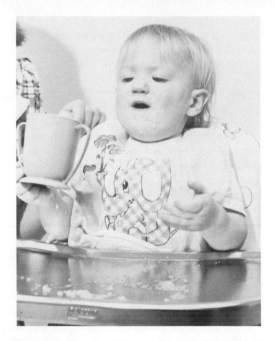

Fig. 16-5. Assessing the steps involved for an 11-month-old child to hold and drink from a cup without spilling much.

history, as well as recording the child's typical feeding behaviors (the seventeen discrete steps mentioned earlier), the child care professional should explore the reasons. Not keeping records can signal ambivalence, difficulty in watching the child eat, or unwillingness to begin a program at this time. Whatever the explanation, it is important to accept the reasons and be verbally supportive. If the parents are unable to proceed with a feeding program, the priority may shift to their personal emotional and psychological needs; the feeding program can be planned for a later, more appropriate time.

If parents are ready to carry out a program, the child care professional should be creative and resourceful in designing it. It is important to remind parents (and siblings or members of the extended family who are going to participate) to limit teaching new behaviors to feeding and not to expect simultaneous progress in other areas such as language or dressing. Everyone involved must clearly understand the goals for the child and for the persons doing the teaching and must appreciate the importance of record keeping. Everyone must also learn to analyze whether consistent approaches are being fostered, whether change is occurring,

whether progress is being carefully documented and monitored at intervals, how each person feels about his contribution to the problem-solving process, and what other options and alternatives can be explored if success and change are not yet visible. The family members who do not participate in the feeding program should be encouraged to be supportive to those who do.

RECORD KEEPING

The record-keeping process can be a valuable learning experience in itself: it can encourage parents to become consistent and systematic in their approach to teaching. In addition, good records allow the child care professional to assess the child's current self-help skills and his readiness to learn new ones and to learn more about the parent-child relationship.

Parents give clues about what they are gaining from record keeping. For example, are they asking questions about what they observe? (Hopefully they are.) Are the questions appropriate? When the observed feeding behaviors are discussed, do their facial expressions become tense? Do they roll their eyes toward the ceiling, grimace, or turn away? Do they show lethargic responses, appear depressed, talk in monotones, and seem more comfortable once the discussion is finished? Are they relieved to be able to discuss some rather normal responses to the feelings they have experienced? Parents often suspect that certain behaviors are occurring and find it helpful to have their own observations validated. A child care professional can give parents immediate, objective feedback such as, "I noticed that he brought the spoon to his mouth twenty-three times."

Keeping records may be difficult for parents for the following reasons:

1. They find it difficult to observe the child's behavior because it has become a source of irritation and anger and is repulsive to them.

2. They are upset or disturbed by the frequency of some behaviors.

3. They are losing hope because certain behaviors are not happening often enough.

4. A behavior is happening so often that they cannot record it accurately.

5. A behavior has gone on so long that they do not think change will occur.

6. They are discouraged.

7. They have observed a behavior so often that they perceive it as normal.

8. They are not ready to institute changes themselves; the pressure for altering the behavior is coming from other sources.

9. They do not feel capable of generating changes.

10. They do not understand how to write, count, or keep records even after they are shown.

Whatever the reason, parents need support for the difficulty they are experiencing in watching and recording behaviors. It is important to help parents overcome such obstacles because reliable records serve as indicators of real progress that is occurring and provide visible evidence that positively reinforces parents for their efforts.

Teaching parents how to keep records is best done during home visits at feeding time. The first teaching-learning session should take place before the child's usual morning meal, since food is a powerful reinforcer for a hungry child for certain spoon-feeding behaviors. During this home visit and at least one more, parents will learn to observe both the child and the teaching environment and to keep records. It may be helpful if they concentrate on a select number of behaviors that occur during feeding; they should not be kept unnecessarily busy, gathering volumes of data. Parents should record the frequency of the selected behaviors, when they occur, and what the parents do in response. As the feeding program proceeds, the record-keeping focus can shift to other specific behaviors as needed. Parents should never be overwhelmed or asked to make too many observations, and they should be given an idea of how long the record keeping will continue (perhaps just for a week at periodic intervals).

Interestingly enough, most parents experience fewer feelings of anger as they begin to keep records. When they are writing down disturbing behaviors, they are ignoring the child instead of inappropriately shouting at him, and they may find that the objectionable behavior subsides simultaneously. Thus they learn that any form of parental attention, even yelling or hitting, reinforces exactly the behavior they are trying to eliminate. As parents begin to notice the effect of totally ignoring unacceptable behavior, the child care professional should explore their feelings about ignoring the child (or even just delaying feeding once or twice to promote hunger if the child does not have any health problems) in conjunction with the teaching process. Such actions may make them feel guilty or rejecting; they should be reassured that these are typical parental feelings and that these actions are necessary for effective teaching. They must also be encouraged to systematically show approval and acknowledge the child when he behaves in a desirable way.

TEACHING APPROACHES

Specific approaches to teaching self-feeding must be creatively adapted to the individual child's and parents' needs. However, the most effective approaches to teaching self-feeding have certain features in common. They all involve consistently acknowledging and approving the child's acceptable feeding behaviors and ignoring the child when he does something that is irrelevant, inappropriate, or undesirable for present teaching goals.

At the outset of a feeding session, the child should be sitting up in a comfortable, balanced position. The mother should gain the child's attention, refraining from offering food until he is looking at the food or the spoon. As the child is better able to use the spoon and bring it to his mouth, parental assistance should be decreased. The mother should praise the child, using social reinforcers such as touch, praise, and smiles as he succeeds with each of the seventeen steps in the feeding sequence. If the child cries, the mother should immediately ignore the crying behavior by turning away and simultaneously

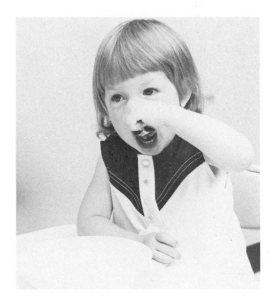

Fig. 16-6. Assessing a 2½-year-old girl feeding herself independently with a spoon.

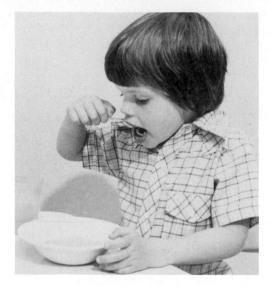

Fig. 16-7. Assessing the independent spoon-feeding skills of a 4½-year-old boy.

removing the child's food. Other unacceptable behavior such as gulping down milk, smearing food on the table, bubbling in the juice, throwing the spoon, or dropping food on the floor should be treated in the same way. The child will soon learn that inappropriate behaviors produce loss of food and praise, affection, and attention from his parents. The parents must learn to relax and be firm, gentle, and patient. The child has a better chance to succeed if he is not pushed and rushed, but he should not be allowed to play games with the parents. Practice sessions are a must, and at each one, parents should remember to teach only one

skill at a time and to watch for even the slightest amount of cooperation, effort, or improvement. As the child progressively succeeds, reinforcement will no longer be on a continuous schedule; that is, the parents will not lavishly praise the child each time he directs the spoon to his mouth and successfully swallows but will make judgments about how often to offer reinforcement (perhaps every two or three bites).

The child care professional must apply similar principles of learning theory to dealing with the parents. Each small success should be acknowledged and as the parents become more capable and the child steadily reaches objectives, the child care professional should offer less assistance. Thus parents will perceive themselves as being skillful in promoting the child's learning, even though they initially had to ask for help.

REFERENCE

1. Powell, Marcene: An analysis of behaviors to promote independent feeding skills. In Nursing in mental retardation programs. Fourth National Workshop for Nurses in Mental Retardation, University of Miami, 1967, sponsored by Children's Bureau, U.S. Dept. of Health, Education and Welfare and Child Development Center.

ADDITIONAL READINGS

Gesell, A., and Ilg, F. L.: Feeding behavior of infants, Philadelphia, 1937, J. B. Lippincott Co.

Whitney, L.: Operant learning theory: a framework deserving nursing investigation, Nurs. Res. **15:** 229-235, 1966.

Zieler, M. D., and Jervey, S. S.: Development of behavior: self-feeding, J. Consult. Psychol. **32:**164-168, 1969.

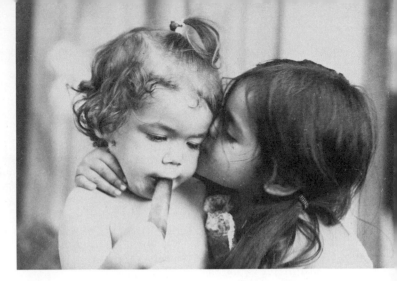

17

PARENTAL
MANAGEMENT OF
SIBLING INTERACTIONS

The addition of a new infant to a family with a young firstborn child presents a unique challenge to parental child-rearing methods. The firstborn may respond to the presence of a newborn in a number of typical ways, most of which stem from the older child's lack of experience in the developmental process of sharing his parents' exclusive attention. Parents can benefit greatly from anticipatory counseling. They can learn to expect changes in the older sibling's behaviors when a new infant is brought home and to explore their readiness to respond to them. The child care professional can provide guidance that will help prevent problems and make the adjustment easier for both the older sibling and the parents.

The child care professional can encourage parents to prepare the 2- to 3-year-old child for the coming birth of a new infant. Parents can use examples from the firstborn's own infancy to describe what babies are like. If parents plan to move the oldest child to another room or to send him to nursery school, they should do so well before the arrival of the new infant. All other changes that will affect the older child should be made several months in advance. Above all, parents should know to anticipate changes in the older sibling's behaviors when the new infant arrives.

CASE HISTORY

Before her new infant's arrival, one mother planned ahead and discussed ways to lessen the number of conflicts, mother-daughter disturbances, and problematic behaviors that the arrival of a new infant would occasion. She described to a nurse her preparation of C, her 2½-year-old daughter, for the arrival of a new infant.

Mother: I started lying down with her to take a nap. We both get a nice rest, which I need too. I just have three months to prepare her for the new one.

Nurse: How do you think she will react to the new infant?

Mother: I really don't know. I'm curious about what her reactions will be. She loves the infants in the newborn nursery. I have taken her to the hospital nursery to see the new infants. Also my sister-in-law had a baby a few months back. She really likes to see T and I've held him and fed him since he was born, and most of the time she likes to be up on my lap or she likes to be close to me. I have some ideas, mostly about bathing time and how she can be included in helping with the new baby, and she has a doll that can be washed when I'm bathing the new baby.

Nurse: It sounds like you thought of some

ways to help her and to make the transition easier.

Mother: She keeps talking about her new baby brother. You ask her where C's baby is, and she points to my stomach. She's talking about it and seems to be looking forward to it. I've even gone away for a period of 2 to 3 days to see how she will adjust to my being gone. She will probably be with her grandmother when I go to the hospital. So far she doesn't seem to mind when I'm gone. She's with people she knows, likes, and trusts.

Nurse: Have you thought of any changes to expect from C when the new baby comes?

Mother: I hope she won't go backward in her potty training. There is that possibility. She sucks her thumb and may even do it more when the baby comes. I really don't know what to expect. My husband and I both have talked about it. I think I'm going to involve her with the care of the baby. I'm planning on breast-feeding I'm going to try to involve her at feeding time. I am going to try to have her as close as possible. When I feed the baby she can be on one side of me on the couch and she will be as close as she wants to be to both of us.

Nurse: Your ideas sound appropriate.

Mother: Yes, they sound good, but until we bring the baby home, I don't know what will occur. I will wait to see what happens. It will have to wait until we bring the baby home and she sees how much attention she will have to share. That is going to be the important thing.

Nurse: You are prepared for a number of possible changes.

Mother: Yes.

Nurse: No one can really tell how a child will react, but it sounds as if you're prepared for change and are anticipating some things to be different. That in itself is important.

Mother: We've even thought of bringing something home for her, something just for her, when we bring the baby home, maybe a little doll for her.

HELPING PARENTS ANTICIPATE POTENTIAL PROBLEM AREAS

An older child may think that all has been lost to him when a new infant enters the household. The parents' attention and time ostensibly shift to the noisy intruder who requires seemingly endless feeding, diapering, bathing, clothes changing, formula mixing, holding and rocking, and kissing or other

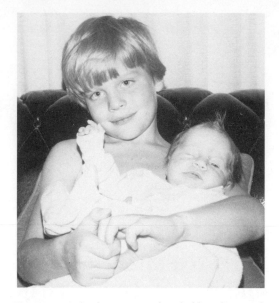

Fig. 17-1. A firstborn young boy holding his newly born sister. (Photograph by C. Spencer Powell.)

displays of affection. All these are extremely visible behaviors to the older child, who is sensitive to the loss of his parents' attention.

The firstborn may find he has to resort to extra attempts to gain even brief parental attention. Some children learn that their parents give them attention when they misbehave or act disruptively in an obviously purposeful way. Others find that whining, fretting, or fussing does not command instant attention, but that an escalated cry or piercing scream, however ill received, will. The older child may show dramatic regressive changes in toilet habits.

It is important that parents be sensitive to the range and variation of cues that signal a child's need for appropriate parental attention. Parents should become alert to the older child's behavioral manifestations such as the following:

1. Increasing attempts at gaining mother's and father's attention whether the new infant is present in the same room or absent
2. Tendency to whine, fret, and cry when asked to do a task that is routinely carried out in a positive way
3. Increased requests for help in undressing, dressing, bathing, and self-care activities
4. Requests for help in getting ready for bed
5. Tendency to resist bedtime preparation;

attempts at prolonging rituals preceding bedtime; getting out of bed

6. Tendency to suck thumb even though habit may have stopped

7. Clinging behaviors such as pulling at the mother's skirts or physically trying to direct her attention

8. Increased attempts at climbing into mother's lap or seeking affection

9. Increased use of "I can't" when asked to do something and more "why's"

10. Increased use of "no" even after the stage of accentuated negative responses

11. Shyness with family members, friends, and sometimes playmates

12. Changes in eating patterns

13. Regression in toilet-training habits

14. Imitative behaviors with dolls that replicate parents' behaviors with the new infant

15. Increased display of nurturing behaviors when playing with dolls

16. Overt signs of trying to get physically closer to mother when she is engaged in caregiving activities with the infant

17. Increases in spilling food

18. Tendency to revert to baby talk or jargon

19. Evidence of wanting to eat when the new infant is being fed

20. Outbursts of crying with tears when mother is observed to display overt signs of kissing, smiling at, laughing at, and talking baby talk with the new infant

21. General increase in dependency

22. Prolonging of time to complete a task

23. Unusual interest in playing with the new infant's toys

24. Attempts at sucking on the baby's bottle

25. Changes in play habits, toy preferences, attention span to toys, and reduced pleasure in playing alone

26. Increased requests for mother and father to play

27. Reference to self as "a baby" or "I'm little"

28. Expressions of questions that imply the child's need for reassurance

29. Reduction of exploratory behaviors

The health care professional can encourage parents to reinforce systematically some (not all) of the older child's usual behaviors such as dressing himself, helping with small chores, and responding to parental requests. These behaviors, previously taken for granted, may deteriorate with the arrival of the new sibling.

Parents should be encouraged to ignore inappropriate behaviors and find ways of planning and giving consistent forms of attention to the child who feels left out.

CASE HISTORY

In this example, the mother is attempting to deal with her first child's response to the advent of a newborn in the family. The older child is a 2½-year-old girl.

Mother: When the new little one came home, L started crying and reverted back to whining again. I was sort of concerned about this, because it was so unlike her, but thinking back on it, the new baby does cry and gets my immediate attention. L's trying this also. L's starting to cry herself to sleep again at night, which is also not normal for her; she now cries instead of going right to sleep. I don't like to have her go to sleep unhappy, but at the same time I'm not going to worry myself about it. I think it will all work out in the long run. L only cries for about 10 minutes. I don't think that's too long.

Examiner: What do you do when she reverts back to crying, whining, and crying at bedtime?

Mother: I try to ignore it. I also ask her to ask for things with the right words instead of baby talk. She thinks about it and goes about her business and comes back and asks for it if she wants it badly enough.

Examiner: It sounds like you are reinforcing her for the appropriate behaviors she had before the infant came home. That sounds very promising. It also sounds as if your ideas on ignoring her babylike behaviors are working too. That must be encouraging to you. Also, as you pointed out, you expected some of these things to occur with bringing the new infant home and expressed that it was not a surprise that these changes in L were inevitable. From what you have described, it sounds as if you're comfortable with your decisions and L is progressively showing signs of coping with the new infant in easier ways for her.

Mother: I think the most difficult thing for me was to try to reinforce her for her usual earlier behaviors which I took for granted before the baby arrived. I'm still trying. It is sometimes difficult for me to treat her like a 2-year-old. I have to remember that she's only 2. It's hard for me. She's still a child too, and that's rough. But I'm continuing to be careful about her needs every day. One of them has to wait while I attend to the other. I'm learning ways to do this.

Examiner: Are you able to find time to spend with L?

Mother: I don't have as much time as I did before, but I do spend at least 2 hours in the morning with L. I find time again just for her in the afternoon. We play with her dolls, and we play at serving tea time. She has an imagination. We pretend a lot, and I enjoy playing with her, and I don't expect any real difficulties. So far, we're doing just fine, and as long as I can find special times for L, I think things will continue to go smoothly for all of us.

Examiner: I agree with you. You have come up with some very creative, helpful ways for all of you.

ASSESSING PROBLEMS BETWEEN OLDER SIBLING AND YOUNGER INFANT

It is common for parents to seek guidance in dealing with some of the behavior patterns that have just been outlined. Ironically parents may have been unwittingly reinforcing some undesirable behaviors.

Some children learn that the best way to attract prompt parental attention is to act aggressively toward the new infant. The child, feeling jealous, does something that makes the infant cry. The mother, startled by the sudden outburst, rushes to the scene. She chastises the offender, telling him that his action was not nice, that he is not acting like a big boy, that big kids should not do such naughty things to helpless little babies, and other similar statements. The older child may be threatened or spanked. The offender may not perceive the parental response as the punishment it was intended to be. Significantly, the mother has established eye contact with him, talked to him, come near him, and perhaps even touched him. What is more, the mother spent more time with the older sibling than with the infant, who is at this moment crying. The parents have allowed a pattern to be established. An escalation of acts of aggression by the older child against the new infant begins. The first child may continue to hit, scratch, slap, or remove favorite objects from the infant. Aggressive behavior has paid off.

A mother seeking solutions to problems of aggression can be asked the following questions: When is the younger infant in distress? Can she leave the two children unattended in a room and feel secure and confident that no

rescue efforts will be necessary? A mother can be queried about when her attention is needed, the times the younger child begins to cry, how often the older sibling is observed to interact with the younger child during a problematic period of time, and how long the problem lasts. The mother also needs to express the measures she has thought of and tried and what response has been most effective in reducing the number of incidents in which the older child uses aggression against the infant.

Parents, if genuinely concerned, willingly keep records to identify the source of the problem to alleviate its future occurrence. An analysis of the record generally indicates when sibling interactions begin to become problems, the rationale for the older child's behavior, and what the older child is gaining. Parents can learn more effective ways to lessen the older child's special efforts to gain parental attention.

KEEPING A SIBLINGS' INTERACTIONS RECORD

A record for obtaining objective, accurate information on the interactions that occur between two or more siblings and parents is desirable before appropriate intervention can be planned.

A record is helpful in obtaining information about one child who displays problematic behaviors toward a brother or sister in his household. The record also points out parents' behaviors in response to children's behaviors. It is helpful to have parents document data on children's behaviors, the times these behaviors occur, the number of times a parent interacts with one sibling, and the length of specific behavioral interactions. The parents should be prepared to record the children's behavior for an entire day, from the time the children wake up until they go to bed, to get an impression of rates of behavior. Parents should ideally record each time that one child hurts or hits another sibling, when one child teases a sibling, and when one child takes food or toys or any possession from another brother or sister. The record should indicate when one child quarreled or fought with a brother or sister, when one child refused to share toys with a sibling, if one child showed jealousy when another child received parental approval or attention, and when one child competed with a sibling for parental attention. In addition, the record should indicate the beginning and end of a temper outburst of each child.

Parents can draw in the following symbols to

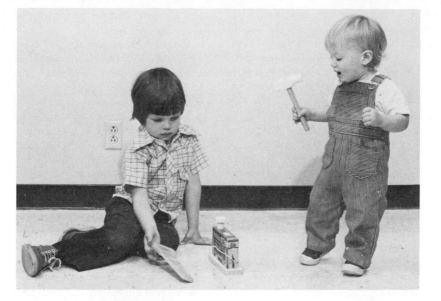

Fig. 17-2 Assessing the social and play interactions between an 11-month-old child and a 4½-year-old.

indicate a happy ☺ or unhappy ☹ face and show perceived mood changes of each child during morning, daytime, evening, or night. The parents' faces should be drawn next to the child's face to indicate mood changes. The parents' faces should be proportionately larger than their children's faces to distinguish differences between the two. Faces should be drawn in when a behavioral interaction is recorded between a sibling or parent.

Parents should be instructed to comment about anything unusual or major changes that occurred for them or their children on the days that the record is being kept.

It is advisable for parents to keep a record for 5 to 7 days to determine if behavioral trends are occurring or if patterns exist before implementing a program of change.

Parents might designate the children as "A" or "B" before beginning record keeping. If parents report that one of two or three siblings has problematic behaviors, this child is designated as "A." The other child with whom the problem child interacts is designated as "B." If there are other children, they should be designated as "C," "D," "E," and so on. Parents can be advised to write in comments that they think are appropriate for consideration in planning ways to alter behavioral interactions.

In reviewing these records with the parents, the health care professional can acknowledge the precise recording of interactions between siblings. Parents receive confirmation that indeed the concern is one that demands attention to prevent it from escalating and becoming more frustrating for all concerned. Generally, a record of aggressive behavior from the older sibling shows that parents are not in the same room at the time of a sibling interaction problem; that the older child disturbs the infant when the parents are not looking; and that when the younger infant does cry out or vocalize distress, the parents rush in and usually interact with the older child first. Once the parents realize that a general pattern of interactions seem to occur, they can begin considering ways of altering their responses or choosing different ways to react to the child's actions. Once the parents begin to observe, keeping records is the opportunity for them to document what they thought was happening.

HELPING PARENTS PLAN APPROPRIATE ATTENTION FOR CHILDREN

After behavioral patterns are identified, parents can be encouraged to express what the child's behaviors mean to them. Parents can contribute to the planning of different and more effective ways of responding to these common behavioral manifestations. They will gain confidence by learning that their child is responding normally if he is receiving less parental attention.

Parents should be supported in their observational efforts. The child care professional can ask what worries them most about the child's behavior and what they have thought of to produce more appropriate kinds of interactions? The parents might admit that they tend to give the child more attention when he is exhibiting undesirable forms of behavior. Once parents have realized that they are contributing to the maintenance of a problem, there is a greater chance of success in giving *planned* parental attention to their children. Those occasions deserving parental attention are when the child is playing quietly and nicely with the younger sibling rather than when is he is grabbing at toys, breaking well-established rules, whining, fussing, demanding attention from the mother when she is talking on the telephone, or reverting to less mature developmental habits such as in toilet training. Frequently, it is necessary to stress to parents that it may be difficult to interrupt routine activities to give a child attention when he is not behaving disruptively. A smile or touch, however, signals definite parental approval for desirable behaviors. Most parents find it effective to plan special times to give attention to the older sibling. The older child gradually learns to share the parents' attention as he has learned to share toys, to wait his turn, and to become increasingly tolerant of delays. It can be helpful to allow the older child to pick out the activity, game, or specific event he

would most like or prefer during his special time with his parents.

Parents can be encouraged to praise the older sibling throughout the day when he does something the parents approve of, even if this behavior previously has been taken for granted. Parents can comment on how quietly the child is playing, how nicely he is picking up his toys, and the fact that he is going to take his nap, or is doing activities to help his mother or father. Occasionally it is difficult, even overwhelming, for parents to ignore dramatic regressive changes such as in toileting habits. Parents may need special preparation and guidance to ignore soiling, wetting during the day, or wetting at night. The degree to which parents can ignore these less desirable and less mature habits while making special efforts to reinforce the socially desirable and positive behaviors the older child continues to show can influence the child's rate of success in adjusting to the new situation.

Parents must believe that they are doing the best they are capable of and are succeeding in preventing problems. Their needs for recognition and reinforcement about their adequacy, parental competence and success should be taken into account.

Most importantly parents must learn to anticipate and to be more accepting, more realistic, and more comfortable with temporary changes

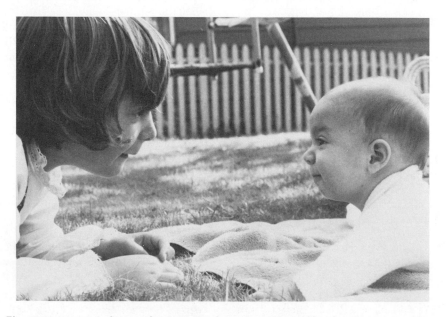

Fig. 17-3. Assessing the social interactions between a 5-year-old girl and her new sibling.

that occur. Parents must be reassured that their child's changes are natural reactions; children are sensitive to a reduction of the amounts of attention, approval, and affection they are accustomed to receiving on an exclusive basis from their parents. Parents should be assured that although it may not be easy to accept, the situation will not last forever. The older child is going through the developmental process of learning to cope and needs feedback from the parents on how well he is doing. The parents may also find it comforting and a relief to be told that they are responding appropriately to a common parent-child challenge. Parents can be encouraged that they are learning appropriate ways to solve new concerns and that change can occur for the benefit of both the parents and their child.

Parents' empathetic responses and sensitivity will help ease the degree of difficulty that the older child may experience. Parents can learn to plan different times that are specifically and specially put aside for the older sibling so that he can be reassured that he is as highly valued, much loved, and cared about as he ever was.

AIDING PARENTS WITH CONCERNS ABOUT SIBLING RIVALRY

There is considerable stereotyping, confusion, and haphazard approaches to what parents and others refer to as "sibling rivalry." The usual, instant, advice received by parents is to give equal time to both children. This is impossible. The care of a new infant requires certain maternal activities at specific times that simply cannot be omitted. An older sibling who is being upstaged by a younger infant needs his mother's and father's extra attention, not equal attention. Giving extra attention requires consideration of the older child's developmental attainments, unique characteristics, and behaviors that indicate when he needs attention most. Can the parents realistically give attention when the older child needs it? Can they keep records if the older child's behavior becomes troublesome, bothersome, or annoying to them, particularly before it reaches unnecessary disproportionate levels such as when the child demands attention regardless of the consequences? Once parents have explored these aspects, they can discuss their degree of concern, decide what response seems best, and respond to both or all children at more appropriate times with specific goals in mind. A reasonable goal under these circumstances would be to respond in such a way that

helps the older child experience a feeling of undivided parental attention and one that is viewed as a positive, nurturing experience for both the child and parent.

Problems with giving adequate parental attentions to a sibling who thinks he is being deprived of parent recognition are often approached in unsystematic ways. Generally, the parents are told to reinforce the older sibling's worth more often, to give equal time, and, most frequently, to give equal attention. Some parents are even advised to have the older 2½- or 3-year-old child help care for the newborn. In reality and in consideration of safety factors, is it fair, safe, or reasonable to impart such advice to parents? Most 3-year-old children cannot assume responsibility for any of the usual caregiving activities required for newborns. What appropriate kinds of activities can a 3-year-old child participate in to care for a newborn? It is important to help parents get away from setting unrealistic goals. It can be unfair to ask a mother to breast-feed her newborn and at the same time

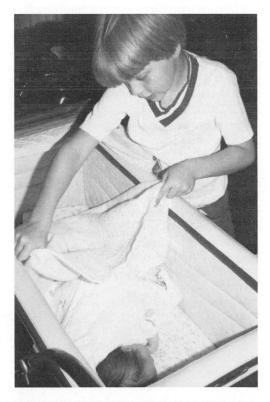

Fig. 17-4. Assessing the sibling interactions of the firstborn with the newborn infant. (Photograph by C. Spencer Powell.)

talk to, amuse, entertain, and give an older sibling attention that he needs. Meeting the needs of both children at the same time simply may not be realistic for any mother.

If parents express excessive alarm, concern, disturbance, anxiety, or frustration with behavioral changes of a child that shift to less mature forms of behavior, it may be helpful for the child care professional to remind and reassure them of the child's previous developmental accomplishments. Parents can be shown the results of the latest DDST, the results obtained from the Developmental Profile, or other assessment results which have indicated that the child is capable of age-related developmental attainments. The child care professional can point out positive features of the older child. The needs of the parents and not the child's changes may be the most appropriate focus of attention. Parents who are experiencing difficulty in accepting less mature forms of behaviors in their children may find it difficult to stop pressing their children to conform in the usual ways. Parents who experience this difficulty need emotional support for themselves; their strengths can be pointed out. The parents may not be able to evaluate their own flexibility. They may find it encouraging to know that they and the older sibling are in fact coping well with the new demands made on them and are responding nicely to new time schedules. They may be surprised to learn they are showing visible signs of coping, making decisions that are appropriate to the problems confronting them, and placing priorities in perspective.

Most importantly, parents should be advised and encouraged to find ways to relax, to meet some of their needs, and to take it easier on themselves and the older sibling. They should learn not to expect so much of themselves during stressful times and to realize that with continued efforts, routines may return to normal. The child care professional can point out that parents can profit from this learning experience. It can be pointed out that they will learn new facets about themselves, discover new ways to problem solve, and may even find that the changes they make are for the better.

Occasionally parents get enmeshed in networks of negative cycles and describe only the difficulties, trials, or frustrating events that occur. It can be helpful to ask the parents if they have experienced anything positive. Have they found a new approach or gained a new perspective? Parents deserve abundant credit for the strengths they demonstrate, the changes they effect, and the investments they make in changing and maintaining more appropriate kinds of behavior.

CASE HISTORY

Following is a mother's account of the experiences and difficulties she encountered and solved with sibling rivalry between a 3½-year-old boy and a 21-month-old girl. Both children were active and well; each had excellent test results with both the DDST and Developmental Profile. Each had reached developmental landmarks ahead of their chronological age and lived in an environment that consistently met their individual developmental needs. The parents were eager to do what was correct for both children at each stage of their development. The children were regularly taken for well-child examinations, and the mother in particular was well read and well versed on the best ways to rear children.

The mother started by telling the child care professional who was counseling her that both her children were bright and active and that she saw no problems with either one. She did have concerns about their interactions, however. She began to describe how much she dearly loved T, her 3½-year-old son: "My main problem with him, I think . . . if I didn't have the two of them, he would be just terrific. The sibling rivalry between the two of them has been rather difficult for me in the past to accept and to understand and, quite frankly, to deal with."

The mother reported that she had tried different approaches and that the sibling rivalry situation was improving. She commented that people "tell me that T will grow out of it and that was about the main hope that I could cling to, that he would grow out of this sibling rivalry."

The mother was asked to define specifically what she meant by "conflict" and "sibling rivalry." Her explanation was that when her 21-month-old daughter R was born, T was interested in her for about 6 to 8 months. Then the mother started noticing that T would push R down and bite her. She emphasized that he was a terrible biter for awhile and obviously jealous of R. The mother was surprised.

The problem began to increase, and she sought help from her pediatrician and a psychiatrist. She remembered that R was 9 or 10 months old and T was about 2½ years old at this time. The child care professional made the supportive statement that the mother had experienced this concern for a long time and that the length of time in itself was a draining factor and had probably been fatiguing for her. The mother agreed. The child care professional commented that it must be frustrating to have tried a variety of techniques without success, and that would be fairly overwhelming, fatiguing, and discouraging for most mothers. The mother agreed heartily.

The mother asserted that T was beginning to grow out of the behavior and was beginning to show love and protection for R. "He's developing concepts of love and protection for his sister," she said, "as we expect children should naturally feel for each other."

She was encouraged because T no longer "sees her as just an object getting in his way." He no longer "sees her as stealing my love and doesn't see her as an object of frustration for him," she added. In support, the child care professional said, "That must be a relief for you, finally." The mother agreed.

When asked to describe how T indicated to his mother that R was stealing her love from him and was an object of frustration, the mother recalled that she had reached her conclusions in a variety of ways. She recalled that she watched him hit R. T would demand more and more attention from her generally when she was busy. He would take toys from R, usually something that she wanted. The mother recounted that she could not leave the two of them in a room unattended and was never comfortable with the idea. T would typically push R down to the floor, bite her, and inevitably hit her with a toy. He would find the perfect time to rush over and push her down and bite her. By that time the mother was fearful of R's safety. She mentioned that 3 or 4 weeks earlier he had broken a large mixing bowl over R's head. However, she was primarily concerned with the fact that he was a biter.

The mother was asked to describe her reaction to the interactions. On seeing T act aggressively toward R, she spanked him. Referring to the number of books she had read on child care, the mother said she had learned that "you just don't let this kind of behavior happen." She had decided to put a stop to it.

After reading the books, she tried spanking T when he hit or hurt R enough to make her cry out loud. She separated the children by placing each in his room and thought that would resolve the problem. "No matter how angry I got or the amount of frustration I felt," she said,

"it didn't make any difference in T's behavior. In fact, one of the things that bothered me the most was that although I had decided this had to stop, it didn't phase T at all. It did not stop the immediate problem." The child care professional replied, "It's difficult to learn that just thinking something doesn't stop, start, or change it. That can be difficult for all of us to accept at times."

The mother described the ways she responded to R when T hit her. Generally, she would just pick her up and love her. But she added, "If I got angry or too frustrated, I would just let her cry, give up, and ignore her." She was asked to clarify what she meant by "ignoring" R. The mother answered that she had to ignore R because the situation happened all the time and if she did not ignore R, she would be holding her all day long.

The mother was asked to recall how often this behavior occurred throughout the day. She replied that the frequency of this behavior depended on how busy T was and what his attention was directed to at any particular time. The mother said he tended to hit R out of boredom, anger, or frustration or if the mother did not pay immediate attention to him. She recalled a variety of reasons for T bothering R in general terms. She mentioned that T's behavior of aggressive acts toward R occurred three or four times in a half hour if he were left to his own devices.

The child care professional said, "I get the impression you have tried ignoring, distraction, separation, spanking, and reasoning with T and R." The mother agreed and mentioned that she had found another excellent book and had become convinced that "my punishment was not going to change things, so I stopped spanking T. Spanking wasn't working anyway. I started putting him in his room, and he wouldn't stay there." When asked if she were comfortable with this approach, she said, "No, because I felt guilty. The book said I should isolate him; it didn't say to lock him in, but I did for about 5 minutes at a time. That seemed to help and I was encouraged for awhile. I felt encouraged because it was something positive I could do. I was no longer frustrated to such an extent as I had been. It was something I could actually do."

The mother added, "I think a lot of this problem is myself, and my feelings were involved. I began to feel badly that I could not stop him from hurting her nor at the same time could I feel I had the ability or strength to turn him into a nice, sweet, loving little brother."

The mother was reassured that these indeed were difficult and painful ideas to think about but that it was natural for a conscientious mother to try everything and end up feeling disappointed, angry, and uncomfortable with little or no change. It was a difficult process for her to experience and a painful one at that. The child care professional pointed out that it was healthy that she could discuss the thoughts and feelings she had experienced. She was supported for her efforts at continuing to try new ideas, ways, and approaches and for her ability to cope effectively with her anger and frustrations. She was reminded that no mother is expected to be perfect and come up with all the right answers and that it was indeed appropriate for her to seek help. She agreed to keep records for 1 week on how often T was observed to hit, push, bite, take a toy, or make R cry. She was surprised to find out that T's aggressive behaviors were occurring as often as fifty-nine times a day.

The mother said she had started using a kitchen timer that she would set for 10 minutes while T was left in his room. She said that occasionally the time in which he was in his room seemed infinite and that the timer helped relieve her thoughts that she was torturing or punishing him excessively. She emphasized that he did not like being in his room and would kick on the door, write on the door with crayons, throw objects all over his room, cry, scream, and hammer on the door until the time was up. The mother was supported for her strength in ignoring the behavior and for expressing her feelings.

She was told that it is difficult for mothers to deal with behaviors such as T was demonstrating, particularly on a long-term basis, and that most mothers do have feelings about taking measures that make both themselves and their children unhappy. The mother was reassured that her feelings were natural, to be expected, and appropriate for the experiences that she and T were working on.

The mother began to share how much more optimistic she had recently become, and she thought that both she and T were progressing. She said that T's aggressive behaviors were decreasing because of some of her own ideas and some that her pediatrician had suggested to her. These suggestions included keeping T busier with games, play toys, and Playdough

that the mother had just purchased. She had some new felt tip pens he could use and mentioned that they were starting swimming lessons.

The mother could not decide whether the improvement had occurred because T was older or because of a combination of measures she had been taking. She thought she had been in a better frame of mind and did not want to blame it on herself. She was supported for not wanting to blame the situation on herself or anyone else and was told that blame did not change or improve the problem.

The mother said that she would think her children were terrible at the end of the day and felt guilty about feeling this way. She did describe, however, how positive she felt toward them in the morning, how she thought they were cute and nice, and how much easier it was for her to tolerate just about anything. She would start yelling at them at about 4 or 5 PM and find it exceptionally difficult to respond in any way but with a loud voice. She was reminded that sometimes mothers are normally accepting and at other times less accepting of their children. It was also pointed out that most mothers get discouraged with children's frustrating behaviors at the end of a day, particularly if the mother has spent all day entertaining them to avoid conflict.

She said it had helped her talk with other mothers of 3-year-old children. She had three or four friends with whom she could talk at length and wished she had more friends to discuss matters with. One friend in particular was helpful to her because she too had a 3-year-old boy. The mother said that when she went to this friend's house, "I find there are boys just like mine, just as naughty, juvenile, and bratty, and it makes me feel as if I haven't failed." She described her 21-month-old girl as easier to take care of and said she was sweet and nice, mentioning that "maybe it's because I ignore her when she's with T." She said that 2-year-old children were frustrating for all mothers. The child care professional said, "It must be comforting to talk with these mothers of similar-aged children and find out that they experience the same kinds of ideas, situations, frustrations, and gratifications that you do with both of your children." The mother's response to this comment was positive, but she did mention how nice it would be if one could be absolutely certain about what one did with her children. One friend acted as if she did not have any doubts about her child-rearing decisions. The child care professional said that most parents want to do the right and best action for their children and find successful actions that they can take credit for. "One of my problems is that my pediatrician complains," the mother said, "that I'm consistently inconsistent." She was asked to clarify that statement. "You're supposed to have rules and I've been very lenient," she said. "I have very few rules."

In response to her statements about inconsistency and the importance of being consistent, the child care professional emphasized that there had been improvement in T's behaviors in the last month. From what the mother had reported, there were definite signs that she was taking measures that were consistent such as placing T in his room, setting times, and keeping him in his room in spite of his begging to be let out. It was also pointed out that if the mother was observing more consistency in T's behavior, it appeared that her expectations were clearer, and that she was increasingly following through with her objectives in reducing T's aggressive behaviors toward R. The child care professional stressed that it seemed obvious that she was improving in communicating to T that there were limits for his behavior, and his decreases in behavior seemed to indicate that her messages of what she distinctly did approve of and absolutely would not tolerate were indeed getting through. Although this still was a difficult learning process for both of them, the child care professional said, "It's sound for mothers to let their children know what is all right and what is not allowed. Children eventually learn that there are rules and that they must respond to these in a gradual and increasingly mature way." It was pointed out that this was a learning experience from which both seemed to be gaining.

There was considerable emphasis given to the process of learning that was occurring. The child care professional emphasized that children generally learn first and in gradual doses what behaviors are permissible, where, and with whom. It was also emphasized that occasionally it is difficult for parents to stand back and look objectively at what is being transacted. The mother agreed.

She admitted that when she was rested and in a good mood or in a good frame of mind, T's behavior was not so distressing to her. Asked if she ever found time just for herself, she admitted that she was getting out at least 3

evenings a week and that exercising was helping her clear her mind. She said that getting out regularly helped take the pressures off and gave her relief from chronic frustration at home. She was strongly encouraged to continue this routine because she had needs of her own that were important. The child care professional told her that her needs counted too and meeting them on a regular basis was extremely important in helping her feel better about herself.

There was a discussion about whether her husband was a source of help, support, and agreement on the approaches that she was trying to decrease T's aggressive behaviors toward R. She enthusiastically responded that her husband was a good helpmate and was supportive of her. He told her that he thought she was around too much, serving as T's playmate too much, and that she was promoting an excessive amount of dependency as a playmate for him.

In describing a typical day, the mother reported that T watched television in the morning and that she took him out between 10 and 11 AM for errands or visiting. They played various games throughout most of the afternoon. The mother added that "he wants to play very badly with me between 4 and 5 PM."

She said, "T is very fond of R in his own way and wants her to play with him. He drags her around, pushes her around, and gives her a lot of directions but essentially shows he wants to include her in his play." She mentioned that maybe he was giving clues that he needs other children of his age with whom to play. The child care professional agreed with the mother's astute speculation.

The mother received acknowledgment for her remark that T and R played together at times. The child care professional said, "So what you're saying is that there isn't a continuous clash between them. That must be encouraging to you. It must be a relief that they can increasingly interact in positive ways." The mother was enthusiastic about this new and recent observation of hers. She also mentioned that the baby-sitter reported how protective T was of R and that made her happy to know that they were not always in conflict and always experiencing unhappy times with each other.

In acknowledging the mother's observations, the child care professional said, "It must be increasingly encouraging for you to see that change is occurring and that the situation you've experienced in the past is lessening and that it is not going to last forever. It must also make you feel better and have more comfort in knowing that you can effectively find approaches to try to change such unhappy experiences, and that as a matter of fact, you dealt with a difficult situation and had the strength to persevere." The mother replied, "I don't want to take all the credit. He's just growing up a little. I've done some things, but I've also been waiting for him to grow up and mature."

The child care professional commented that there had been at least a year of waiting for change to occur and that it had not been easy for either T, the mother, or R. In fact, at times the experience had worsened and had become increasingly difficult.

Again the child care professional emphasized that children and parents learn together. Parents find that there is a process involved in adjusting to each other's needs. They learn that they have more strengths than they generally acknowledge. Being a parent is not always an easy task. Children are individuals and respond in different ways to situations that parents arrange. It was agreed that T had learned how his mother responded to him, and she had learned new and better ways to interact with and respond to his developmental need for firm, consistent follow-through with limit setting. The mother agreed that up to now the most important discovery she had made was that she was getting ideas about how to carry out something once she defined it as an objective.

The mother said she did not enjoy having to chastise T constantly and pointed out that "he's fun to play with and he's not always beating R up." She emphasized that she has tried to show him that she enjoyed playing with him.

The mother was asked how often T had been placed in his room in the previous 4 days, and she reported a significant number of incidents that were incompatible with the positive report she was giving. Since his rate of being sent to his room was as high as twenty-two times a day, the mother was asked if she would be willing to try another approach that would involve a systematic effort and a consistent attempt to ignore T for any undesirable behaviors such as taking R's blanket or toys, touching, hitting, or any act of aggression toward her. The mother agreed to comply with the new behavioral approach.

In reviewing the mother's report of progress to date, it should be remembered that this mother recorded fifty-nine incidents the first day of T's either pushing, hitting, touching, pulling hair, biting, grabbing toys, knocking down, or hitting R with hard-surfaced objects.

The number of incidents toward R decreased gradually. When asked to carry through with a new program, the mother was able to do the following:

1. Ignore T completely when he exhibited aggressive behaviors toward R, with no looks in his direction, and to go immediately to R to soothe her, comfort her, lavish her with kisses, embrace and hold her, and walk about the room with her, making no mention of broken toys, glass, or furniture or the event that had occurred

2. Not to talk with T after the aggression toward R occurred, to offer no threats, to refrain from trying to reason with him, or to threaten isolation in his room

The number of aggressive acts dropped dramatically to fifteen per day and further downward to an average of nine acts per day.

The mother found the improved atmosphere easier to cope with but thought it easier to follow through immediately by sending T to his room and setting the timer. Twice the mother went in, talked with him, and apologized for having to put him in his room. Each time the disruptive incidents increased rapidly.

Finally, the mother found it easiest and most effective to remove herself completely from both children for 10 to 15 minutes. This proved the most successful strategy that she used. The number of aggressive incidents toward R dropped to zero for periods as long as 5 days. On one occasion, the mother simply walked away and out of sight of both children. Both stood and watched as their cherished, most treasured, and choice supply of reinforcers moved precisely and determinedly away from them.

T watched as his mother left. She did not look back. This turned out to be effective in teaching him that he had a number of valuable reinforcers to lose simultaneously. These included his mother's soothing voice pleading with him to be a sweet, loving, nice brother to his little sister; her smiles and praises when he made efforts to play with R; and all the attention he was accustomed to receiving when he was behaving or acting in unsafe, aggressive ways toward his little sister.

In reviewing the situation from beginning to end, the mother commented that she had learned that spanking does not work except to get a child's immediate attention if he is stepping in front of a car or balking at attempts to dress him. This mother thought that isolation was the best solution to interrupting, disruptive behaviors between children. She also concluded that yelling, talking, reasoning, and spanking were not effective with T. However, being cut off from his mother's attention "did get to him."

The child care professional and mother also discussed the value of documenting behavior. The child care professional asked the mother, "In what ways was writing helpful to you?" The mother replied, "I get ideas but it's difficult to pinpoint exactly when or how often something happens unless you write it down. If you're in a bad mood, it seems that things are happening all the time. There's nothing you can do to stop it. When you're in a good mood; it seems easier to tolerate and it's easier to write it down. The doctor said you should write down rules too. The first time I wrote it down I had no idea it was as bad as it was. It happened fifty-nine times. To see it on paper in black and white, it helps give a gauge of how often it happens. If you ask for help, you only have a subjective way of describing it. You can't be as objective in describing it as you can with numbers, You think you're consistent, but if you see it in black and white, it's not that way at all."

The child care professional responded to the mother's statement as follows: "It is my opinion that you used isolation appropriately because you tried a variety of techniques over a long period of time, and, furthermore, it worked in helping both T and R." When the child care professional said, "You were concerned about R's safety," the mother answered, "Yes, she had bruises all over her from his hitting her and biting her." The child care professional continued, "You tried a number of techniques and gave several alternatives to your young boy who was hurting his sister on a high-frequency basis. His behavior had reached a point where he was biting and you were fearful. He escalated his behavior also as you tried to reason with him. You eventually found approaches that worked for him as well as for yourself. I have the feel-

ing that you're feeling better about the changes; that you are encouraged with progress. You learned that the behavioral problems were something you could successfully deal with. You learned that a concern doesn't have to go on forever. You feel encouraged; you feel secure about it; you feel positive about what you've accomplished. You learned to spend more appropriate time with him, such as playing with him. This is a common experience that happens with children of R's and T's age."

The final discussions about these behavioral interactions focused on the mother's perception's of the steady progress that had been made. She emphasized that she found it helpful to realize that "he's growing up, which is something I never thought was forthcoming." The mother accepted the child care professional's statements that, "You probably have learned you can find effective ways of responding to his unique needs and at the same time find it positive to know that you are making correct and accurate decisions based on facts which you gathered. You can also look forward to doing things that are effective, successful, and are positive approaches to the different needs he will experience with increasing chronological age, experiences, and successes with different tasks and events."

The mother closed by commenting, "One of my girlfriends was so surprised to learn for herself that you have to be more than just nice to your children. You can't just love them. You also find out that you have needs of your own to meet, and it's OK to find ways to meet them."

SUGGESTED READINGS

Cecil, Henry S.: The preschool age. In Green, Morris, and Haggerty, Robert J., editors: Ambulatory pediatrics, Philadelphia, 1968, W. B. Saunders Co.

Prugh, Dave G.: The pre-school child. In Stuart, Harold C., and Prugh, Dave G.: The healthy child: his physical, psychological, and social development, Cambridge, Mass., 1962, Harvard University Press.

Smart, Mollie S., and Smart, Russell C.: Children: development and relationships, New York, 1972, The Macmillan Co.

Spock, Benjamin: Baby and child care, New York, 1972, Pocket Books.

18

HELPING PARENTS
SOLVE SLEEP PROBLEMS
OF CHILDREN

Sleep problems, like other concerns that parents present, require the documentation of behaviors of the child and parents. Since sleeping can be observed, measured, and recorded, it can accurately be described in rates and cycles. It has definite patterns that emerge and change usually in response to environmental events. Sleep problems are increased, decreased, or eliminated on the basis of their cause. Parents need to learn that their general responses to problematic behaviors exacerbate or minimize their child's sleep problems.

The start of a sleep problem can stem from physical, physiological, environmental, or behavioral causes or from expectations and attitudes conveyed by caregivers. Whatever its cause, the sleep problem can quickly escalate to unnecessary levels.

ANTICIPATORY GUIDANCE
ABOUT SLEEP PROBLEMS OF INFANTS
AND CHILDREN

The solving of a sleep problem can be influenced by anticipatory guidance that takes into account the parents' realistic expectations of the child's abilities to change or conform, their knowledge of the range of sleep periods that are characteristic of certain age periods, and their

ability to collect objective data on an individual child's behaviors related to sleep.

The preparation that parents receive before problematic behaviors occur greatly enhances their ability to deal with them. Parents who know in advance what to expect from a child feel more adequate and certain about how to respond appropriately to their children's behaviors associated with sleep. It is important that parents be supported for every effort they make to assess their child's needs, to attend to these needs in a brief manner, and then to cease further parental attention once the child's safety is assured. It is vital that parents not inadvertently reinforce sleeplessness.

SLEEP CHARACTERISTICS OF
INFANTS AND CHILDREN

During the first eight months, an infant devises his own methods of falling asleep. The infant may suck his thumb or rock in his crib. Usually a bottle before bedtime or being held in a parent's arms is sufficient in helping an infant go to sleep. During the first year, it is common for infants to awaken during the night. Some infants amuse themselves and readily go back to sleep. Generally, parents do have to intervene to help an infant get back to sleep.

If an infant requires attention during the night, it may be due to colic or an unusual change in a family's routine. The infant may need to be consoled under these circumstances.[1]

By 2 years of age, children go to bed but may make a number of requests once in bed. It is reasonable that a certain amount of the child's requests be attended to, but parents must set limits to avoid having the situation get out of hand.

The rapidity of success in reducing the amount of the child's requests that are attended to, the number of rituals that are carried out, and the length of time the child prolongs the parent's attention depends on the degree to which both parents expect postbedtime demands. Parents must be able to carry through consistently with their plan to ignore the child's unreasonable demands once they have given attention to certain rituals and requests agreed on in advance. Battle[1] suggests that if parents are not prepared sufficiently for this expected behavior, they may view the child as "bad." Parents may blame themselves because the child needs extra attention.

By the age of 2½ years, children may make increased efforts at prolonging the bedtime ritual.[1] This is a sign of protesting change. It is important that parents allow a certain amount of time for rituals, knowing in advance that the child's behaviors may occur, and decide that they are going to be decisive about withdrawing their attention at a certain point. Otherwise the child can quickly increase the number of rituals he practices.

After the age of 3 years, there are fewer problems with children resisting bedtime preparation and getting to sleep. The occurrence of night awakenings, however, is not unusual. Night terrors may cause the child to sit up and call for his parents, but he will not necessarily recall what he dreamed about.[1] He will go back to sleep. There are variations in how a child may behave. He may lie quietly, get up, or seek parental comfort.

Nightmares are dreams that frighten and awaken children at night. They are associated with fears that the child may have during the day. The child usually remembers the dream but can be distracted from the discomfort of its memory.

Head-banging or rocking between the ages of 1 and 4 years is not uncommon and may be related to tension releases.[1] Both behaviors usually occur as the child is going to sleep and

are related both to age and individuality of children.

Waking once a week or more between midnight and 5 AM constitutes a sleep problem, according to Battle.[1] Ordinarily a sleep problem is defined by the number of times the child awakens during the night. It is important to determine if the parents are overanxious due to previous experiences with trauma related to sleep.

Parents require information that children's sleep needs are highly individual. Children's sleep needs change with increasing age. Children give readily identifiable clues about their fatigue levels that indicate the need for bedtime or a nap. Parents can learn to recognize and respond to each child's need for sleep.

Parents can be counseled about sleep difficulties on the basis of environmental events. Frequently, parents express the concern that the cause of a sleep problem originates with the child. It is important that parents learn that the environment plays a major role in promoting or decreasing difficulties that are experienced by young children. Parents also need to recognize that sleep problems can be modified as events in the environment are changed. Parents can be encouraged that their changing responses to a child's sleep patterns can result in the disappearance of the problem. Rearrangement or change of the environment can be a powerful force in reducing sleep problems.

There is increased awareness of the need to build up and maintain the self-confidence of the parents about their ability to set limits. Parents need encouragement for their attempts at setting reasonable limits; they can benefit from discussions on how setting reasonable limits affects them. Do they see themselves as too permissive or not permissive enough or too rigid and expecting too much? Have they been successful with setting limits on other kinds of behaviors?

RELATIONSHIP OF SLEEP PROBLEMS TO PARENTAL RESPONSES

Most sleep problems, according to Illingworth,[2] are related to parents. Illingworth relates that parental overanxiety in general and overpermissiveness specifically are closely related to sleep problems of the older infant and child. The concept of providing the infant and child with an abundant supply of parental love, appropriate attention, and trust in the environment can be encouraged. Illingworth stresses the importance of curbing parental overreaction to a fussy infant or responding to the slightest whimper in an infant. He states that parents are prone to respond to the first sounds and act too quickly with consolation measures, possibly overreacting by picking the infant up, rocking, holding, and taking the child into their bed. Parents may report that the infant or child does not sleep well, but an in-depth inquiry may reveal that they wake up to check the infant and keep the child awake by constant checking.

Illingworth[2] states that parents tend to try a variety of methods to entice a crying child to sleep. As the parents' efforts escalate, so does the infant's or child's efforts to keep the parents' attention. The parents may sit and read stories, play games, lie down next to the child, and eventually end up with the child in their bed after all other efforts have failed.

According to Illingworth, parental over-anxiety is connected with a number of factors that were present before the child's birth. Some factors might be the parents' personalities, a long wait until marriage and conception, advanced maternal age, or difficult labor or delivery. Parental overanxiety is not uncommon in the case of an only child or a delayed yet unplanned second child conceived long after the last child. Parental anxiety may also be generated by worrying about the child considered delicate due to premature birth.

IMPORTANCE OF PARENTS' AND CHILDREN'S HABITS AND THEIR EFFECT ON SLEEP PROBLEMS

Habit formation is a major contributing cause of most sleep-related problems. The child originally may have experienced some physical distress and was picked up and consoled. The child makes the connection between crying and being held and continues to be successful in generating and perpetuating pleasant consoling measures by his parents.

Parental attention, given with appropriate consideration of the child's needs to learn acceptable habits, and reasonable loving discipline constitute the major ingredients for reducing and eliminating sleep disturbances. Picking up a child at the first whimper is not encouraged. Illingworth[2] does point out that when a child wakens with a sudden scream, it could signal physical distress, vomiting, strangling, or nightmares and demands immediate attention. According to Illingworth, parents frequently fail to allow their children a chance

to go to sleep. They play with the child, sit with him, visit his room, and thus prolong the child's wakeful state. It is unequivocally an error, Illingworth states, for parents to take the child into their room as a measure to get the child to sleep. He emphasizes the constructive use of firm and positive limit setting to reduce sleep problems that could have been created by the parents originally.

ASSESSMENT OF PARENTS' NEEDS

If parents experience anxieties about bedtime problems or management, the child care professional should explore their needs, feelings, and views rather than focusing on those of the child. Are the parents asking for help? Have they initiated any change? What is most distressing to them? What are their expectations in regard to the length of time it will take to decrease and terminate the concern? Are they trying to solve other problems concerning parent-child interactions concurrently? What would they prefer to see changed first? Can they describe some approaches they think might work? Are both parents in agreement about alternatives to change interactions with the child at bedtime? Is this a convenient time to attempt changes? Are major stressful events occurring in the family's life? Can the parents see their own strengths in identifying concerns and in being able to discuss them openly and frankly? Are the parents willing to keep records of both the child's behavior and their own responses? It is important that parents learn to feel comfortable in ignoring a child who is presenting certain sleep problems. Instead of checking the child every 20 minutes, could the parents stretch out the time period, and peek instead of going into the room or picking up the infant? What kinds of precautions have the parents taken to assure the child's safety during the night? Does a problem really exist for the child? It is necessary to clearly delineate between problems of children and those of their parents.

DEFINING AND ASSESSING SLEEP PROBLEMS

What constitutes a sleep problem is usually determined by the child's parents. The degree to which behaviors related to sleep have become problematic can be described by the parents, depending on when they began to observe and identify the need for decreasing certain behaviors. Sleep problems vary in the time they start, what coincides with their beginnings, how long they last, and the degree to which they become bothersome or problematic to both child and parents. Behaviors related to sleep problems typically vary in the amount of disruption they present to family members. The degree of disruption and length of time needed to cope with problem behaviors associated with sleep usually determine when outside help is sought. Frequently, sleep problems of children can be determined by how much sleep the parents miss. Concerns about a child's sleep also can be determined by the time spent, either in minutes or hours, to decrease behaviors. The frequency of time devoted to a child's problem with sleep may range from once a week to more often.

IMPORTANCE OF AN ACCURATE HISTORY OF THE SLEEP PROBLEM

A successful approach to satisfy the needs of the child and parents requires an accurate, in-depth history about beginning clues of the sleep problem, the duration of the behavior, how long the parents have attended to the child's demands and requests, and what they have tried. Do the parents think their interactions with the child have contributed to reducing the frequency of duration of the problem under consideration? What interactions or events have increased the problem as judged by the parents? What do they think is the most appropriate way to start reversing the problem? What do they judge is the most appropriate way for them to change their customary responses? A problem around sleep can occur once or twice, be repeated over a period of time, or come and go. It may affect one parent more than the other and can be traced to a number of reasons.

It is essential to define the parents' immediate concern. What is their principal worry about the child? Are they concerned about the child's health as a result of lack of sleep? Are they willing to keep records now? Is there a better time to keep sleep records? Are there any major life changes occurring in the family? Has the family moved? Is the child adapting to a new sibling? Are there other stresses that the parents are trying to reduce? What do they suspect is the reason for continuation instead of termination of the problem?

If there are other behavioral problems such as the child's getting into the parents' bed, awakening another sibling, or getting up and going to off-limits areas while the parents are sleeping, can the parents rearrange the child's physical sleeping arrangement? Can both parents agree to set limits on the child and not allow him in their bed? Can they at least begin to consider not allowing the child into their bedroom?

HELPING PARENTS PLAN FOR CHANGE

Parental guidance about a child's escalating behaviors requires a consideration of parental feelings. Parents may need to discuss their feelings of discomfort in allowing a child to cry or their belief that they are allowing their child go to sleep unhappy. They may think that they are rejecting the child and may perceive themselves as mean or bad if they do not respond to his crying at bedtime. Generally, it is the crying of the child that they are attending to, once the problem has reached inappropriate proportions of time spent in consoling, bribing, or giving parental attention to the child. What percentage of time are the parents spending every night in response to the child's behaviors?

In planning more suitable responses to the child's behavioral patterns related to sleep, one must take into consideration environmental changes. Planning for change depends on objective information concerning parents' behavioral responses to the child. The rate of success and time involved for a suitable solution to a defined sleep problem depend on the collection of data or information about the child's current sleep and awake periods, as well as information about the parents' interactions with the child. It is actually the absence of sleeping behaviors of a child that is frustrating to parents.

RECORD KEEPING OF SLEEP BEHAVIORS

Sleep records kept by parents are useful for different reasons. One reason is to determine developmental patterns of sleep at one age period as compared to an earlier developmental period. Another reason is to determine the frequency, duration, and length of time of occurrence of a sleep problem, as well as its intensity or escalation of severity. These data are helpful in determining probable reinforcing events or responses, which tend to perpetuate and sustain the behaviors that the parents are attempting to eliminate. In addition, record keeping assists the parents in defining sleep behaviors that they are desirous of changing. Different data are necessary according to when problems occur, whether during the night, naptime, or at bedtime preparation. They are also useful in determining what kind of support and encouragement seems advisable for the parents.

Parents can be asked what they have gained from their efforts in keeping records. Are they learning anything about the child or themselves that is beginning to represent clues to which they can respond in more consistent, definite, and appropriate ways? Parents may be discouraged. They may find by keeping accurate records that a majority of their time is spent in responding to the child's requests at bedtime. They may experience frustration at not having instant success in reversing a problem of chronic duration. They may also need to express their frustration at having allowed the problem to start in the first place. They may be experiencing sleep deprivation. They may have feelings of anger about a frustrating situation. They need to be reminded that the problem is not permanent, that their feelings of frustration are to be expected, and that they have the capacity to respond in new and more appropriate ways.

Assessment of behaviors and interactions related to resistance to bedtime preparation

The following data are important in determining an appropriate approach to bedtime management:

1. The exact time at which the parents started to prepare the child for bed
2. The exact time he is placed in bed
3. The child's response to being placed in bed and the parents' responses to the child's behaviors (note time for both child's activities and separate time for parents' responses)
4. The exact time that the child is asleep

Can parents objectively describe the child's typical behaviors that indicate his readiness for sleep at night such as fussiness, irritability, and fatigue? Is the child being put to bed for sleep at night when he is ready? Or is he being placed in bed when the parents are ready? Are his needs being attended to, or are the parents' needs receiving greater priority? Is the child put to bed at the same time every night? Parents can be asked to record the time at which the child was involved in routine pre-bedtime activities. This record should indicate the number and length of time the activity was carried out. Parents should also record the time the child was settled in bed after pre-bedtime activities and record each time the child asks for water, food, bathroom, playtime, toys, stories, parents,

or rituals once settled in bed. Parents should indicate each time they grant the child's requests. Parents should record the number of times the child gets out of bed once settled. Parents should also record the number of times they use negative parental persuasion such as scolding, threatening, or spanking. Parents should also record the number of times they use positive parental persuasion such as praising the child, promising privileges, promising special activities, or concretely rewarding the child's conformity to stay in bed. Positive persuasion would also include reasoning with the child or explaining the necessity of bedtime. Parents should also record the time when the child ceases resisting bedtime and sleeps. Parents can be asked to draw a happy face ☺ or an unhappy face ☹ to show perceived mood changes of the child or parents to correspond to each event or activity they have recorded. Parents can be reminded to comment if there is anything unusual or if a major change occurred for the parents or the child on the days or evenings that the records are being kept. A record kept for 5 to 7 evenings is most helpful in planning a successful management program for both the child and parent. Records of specific behaviors, attitudes, and activities can be valuable in pinpointing the exact number of times a sleep problem is occurring; the number of times a child acted in a certain way; and the number, length, and duration of parents' interactions with a child at sleeptime.

Keeping records of naptime behaviors

Data are required around events at naptime. It is important for parents to observe the activities preceding the child's typical behavioral signs of fatigue or irritability that signal the need for sleep. Have parents noted differences in the child's behavior that signal the need for rest? Are activities preceding sleeptime low-key? Is the child helped to slow down; that is, are noises reduced and tempo of activities structured in such a way that the child is helped to slow down gradually before being expected to fall off to sleep immediately?

At what time was the child placed for a nap? How did the child respond? How many times did parents respond to the child's behavior? How much time was spent in appealing to the child to go to sleep? Data are necessary to determine amounts of sleep the child is receiving according to his age and whether it is reasonable for him to be taking a nap. Occasionally children show signs of needing a nap and are not encouraged to take a nap. At other times there are no indicators that a child needs a nap, and parental expectations should be altered. The child simply may be outgrowing the need for a daytime nap. If a child is sleeping excessively throughout the day, it could signal the need for a medical examination, or it could indicate that the parents are unreasonable in their expectations that the child go to sleep immediately at night. The last nap may be too near bedtime, and the parents may need to review the unreasonableness of their expectations.

Obtaining information on child's and parents' behavior at night

In obtaining data regarding awakening at night, it is significant to note who is awakened first—the mother or father. Is the child crying? How loud? How soon does the crying begin? Does the child cry every time he awakens? Does the child play in his bed with toys at this time? Is he encouraged to get into the parents' bed? Is he customarily fed? How soon does the child go back to sleep? What is the exact time? How much actual time was spent in interacting with the child? How soon were the parents able to go back to bed and fall asleep? Is there a difference in the amount of time that it takes to get the child settled down when one parent responds to his needs in comparison with the amount of time that it takes with the other parent? Do parents use similar approaches and interactions? Do they express similar comments? Is one parent acting differently from the other? What seems to account for the lesser amount of time that is spent by one parent?

HELPING PARENTS FORMULATE REALISTIC EXPECTATIONS FOR THE CHILD

In helping parents formulate more realistic expectations about sleep behavior, it is important to discover if they know the average amount and duration of sleep that infants or children of their child's age usually receive. The average number of hours infants and children sleep was reported by Traisman and associates.[3] These investigators conducted a longitudinal study of sleep patterns of infants and children up to 2 years of age and found the following trends during the first year:

1. At 1 month of age, total sleeping time averaged 17.31 hours a day.

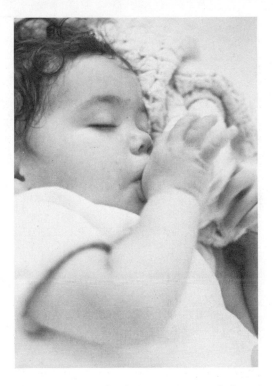

Fig. 18-1. Assessing the sleep environment of a 2-year-old girl.

2. At 8 weeks, infants averaged 15.30 hours a day.

3. At 1 year, infants slept 14.30 hours a day.

4. Naps decreased from three to two a day during the first year of life.

5. Total daily naptime was reduced by 4 hours during the first year. The longest sleeping period a day increased from 8.71 for the 8-week-old infant to 11.94 hours for the 1-year-old child.

The following trends were noted during the second year of life:

1. Total sleeping time was decreased.

2. Total naptime decreased by 0.5 hour a day.

3. Total number of naps became less frequent; most infants were taking one nap a day at 18 months of age.

4. The longest sleep period increased slightly so that by 24 months of age, infants averaged 12 hours a day.

It is important that parents know what to expect with regard to typical sleep characteristics of infants and children. The sleep section from the Washington Guide for Promoting Development in the young child follows.[4]

SLEEP*

Expected tasks	Suggested activities
1 TO 3 MONTHS	
1. Night: 4- to 10-hour intervals	1. Provide separate sleeping arrangements away from parents' room.
2. Naps: frequent	2. Reduce noise and light stimulation when placing in bed
3. Longer periods of wakefulness without crying	3. Have room at comfortable temperature with no drafts or extremes in heat
	4. Reverse position of crib occasionally
	5. Place child in different positions from time to time for sleep
	6. Alternate from back to side to stomach
	7. Keep crib sides up
4 TO 8 MONTHS	
1. Night: 10 to 12 hours	1. Keep crib sides up
2. Naps: 2 to 3 (1 to 4 hours in duration)	2. Refrain from taking child into parents' room if he awakens
3. Night awakenings	3. Check to determine if there is cause for awakenings: hunger, teething, pain, cold, wet, noise, or illness
	4. If a baby-sitter is used, attempt to find some person with whom infant is familiar. Explain bedtime and naptime arrangements
9 TO 12 MONTHS	
1. Night: 12 to 14 hours	1. Short crying periods may be source of tension release for child
2. Naps: 1 to 2 (1 to 4 hours in duration)	2. Observe for signs of fatigue, irritability, or restlessness if naps are shorter
3. May begin refusing morning nap	3. Provide familiar person to baby-sit who knows sleep routines
13 TO 18 MONTHS	
1. Night: 10 to 12 hours	1. Night terrors may be terminated by awakening infant and offering reassurance
2. Naps: one in afternoon (1 to 3 hours in duration)	2. Check to see that child is covered
3. May awaken during night crying (associated with wetting bed)	3. Avoid hazardous devices to keep child covered, including blanket clips, pins, and garments that enclose child to neck
4. As he becomes more able to move about, he may uncover himself, become cold, and awaken	
19 TO 30 MONTHS	
1. Night: 10 to 12 hours	1. Quiet period of socialization prior to bedtime— reading child book or telling story
2. Naps: one (1 to 3 hours in duration)	2. Holding child—talking quietly with him

*From Barnard, Kathryn E., and Erickson, Marcene L.: Teaching children with developmental problems: a family care approach, ed. 2, St. Louis, 1976, The C. V. Mosby Co., pp. 80-81.

SLEEP—cont'd

Expected tasks	Suggested activities
19 TO 30 MONTHS—cont'd	
3. Doesn't go to sleep at once—keeps demanding things	3. Ritualistic behavior may be present; allow child to carry out routine; helps him overcome fear of unexpected or fear of dark; for example, child may wish to arrange toys in certain way
4. May awaken crying if wet or soiled	4. Explain bedtime ritual to baby-sitter
5. May awaken because of environmental change of temperature, change of bed, change of sleeping room, addition of sibling to room, absence of parent from home, hospitalization, trip with family, or relatives visiting	5. Give more reassurance, spend more time before bedtime preparation
	6. Provide familiar bedtime toys or items
	7. Allow crying-out period if he is safe, comfortable, and tucked in
	8. Place in bed before he reaches excessive state of fatigue, excitement, or tiredness
	9. Eliminate sources of stimulation or fear
	10. Maintain consistent hour of bedtime
31 TO 48 MONTHS	
1. Daily range: 10 to 15 hours	1. TV programs may affect ability to go to sleep; avoid violent TV programs
2. Naps: beginning to disappear	2. Anxiety about going to bed and desire to stay up with parents—requires limits
3. Prolongs process of going to bed	3. Regularity and consistency important to promote good sleeping habits
4. Less dependent on taking toys to bed	4. Reassurance—night light or leaving door ajar
5. May awaken crying from dreams	5. Don't use bedtime or naptime as punishment
6. May awaken if wet	6. Encourage naps if signs of fatigue or irritability are evidenced
49 TO 52 MONTHS	
1. Daily range: 9 to 13 hours	1. Encourage napping if excessive or strenuous activity occurs and child is overly tired
2. Naps: rare	2. Explain to child if sitter will be there after child is asleep
3. Quieter during sleep	

SUMMARY

The child care professional should keep the following in mind when preparing parents for planning different approaches to sleep management. First, the child care professional should acknowledge that a child's sleeping behaviors are a concern as described by the parents. They can be supported in knowing their concern is valid in nature.

It should be acknowledged that sleep problems may result in fatigue for both the child and parents. The child care professional should be supportive by assuring parents that sleep problems can present frustrating experiences.

Parents should be reinforced for naturally wanting to do what is best and right to correct and/or eliminate problems. The child care professional should acknowledge the number of times that parents have attempted to solve their concern; they need to be reminded of their creative efforts and resourcefulness in dealing with the problem. Their good ideas require reinforcement, particularly if they are appropriate to the child's level of development and age.

The child care professional should ask parents if they are willing to keep records on the child's behaviors and their responses to the child. They should be asked if they are willing to try to put the child to bed at the same time each night. If the child tries to talk his way out of the situation and prolong the parents' interactions, can they be firm and set limits on the amount of time they will and will not spend with the child?

The child care professional should teach parents to ignore how "cute" the child is and to respond increasingly to behaviors that are more compatible with reasonable goals they have initially set for the child and themselves.

Parents can be offered reassurance that they are off to a good start in reaching an appropriate solution to management of problems when they are able to do the following:

1. Keep accurate, up-to-date and night-to-night or day-to-day records for at least 5 to 7 days
2. Attempt to change their own responses
3. Show signs of being able to follow through
4. Be consistent about limits they have decided to set

5. Show more appropriate kinds of parental responses in accordance with the child's behaviors once a program has been decided on
6. No longer attend to the child's requests once prebedtime activities are completed
7. Report relief and satisfaction with accomplishment of beginning success in achieving realistic goals
8. Get more sleep

Other important indications that the problem is being solved are that the child is decreasing requests and demands for parental attention at bedtime, is consistently going to bed at the same time each night, and is getting more sleep.

REFERENCES

1. Battle, Constance U.: Sleep and sleep disturbances in young children: sensible management depends upon understanding, Clin. Pediatr. **9:**675-682, 1970.
2. Illingworth, R. S.: Sleep problems of children, Clin. Pediatr. **5:**45-58, 1966.
3. Traisman, Alfred S., Traisman, Howard S., and Gatti, Richard A.: The well baby care of 530 infants, J. Pediatr. **68:**608-614. 1966.
4. Barnard, Kathryn E., and Erickson, Marcene L.: Teaching children with developmental problems: a family care approach, ed. 2, St. Louis, 1976, The C. V. Mosby Co.

19

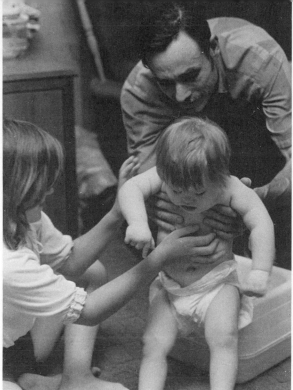

ASSESSMENT AND MANAGEMENT PRACTICES WITH PARENTS OF CHILDREN WITH MENTAL RETARDATION

Mental retardation is one of the most misunderstood, mistreated, misdiagnosed, mishandled social and emotional problems as well as one of the most prevalent handicapping conditions that plagues the United States today. Ehlers and co-workers[1] estimate that more than 6.5 million persons—3% of the population in the United States—are afflicted with mental retardation. An estimated 126,000 infants who will be mentally retarded are born each year. The majority of the mentally retarded, nearly 5.3 million persons, are classified as mildly retarded. Approximately 360,000 individuals are classified as moderately retarded, and another 210,000, as severely retarded. Since the majority live within their home community, at least 20 million persons in the United States are affected by the problems that this handicapping condition presents.

This is a problem of tremendous magnitude and one which is receiving increased national attention. In recent years the federal government has passed legislation guaranteeing the rights of mentally retarded individuals to legal

protection, treatment, and education—basic rights formerly denied them. An increasing number of state governments have required local school districts to provide suitable educational programs for mentally handicapped youngsters. This is an overdue acknowledgment that although these children have unique learning needs, if provided with the opportunity, they can learn. There is also a growing awareness that mentally retarded children benefit from early teaching in the home, not only in the area of basic life skills such as eating, toilet training, dressing, and playing but also in the development of language, social, and fine and gross motor skills. In the past, parents were encouraged to institutionalize their children with mental retardation before they reached 6 years of age. Responsibility for the child's learning and development was left to a variety of child care professionals. Today, parents are encouraged to keep their children at home and to assume more responsibility for their learning and development by working in partnership with child care professionals. Parents are also expected to participate more fully in teaching their children in the home.

These new attitudes and approaches to dealing with the problems of mental retardation have important implications for all child care

---

professionals, parents, and children. Since the majority of mentally retarded individuals live in their home community, more are using community programs and services. Parents with mentally retarded children at home often need help with the complex and difficult problems associated with responding to their children's needs. Parents are learning to work with professional care providers and expect to participate fully in planning, caring, and teaching of their children. Child care professionals must be prepared to help parents in the newer, demanding roles that parents are assuming with their children. Nurses, in particular, are in a strategic position to help coordinate, monitor, and manage problems presented by parents of mentally retarded children who live at home and who use locally available services and programs.

COMMON MYTHS ABOUT MENTAL RETARDATION

Those who are concerned with the dilemma of mental retardation have long been plagued with the problem of defining it. In spite of centuries of concern, uncountable clinical observations, and thousands of empirical studies, health care professionals are no closer to a final and best definition of mental retardation. Hobbs[2] reports that ninety-three experts from different disciplines submitted working papers and policy proposals to define the concept of mental retardation. Grossman[3] probably comes the closest to providing a generally accepted definition: "significantly sub-average general intellectual functioning existing concurrently with deficits in adaptive behavior, and manifested during the developmental period."

Lack of a precise, commonly accepted definition has made it even more difficult to eradicate common myths and misperceptions about mentally retarded persons. In the past, the orientation of child care professionals to interacting with and planning care for clients with mental retardation was based on some archaic, destructive models and concepts. It is important to examine these misconceptions and how they have affected professional attitudes if child care professionals are to respond optimally to the needs of mentally retarded individuals and their care providers and parents.

Wolfensberger[4] points out that the individual with mental retardation has been perceived as a subhuman organism, lacking many of the needs, aspirations, feelings, and sensitivities of other human beings. This view supported the assumption that these people could not benefit from the same experiences as others—or from life itself. This perception is also the basis of four common myths about mental retardation: the menace, the object of pity, the eternal child, and the diseased organism.

The menace. Mentally retarded individuals were believed to have criminal tendencies and to be capable of reproducing only defective children. To protect society from this menace, they were housed in prisonlike institutions where they could be controlled.

The object of pity. Mentally retarded individuals were seen as suffering, totally dependent beings who needed to be lovingly nurtured and protected. Overprotection often imposed retardation upon retardation. Institutions that house persons with mental retardation too often continue to reflect this view. For example, by always turning on a light for them, the individual is even denied the opportunity to learn this simple self-help task.

The eternal child. Mentally retarded individuals were believed to be perpetual children who could not be held accountable for their behavior. Their caregivers' role was to keep them happy.

The diseased organism. Mentally retarded individuals were perceived as sick. Dependency, safety, and cleanliness were stressed with emphasis on medical services and custodial care. Needless to say, little attention was given the person's growth and development.

These myths and the misperceptions associated with them persist today. Mentally retarded children are often described as being incapable of feelings such as affection, embarrassment, or shame. Too many persons still believe that even mild retardation renders an individual incapable of understanding the simplest directions or of comprehending what is said about him or done to him. Some people fail to acknowledge his capacity to feel hurt when insulted or ridiculed. The behavior of mentally retarded children may be considered bizarre and their emotional reactions inappropriate. They may be often incorrectly judged as incapable of learning self-care skills, the simplest social graces such as table skills, or social interaction skills.

The mentally retarded child may not find it easy to live, interact, and learn in an environment that places such great values on industry, beauty, achievement, and getting ahead. In the past, society has found it difficult to tolerate deviancy from its well-established norms. Child care professionals today must struggle with feelings of discomfort in the presence of "differentness."

IMPLICATIONS OF DEALING WITH MYTHS

The prevailing negative attitudes described earlier inevitably influence the way others, such as social workers, nurses, and physicians, respond to the child who is mentally retarded as well as to his parents. Professionals may have to learn to work through their own feelings about children who are different if they are to respond positively to the mentally retarded child and become sensitive to the needs of family members. Nurses, social workers, and other child care professionals must avoid stereotypes and generalizations. All child care professionals must begin to use the developmental model, the educational model, and the strengths model in looking for change and assets rather than focusing on a child's deficits. It is important that child care professionals consider that the caregivers, such as parents of a mentally retarded child, may *also* perceive the child as different, helpless, passive, and lacking feelings. It is a valuable step forward to recognize that attitudes and feelings about mental retardation may influence how one interacts or works with the person who has mental retardation. It may be important to encourage parents to discuss how they view mental retardation, the learning-teaching process, and their expectations of their child's learning progress.

Most parents in this society take it for granted that their parenting skills will be adequate to promote their children's developmental tasks. Parents assume that they are going to have success in teaching tasks such as feeding, walking, communication skills, undressing and dressing, appropriate limit setting, play with toys, appropriate play with peers, adaptive behaviors, independence in activities of daily living, and socialization skills.

In this culture most parents are oriented to the "better-than-average" achievement of their children. They tend to see their children's abilities as a reflection of their own caregiving capabilities. Children are perceived as an extension of the parents' egos.[5]

Parental skills that are necessary for helping children master their developmental tasks seem to include making accurate observations of the child's behaviors and interactions with others; interpretation of a child's behavioral responses; and giving appropriate responses to children's behavior when it occurs, not later.

MEETING THE NEEDS OF PARENTS

Parents of children who are mentally retarded may lack role models to respond effectively to their children and to teach them the basic developmental tasks. They are not generally prepared to teach mentally retarded children. In fact, it is not known what these parents teach their children or from whom they learn how or what to teach. In the United States cultural expectations require mothers to teach and socialize infants and children in the customary activities. Mothers of mentally retarded children may seek help from child care professionals in such areas as teaching children how to suck from a bottle, drink from a cup, eat solid foods, go to the toilet independently, undress and dress, and play appropriately with toys and with peers. Parents often seek help in teaching their child receptive and expressive language skills.

The personal resources available are inadequate to meet the unique needs of parents of mentally retarded children. Parents can no longer expect to give their child to a professional who will "fix him up" and return him to the parent. Today more emphasis is placed on the mutual participation model, whereby parents are expected to participate and are actively included in observing a child's behavior, solving problems and making decisions that must be made for the child's benefit. Parents are assuming increasing responsibility for the learning and developmental outcomes of their mentally retarded children. Nurses are assuming a more strategic and critical role in assisting parents in these areas.

Incidence figures suggest that the majority of persons who are diagnosed with mental retardation live in their own home communities. Child care professionals such as nurses must be prepared to respond to the vast and challenging needs presented by the unique needs of these infants and children. Nurses, in particular, are in a strategic position to assist care providers to coordinate, monitor, and manage successfully those problems presented by mentally retarded infants, children, or adolescents.

Parental skills

Parents should have the following skills to help their children master their developmental tasks:

1. The ability to observe the child's behaviors and interactions with others accurately

2. Skill in interpreting a child's behavioral responses
3. The ability to respond appropriately to a child's behavior at the time it occurs

Parents need to recognize their child's readiness to learn, to change, or to master a new developmental task. They also need to recognize their own readiness, willingness, and ability to respond to their child's learning needs. Parents need to provide and regulate a teaching environment that is successful for them as well as for their child. They must be able to monitor animate and inanimate stimuli that the infant or child receives at different stages from the newborn period into the preschool and early childhood periods. They must also evaluate the appropriateness of their own actions and determine if their responses are consistent and are promoting desired changes in the child's behavior. Parents need to be able to consider alternatives in responding to a child. They need to know that there is more than one way to help a child learn a new skill or master a complex task. Parents also are responsible for communicating clearly with their children so that the children learn what is expected of them in a clear, predictable, and consistent way.

Parents of handicapped children have unique needs and face unique demands. They often need to modify their expectations and ways of helping children master a developmental task. Parents may experience confusion, puzzling experiences, struggles, chaos, stress, and frustration that other parents do not experience on a daily, hourly, or even momentary basis. It is not easy being a parent of a child who is different. Such a child challenges his parents with demands for which there are few sure ways to respond. Parents feel a lack of support, leaving most of them insecure about their parenting abilities. They believe that their infant's outcome is to be shaped by them and by their parenting; at the same time there are few stable cultural practices on which they can rely for guidance in setting their course as new parents. These parents feel disproportionately insecure in their roles and usually extremely inadequate. They often are burdened, tense, and anxious about themselves and what they are doing with their children. It is important to realize that parents have actually lost the ideal child whom they dreamed about and for whom they prepared for so long. Now they must adjust to the real child's special needs, whether the result of minimal brain damage, mental retardation,

or something else. Somehow child care professionals may make the parents feel that they are not accepted, that they are not a part of the health care team, that they do not know enough, and that they cannot handle the child. Thus the professional staff becomes another obstacle with which the parents must cope.

In the long run it is not so much the handicap itself or the mental retardation that affects the child's developmental learning or social outcomes, but the family members' abilities to cope with the problem of the handicapping condition. Thus child care professionals must develop long-term, comprehensive, systematic, family-centered techniques to respond to the infant, the parent, and family members to ensure maximal favorable outcomes.

There is no question that parents need to learn how to handle the day-to-day needs of their children. At the same time they must learn how to sort out behaviors. They must be able to learn the positive traits of their infants and to distinguish between those behaviors which they like and those which they find difficult to accept. From an early period they must learn how to reinforce the desirable behaviors and to withhold reinforcement of maladaptive behaviors. Parents often wait to seek help in modifying inappropriate, undesirable behaviors until the child is older. It is incumbent on child care professionals to respond to parents' observational skills when the child is young so that parents can reinforce the desirable behaviors in infants and children before they reach school age. Parents definitely need models to imitate. From the time a child is born, a parent can learn to help the infant in behavior such as sucking, swallowing, taking formula, or feeding from the breast. The parents may need assistance in learning how to touch, approach, console, talk to, cuddle, and provide appropriate animate stimuli for the infant.

It is especially important for parents to identify the needs of the child and to realize that he has many positive aspects. Sometimes it is difficult for parents to recognize that their handicapped child does have strengths and appealing features and behaviors. The fact that the child cannot function as other children do does not lessen his right to have parents and other caregivers who will meet his needs in the most appropriate way possible. It is extremely important that child care professionals learn to help parents become acquainted with their infant, whether or not the child is handicapped.

Professionals can convey to the parents that their child is a child first and that the handicap is secondary to the child. The child care professional must have a modicum of skill to convey his own acceptance of the infant and should model this acceptance for the parents by holding, talking to, and touching the child and making positive remarks about individual features and behavior.

At the same time it is the responsibility of the child care professional to support parents in their own endeavors to reach out for, attach to, and enjoy their new infant. Child care professionals can be attuned to parental behavior which shows that the parents really are becoming acquainted with and growing closer to their infant and that they actually see the infant as a person rather than a handicapping condition. Parents of handicapped children need a great abundance of anticipatory guidance. For example, an infant may be more demanding if he needs more feeding. The infant might be less responsive than the mother expects. The child care professional must keep in mind that the mother-infant relationship is at great risk and both are vulnerable in their relationship when they are getting to know each other. More than anything else, the parents need information about what to expect from their infant to help them through each period. They may need to learn that their infant, for example, will sleep and eat more often. Such predictions of the infant's behavior should be based only on systematic and documented data. The child care professional is in an optimal position to interpret and discuss the infant's behavior for the parents so that they can understand him and learn to be more accepting. Somehow, in the past, child care professionals have observed, anticipated, and recognized only the weaknesses themselves rather than the total child. Professionals really must be attuned and more sensitive to development as positive and ongoing, and they must help parents see the infant's strengths. They have relied too long on the pathological and deficit model.

Tremendous attention appears to be given to the technological aspects of a child's health and well-being, whereas the child's personality and the needs of the parents and other family members seem to be neglected. It seems that once the diagnosis is made, the child's development, adaptation to the environment, functional levels, and behaviors that are occurring or lacking are overlooked. Also neglected is the adjustment of the parents, siblings, or other members of the extended family. Child care professionals need to help families communicate their questions and concerns about their strengths and weaknesses and to help them discuss the significance and implications of these concerns for the family. Parents of handicapped children cannot assume they will be successful in their parenting tasks. These parents need additional support. Professionals should be available to them because mentally retarded children do not automatically learn developmental tasks nor are their parents automatically successful in teaching tasks. Parents may be confused in interpreting their children's behavior, and thus they may feel inadequate to respond. One study found that mothers of severely mentally retarded children had difficulty interpreting their children's cues and tended to respond in one of two ways. Either they increased the diffuseness with which they responded to the child or they increased the amount of structuring and directions they gave the child.

Parents may not recognize the best time to implement change because they are with the child 24 hours a day and tend to lose their objectivity. Child care professionals can respond to the needs of parents by providing objective input, by helping parents make systematic observations of the child's behavior, and by commenting on the observed interactions. In this case the parents benefit by receiving immediate feedback on their interactions.

There are few prescriptive models for parents to follow. Parents of children with developmental problems lack automatic rules, direction, and precedence or role references to imitate.

Parents may not even realize that changes are possible, that there is hope, and that they themselves are the best resource for any changes they wish implemented. It is usually when parents experience the lack of a ready-made feedback system that they begin to seek help from child care professionals.

When parents seek help from professionals, they basically are seeking reassurance. They are asking, "Am I okay? Am I competent? Will I be up to these tasks? Will others see me as a failure? Will I do what is right and best? Will my child survive? Will I survive?" Parents may not openly and readily verbalize that these questions are what concern them most, but they underlie each professional-parent interaction. Most parents experience varying degrees of,

"I'm confused, frightened, unsure, disappointed. I've never done this before. Will I make it?"

It is unequivocal that parents of handicapped children need to experience success, positive feedback, and acknowledgment for the adaptations that they make as early as the infant is born. They need acknowledgment and feedback on the long- and short-term goals they set, the priorities they choose, the problem-solving methods they use, and the approaches they try. They definitely need praise for the tasks that they master with their child. It is interesting that the literature often discusses the infant at risk but rarely addresses the parent at risk. The parents of the mentally retarded child encounter numerous challenges. First, they must develop a relationship with their infant. Second, they face challenges in the relationships they do or do not have with each other as husband and wife, with their parents, with the infant as he does or does not grow and develop, and with other siblings in the household. Third, they must deal with relationships with children they will have in the future. Fourth, and most importantly, they will be challenged with the way they accept their own values, feelings, and strengths; ways of learning and of discovering new things about themselves; with their ability to cope and to accept their strengths as well as difficulties they may encounter. In addition, parents may have difficulty with their self-image, the ways they cope with stress and conflict, and the way they react to pain. For example, do they suppress their feelings of anguish, or do they express such feelings in appropriate ways that assist them in their own adult development?

Universal parental reaction

Parents of mentally retarded children need help in moving through the classic stages of shock, denial, anger, bargaining, depression, grief and mourning, and unfinished business. During the period in which parents are in shock from learning that they have given birth to an imperfect child, it is important that the child care professional monitor the quantity of information the parents receive. The parents may not hear what is being said to them while they are in shock. Thus the information may need to be repeated at a later time. Parents may need to be asked, "What were you told? What did this information mean to you? What did it mean to you at the time you were told? What does the information mean to you now?" In manifesting shock, parents may show helplessness, cry, or withdraw. A sensitive observer can see from the expressions on the parents' faces that they disbelieve information, are experiencing pain, and are absorbing crucial information which is a tremendous blow to their egos.

The next stage, denial, is not an exclusive coping mechanism for parents. It is also used by professionals, children, and parents who are undergoing other kinds of stresses. In this stage, parents behave as if this misfortune could not have happened to them. They may reject the diagnosis at this point and shop around for other opinions. In looking for other services, parents may be searching for the magic cure. The question that health care professionals need to ask themselves is, is this response so undesirable? Denial is a coping mechanism that allows parents to cushion the shock. They are dealing with painful information at their pace, not at somebody else's, and they should be allowed to deal with their own responses to pain and be supported by nurturing persons. Child care professionals who are sensitive to the behaviors of denial must be careful not to impose further information on parents when they are not ready to hear it.

Parents also experience anger, and during this time they may be asking the eternal question, why did this happen to us? They are angry because they seem to have been singled out by fate to have had a child with a handicapping condition. They may not be aware of their anger, and it may become suppressed. If parents show anger, it may mean they are not denying the situation and are dealing with the facts in a more appropriate way. Health care professionals should encourage parents to express their anger openly, convey that they expect such anger, and not be defensive when parents show anger. Dealing with anger can be frightening for parents who may believe it is unacceptable to show such emotion. But anger is acceptable and desirable, allowing the parents to deal with the conflicts they are experiencing. The sensitive professional can show by his behavior that it is safe for the parent to express anger, that the professional expects it, and does not take the anger personally.

Parents may show signs of bargaining when they say things such as, if only my child could make it through high school, be put in a regular classroom, be accepted into a normal school, or could learn to live independently—then I would be happy. The parents' expectations for the future may not be compatible with the child's current level of functioning. However, professionals must learn to accept this stage in which parents bargain for something better for the child. It is a natural, healthy response.

Parents may also show signs of depression in which the anger is turned inward. They may show signs of withdrawal. This depression can be managed by a sensitive professional who recognizes depression for what it is, offers support to the person, and makes it clear that he will always be accessible whether the parent is happy or depressed. Parents classically go through stages of grief, mourning, and sorrow. They mourn the loss of the idealized child and grieve over the imperfect child. Olshansky[6] reports that professionals belabor the fact that parents feel chronic sorrow in accepting mental retardation in a child and should accept mental retardation, when it is doubtful that it is appropriate to expect such acceptance of parents. Few, if any, parents really ever accept a mentally retarded child. Parents may be dealing with "unfinished business," which means withholding some feelings from their awareness. If child care professionals respond to parents experiencing the different stages of grief, mourning, shock, and sorrow and help them openly and actively deal with their feelings, parents are helped to put closure on the conflict, stress, and pain that should have been dealt with long ago. Unfortunately, parents come to child care professionals when children are of school age, and it is evident that they still have unfinished business. They talk, for example, about how the diagnosis was handled at birth, the way they were told, the inadequacy of the literature, the ways that professionals treated them, how schools discriminated against them, and the fact that their children could not get into a particular program.

Child care professionals, particularly nurses, must be attuned to the need for anticipatory guidance during periods that they know are stressful for the parents rather than intervening when a problem reaches crisis proportions. Certain periods during the growth of a child are known to be stressful to parents. Professionals need to recognize these times and to help parents deal with them before they happen rather than after the fact.

The first expected stress period is when the parents first learn about or suspect a handicap in their child. The next stress period is during diagnosis. Until the parents' anxieties are dealt with by a full assessment and an explanation of the child's behavior and development, the child represents many question marks. The next stress period is when ordinary child-rearing practices do not work, when nothing seems to work even though parents are trying everything, accepting advice from friends and neighbors, working things out on a trial-and-error basis, and feeling frustrated with their lack of success. They are not equipped to respond to the learning needs of a mentally retarded child. Another stress period can be when a younger sibling bypasses the handicapped child. The next period is when parents must decide whether to send the child to ordinary schools.

Puberty creates the next stress period. It is important that the professional not wait until the child's puberty to begin giving information but answer parents' and the child's questions when the child is very young. Health care professionals must attempt to reduce fears and anxieties about sexuality and reproduction when parents are ready. If parents do not show signs of readiness, it is appropriate that the child care professional provide appropriate opportunities for the parents to discuss issues concerning sexual development. There is a high correlation between the parents' comfort with their own sexuality and the way they respond to the needs of their child and prepare him or her regarding sex and sexuality.

Another stress period is when the handicapped person finishes school and parents must decide what to do next. Anticipatory guidance for vocational plans must be considered for the mentally retarded person. Intervention and information is not necessarily received well or effectively on the day that the child graduates. Another stress period is when it is uncertain if the handicapped person will be able to work. It does not have to happen the first time that the handicapped person goes looking for a job and is unsuccessful. This fact should be considered at an appropriate age, when vocational plans should be made.

Stress occurs again when the parents become older and are unable to care for their handicapped child. Advice and reassurance about what will happen should be given when the handicapped person is a child and these questions are occurring to parents. Another stressful time is when institutionalization or removal of the handicapped family member is being considered. At this time parents need additional support and need their questions answered. Sometimes it is beneficial if a nurse is available to help them visit different residential facilities, special care programs, foster care homes, group homes, or intermediate care facilities. Parents need to know that placement in a residential facility is not a last resort, a jail, or a punishment but represents a continuum of care when other environments are not optimal for the handicapped person and his family.

Major concerns of parents

Reactions at time of diagnosis. Child care professionals must be ready to respond to parents' needs to discuss critical issues they have experienced in their lives. For example, they may recall their experiences with the child's birth. Unless these feelings have been effectively dealt with at birth and resolved, they may interfere with activities such as planning a feeding program for a 7-year-old child. Parents may need to discuss their reactions at the time of the diagnosis. The professional needs to be able to find out how the parents reacted at the time of the diagnosis, how and what they were told, how they feel about it now, and whether they think they would have reacted differently if it had been approached differently.

A serious management problem for the professional is that of informing the parents. It appears from the literature that there are a number of conflicting opinions about the best time to inform the parent who has given birth to a handicapped individual. It seems that parents prefer to be told as soon as possible. If the diagnosis is made at birth, parents prefer to be told during the first week. The rationale for this is that parents do not like to tell others that the child is retarded once they have said the child is normal. Telling parents early helps them deal with anguish and excessive concerns when they see there is something wrong. Parents also assert that they have a right to know as soon as the physician is aware of a problem. It is also evident that parents prefer to be told together when possible rather than one spouse bearing the burden of having to tell the other. Parents have made it fairly clear that the person who tells the family should not be a stranger. Mothers have indicated that it is difficult to be told by the pediatrician with whom they have not had a relationship rather than the obstetrician, whom they have come to know. Ideally, it seems best that the physician who delivered the baby and the pediatrician tell the parents together.

Parents emphasize the need to be told in the right way. An example of the wrong way is the case of two parents who related angrily how a professional came to them and told them to institutionalize their infant or consider putting him in a foster home since he was not going to grow and develop normally. Other parents have commented that the pediatrician or obstetrician said that their child was a child first and needed to be loved, cared for, held, caressed, and diapered just like any other baby; that his future development could not be predicted at this point; that the parents should take the infant home and learn his unique behaviors and ways of responding; and that they should not make any decisions about the child's future care.[7]

SUPPORTING THE PARENTS AT THE CHILD'S BIRTH

The child care professional should be particularly responsive to the needs of parents at the time a handicapped child is born. The common response is to leave the mother alone and not talk to her about her infant or question her about her concerns. Such mothers are often avoided or left alone when they begin to cry. Because of this behavior of nurses and physicians, professionals need to examine their own feelings of loss, mourning, grief, and pain. They need to explore what the birth of a handicapped child means to them so that they can become aware of their own feelings and ways of coping with pain and grief and hence be in a better position to respond to the parents' needs. If professionals can be more comfortable with their own feelings, they can help the mother express grief at the time she feels it, not later. Professionals also need to respond to fathers as they also cope awkwardly and try to grasp at the reality of the situation. A father is trying not only to meet his own needs and deal with pain and loss but is trying to support his wife and the family members at home. It is vital that the professional be present when the young infant is brought to the mother's bedside where the mother can examine the infant, look at surface features, and talk about what these features mean, particularly if there is an aberration. The child care professional must also be present when the father comes so that they can discuss their reactions.

Child care professionals need to be accessible so that parents can ask questions over and over again, even though the professional may have answered the very question that same day. Nurses, physicians, and social workers need to be in a position to observe the mother-infant interactions and the beginnings of attachment behavior towards the infant. They must see if the mother makes statements that show she likes the infant, that the infant's behaviors appeal to her, that she individualizes the infant, and that she sees the infant as a person rather than a syndrome of some kind. It is important to be with the mother to acknowledge her concerns about the infant's behavior, particularly if the infant seems drowsy or lacks mobility. The child care professional needs to comment and help the mother perceive and attend to the infant's appealing traits and behaviors. Before the mother and infant are discharged, the physician, social worker, or nurse should check the mother's perceptions of the infant, help her clarify what the infant's behaviors mean to her, and answer any questions about the early period of infancy concerning feeding, bathing, or playing with the infant. Sometimes parents have misconceptions that because the infant is handicapped, he will be inattentive. They may tend to be too protective of the infant or think that he is too fragile or should not be bombarded with too many stimuli. Parents thus may inadvertently neglect the child's needs for early handling, holding, and face-to-face contact.

THE CHILD CARE PROFESSIONAL'S ROLE IN THE INFORMING INTERVIEW PROCESS

Nurses are becoming more comfortable in assuming increased responsibilities in child care management. They collaborate with other members of an interdisciplinary team to provide the most comprehensive care for children and parents. They assist in early case finding, in assessment procedures, in the diagnostic process, and in management of children with mental retardation. They may be case managers who are responsible for directing the informing conference after the diagnostic workup. It is no longer simply the province of the physician, the psychologist, or the psychiatrist to conduct the informing interview. For this reason, nurses need to know some helpful hints in conducting a parent-informing interview, which is not an easy task. Nurses are increasingly responsible for conducting the interview in which they explain to parents their child's mental retardation or developmental disabilities. They are responsible for the conduct of professionals

during the conference, for what occurs during the conference, for providing follow-up letters, and for relaying to appropriate agencies recommendations that have been made during the conference. The nurse needs to keep the parents' agenda in mind if she does nothing else.

The child care professional, such as the social worker or nurse, should encourage parents to be together when they are informed of their child's condition. This will avoid the problem of one parent's having to interpret complex findings and deal with the initial emotional reaction of the other, as well as giving the child care professional an opportunity to observe the interaction between the parents while they are confronted with the tragedy of finding mental retardation in their child. The professional person should remember that because of its social and emotional implications, the concepts of mental retardation are extremely difficult to convey to parents, and this task requires tremendous patience and increased sensitivity. The professional must also be both realistic and cautious, stressing that mental retardation refers to a description of the individual's level of functioning in intellectual and adaptive skills at a given time. *The child care professional is discouraged from presenting numbers only.*

It is important that the nurse or other child care professional answer the parents' questions as they arise. She is responsible for ensuring that the parent understands information and for arranging additional conferences to answer any questions that may have arisen during or after the informing interview. The professional must be able to provide information in a smooth-flowing, comprehensive manner that is tailored to the needs of the parents. The information about the child's behavior should be positive. It is important to avoid a "hit-and-run" approach. In other words, material should be presented according to the parents' readiness to receive more information about their child. The child care professional should not present a great deal of information to the parents and then abandon them to struggle with the trauma of hearing disappointing and painful news. Thus the nurse and other child care professionals must support the parents in the information interview as they need it. Parents are simply overwhelmed, not only with the quantity of information presented but with its seriousness and devastating nature. It is for that reason that the child care professional should be prepared to present comprehensive information but should avoid reading long lists, giving technological information, and trying to impress parents with the comprehensive nature of the diagnostic workup. Parents realize that the diagnostic workup has been extremely comprehensive. They have answered many questions from professionals in different disciplines.

As the child care professional proceeds with the informing interview, it is important that she checks to see if the parents are grasping what is said. One way to ensure this is to ask simple questions such as, "Do you see what I mean?" She should ask the parents to repeat what has been said and to interpret it in their own way. It is at this point that the professional should make any necessary clarifications, interspersing the information with questions such as, "Do you agree with these observations?" "Have you made similar observations?" "Have you seen this kind of behavior at home or in school?" "Are these the observations that you were hoping we would make about your child?" "Is this information making sense to you?" "Do you have any questions?" Then, even though it may appear that a long silence is occurring, the professional should wait for the parents to think about and to comment on what they have just heard.

The child care professional can make the informing interview a highly successful and positive experience if she remembers that an interaction model is much more desirable than the virtuoso model. In the case of the latter, the professional simply awes and finally intimidates the parents with the amount and seriousness of the information. It is time that nurses and child care professionals relinquish archaic and destructive models and use interaction models that permit a reciprocal give-and-take. Parents need an opportunity to provide input, ask questions, and make recommendations. Health care professionals have often failed to seek this from parents. When parents bring children to a diagnostic workup, they obviously have thought about their child's present and future. It is likely that they have creative ideas about the kinds of activities that could be planned to help their child's development. Professionals must learn to use the interaction model not only during but after the diagnostic workup and need to continue including parents in planning for their child. It is important that rapport be established from the beginning of the diagnostic workup and continue through the completion of the informing interview. This will provide a basic, supportive, and constructive relationship that will en-

able future contacts with the same parents and their child to be mutually beneficial. If during the diagnostic workup it seems appropriate for the child to be present at the informing interview, he should be included and asked if he agrees with the suggestions and observations. It is extremely important to accustom the handicapped person at an early age to being included and to having a voice in future plans. Professionals should not perpetuate the archaic stereotype that the child is helpless and has nothing to contribute.

Parents may experience a variety of emotions during the informing interview. If they are learning for the first time that their child does have a problem in adaptive behaviors and is functioning at a significantly low level in intelligence, they are likely to be sad, express gloom, and experience shock. They may show despair and a feeling of hopelessness. The child care professional needs to be sensitive to the expressions on their faces and the times that they look down. She should notice their ability to maintain eye contact with the professional person and should be alert to other behavior that shows they are avoiding what the professional is saying. When the child care professional does perceive changes in the expressions of the parents' faces, she needs to check with them with statements such as, "I can see that this is very difficult for you." "This seems to be pretty overwhelming to you." "This seems to be some very serious information that is difficult for you to be hearing. Am I right?" She can also say, "I can see that this is very disturbing news to you and seems like a lot of information to handle at one time. I can see that you are sad or that you are finding this hard to believe right now." The child care professional needs to be sensitive to all of the parents' signals that show how well they are following what the nurse or other child care professionals are saying.

At this point, parents often are no longer listening to or looking at the child care professional but are preoccupied with trying to keep their own emotions under control. If they do not succeed in controlling their emotions, parents may cry or make angry statements. The professional person needs to accept these feelings at the time the parents are experiencing them and should not try to cover up the situation by telling parents not to worry, that the situation will pass in time, or that she knows this is difficult to take. It is not enough to say, "I know this is difficult to take."

The nurse needs to stop giving information

at this point and to attend to and acknowledge the parents' emotional needs. The child care professional can offer emotional support by having tissues ready for when a parent may cry. She can reach out and touch the parent and show support through her facial expressions and body language. She should not present the information and leave the parents in a disturbed state in which they need support for the anguish they are experiencing. It is wise (and the sensitive professional person will keep it in mind) to ask the parents if they wish to continue this conference. It is seems that the information is too overwhelming and the parents are too sad or angry to absorb more, the child care professional should ask the parents if they feel there is a better time to continue the discussion. It is far better to help the parents resolve the difficulties they are experiencing because it is likely that if they do not resolve their sorrow and anguish then, they will present the same kinds of behavior to the professional in the future. It is the obligation of the child care professional to attend to the emotional needs of parents, to help parents express their feelings, and to respond empathically.

The informing conference can also be a time for the parents to learn of some of their child's strengths, appealing behaviors, and problem-solving abilities and characteristics. It is vital that the informing interview begin with a presentation of the child's strengths and assets rather than deficits. The parents can be asked to describe the appealing behavioral traits of their child. It is important that they be given this opportunity. In a planned approach parents seldom are asked to verbalize openly so that they can hear their own ideas on their child's strengths and positive behaviors. It is extremely important to realize that parents are seeking input about things such as the best ways to respond to their child or the best community programs or services that might be available for their child. They may ask for specific help with language to encourage the child to feed himself, to toilet train independently, or to learn how to dress himself. They may want to know how to teach the child to play in more appropriate ways, how to respond to limits more quickly, and to comply with requests that are made. It is important that parents be given an opportunity to describe their concerns, but the child care professional must also find out precisely what help the parents want and not assume they know the parents' priorities. Parents do come with priorities and concerns that simply may not match those of the child care professional. It is important that the parents' priorities be considered, otherwise even the best designed programs may fail because the parents' needs and concerns were essentially bypassed.

PREVENTING DISTURBANCES IN THE ATTACHMENT PROCESS

Gayton[7] discusses preventing potential interference with the development of attachment. As he explains it, attachment is a term that describes the affectional tie between a mother and her infant. As Gayton[7] points out, research suggests that attachment serves many important functions including providing the infant with a sense of security that allows him to explore the environment and that such exploration is highly related to later cognitive development. He further emphasizes that when mental retardation is diagnosed at birth, it creates a highly vulnerable relationship during the infancy period.

The potential for interference with the development of an adequate mother-infant relationship is apparent. A mother may experience severe loss of self-esteem, feelings of inadequacy, and depression that can make it extremely difficult for her to respond to her baby's needs at the time he needs his mother's care and attention. Because of the danger of this happening, the child care professional should make frequent home visits over a period of time to observe the quality and quantity of the infant-mother relationship and be alert to any disruptions in the relationship.

In addition to observing how the mother talks to the infant, holds him, feeds him, attends to him when he cries or responds when he is not signaling any needs of attention, the professional could use the Home Observation for Measurement of the Environment (HOME) an instrument developed by Dr. Bettye Caldwell.[8] The HOME is helpful in measuring the quantity of physical, social, and emotional support that is available to the child in his early environment (Chapter 8). The instrument was developed to detect signs of children at risk before 3 years of age. The child care professional should use standardized screening tools to make serial, objective, and systematic observations of the child's development and should also be prepared to measure the child's head, obtain dietary histories, record sleep patterns, or consider any behavioral concerns that the mother may bring up.

It is important that the child care professional include the mother early in problem solving in a mutual participation model by having her keep records of her concerns. These might involve the infant's crying too much, eating too little, sibling interaction problems, temper tantrums, thumb sucking, or problems with toilet training. The professional needs to emphasize to the mother the importance of obtaining documented, objective information about a child before intervention can be planned. Professional observations of the mother-child interactions, of the appropriateness of the environment for the child's development, and of the developmental status of the child should emphasize strengths rather than deficits. The mother should first be told the child's strengths, encouraged to state whether or not she agrees with the observations, and then told about those tasks or items that the child did not perform well.

A number of standardized assessment screening tools would be appropriate in early infancy, during the preschool period, or during the child's school-age period. These include, during the first month of life, the Brazelton Neonatal Assessment Scale, which can be a helpful instructional and assessment tool for the parents and has wide implications for teaching or interacting with the infant (Chapter 3). The Neonatal Perception Inventory, developed by Dr. Elsie Broussard, can be effective in determining infants who may be at risk for subsequent problems in development, particularly if the mother rates her infant as not better than the average infant (Chapter 4). During the 4- to 8-month period of life, the Carey Infant Temperament Questionnaire can be given to the mother (Chapter 6). If she perceives the infant to be having problems with adaptability, rhythmicity, temperament, persistence, or other characteristics, prompt intervention based on documented data should be planned. If a mother is complaining of temperamental difficulties of the infant, this is a serious cue that the child care professional must attend to, and one which may necessitate a change in the environment. It is important, however, that the professional perceive the uniqueness of the individual infant's temperament rather than concluding automatically that parental mismanagement is causing the problem.

CONSIDERING ALTERNATIVE METHODS OF CARE

When parents consider institutionalizing their child, they need to learn not to feel guilty about such thoughts. They need to know that other parents have had painful experiences in institutionalizing their children and that this is a real alternative which may relieve problems with sibling or other family disruptions. If institutionalization is sought, it should be done systematically. Parents should have an opportunity to visit and compare different care facilities. They need to be aware of standards of care and judge whether institutions meet these standards. They need to see other children who live in institutional settings.

SUPPORTING PARENTS THROUGH ANGER

Child care professionals may experience anger from parents. One reason for this is because professionals are safe targets. The parents' anger may be justified, and the professional in this case should respond by reinforcing the parents' assertiveness and ability to discuss the things they do not like. Parents will ask health care professionals how to promote the child's development. The best way to respond is to systematically and objectively assess the child's current capabilities by observing the child in his environment. The professional should ask the parents what they have done so far to help the child develop, what has worked, and what progress has been made. The professional should find out if the parents are satisfied with what they have been doing and if they have considered other methods. The child care professional can advise the parents on the appropriateness of their actions.

ANSWERING QUESTIONS ABOUT THE CHILD'S FUTURE

Often, health care professionals are asked about the child's future. They should reassure the parents that these are good questions. The professional might say: "I can see that you are concerned about the child's future development, and I am encouraged that you have been thinking about ways to enhance his future. At the present time, however, I cannot predict what his future behavior or IQ will be. We do not know that much about children to predict what they will be like 5 or 10 years from now. I understand that you probably have asked this question many times before, and it is probably very frustrating for you to hear such an answer, but if I were to give you information about the child's future, I would be doing a disservice to you. However, I can make some comments about your child's present capabilities, how he is functioning, and how he is relating to other people in his environment. We can share our thoughts about how your child is doing in his gross motor development, his fine motor development, his language, his personal and social skills, his preacademic behaviors, his academic behaviors, or his prevocational skills. We can also discuss those behaviors which you think are desirable and wish to see more of and those behaviors which you feel are inappropriate and you do not wish repeated. I would like to share with you also the strengths that I see in your child. Your child has certain skills that have come along and obviously have been worked with. He has initiated some effort. He has tried. He has had some successful experiences in these different areas. On the other hand, some areas have not been so easy for him. These seem to be fine motor, language, and socialization skills."

The important point here is that child health professionals do not tell parents *not* to worry about the future. Instead, the professionals acknowledge parental concerns as valid and convey sensitivity about them. But professionals need to help the parents shift their attention to the child and emphasize his current levels of functioning within the environment. Professionals need to look for signs of readiness for the child to master new developmental tasks and can also comment on what the parents are doing currently so that he makes progress which can be built on the future. In other words, professionals must convey to parents that what is happening now will influence the child's future in a highly significant way and that they have a major part to play right now.

Parents may also express their difficulties in being unable to accept developmental problems or mental retardation. Even though the child may be 5 years old and the parents were told that he was mentally retarded when the child was 3 months old, the professional must show acceptance of these feelings. The professional must convey that these feelings are normal, that parents are not bad parents for feeling them, and that it will take time to resolve the anguish of accepting delays in a child's development. The professional must not convey feelings that the parent is incompetent or inadequate because he cannot accept his child's mental retardation.

SUPPORTING GRANDPARENTS

Health care professionals also need to respond to the conflict that occurs between grand-

parents and their grandchildren. Gayton[7] discusses how grandparents often deny mental retardation and say things such as, "She will catch up" or "You must have been told the wrong information." Professionals must be attuned to the needs of grandparents. They should be invited to child health conferences and included in making observations. Their input should be considered, and they themselves should receive progress reports instead of hearing them secondhand. At the same time, if the grandparents are a source of anguish for the parents of the retarded child, a professional can be an intermediary and provide counseling for the grandparents. Essentially, however, health care professionals have forgotten that grandparents play a vital part in the lives of mentally retarded children. Professionals need to bring themselves up to date, meet the needs of grandparents, and make them part of the team. They, too, should be included in a mutual participation interaction model. Professionals should listen to what grandparents have to say, since they may feel helpless and uninformed and may need to ventilate their own feelings of anger, grief, and sorrow.

INCLUDING FATHERS IN ASSESSMENT AND MANAGEMENT

It is evident that health care professionals have failed to systematically include fathers in the assessment process, in the diagnostic workup, or in planning care approaches for an infant or child. In the past professionals have tended to focus on mothers and their reports about the mentally retarded child rather than actively seeking the father's input and participation. The time has come when professionals must make the father feel that he is an extremely important part of the decisions that are made about his child. They must help him make observations of his child, share his opinions of the child's behavior, and share his preferences. He must be included in the problem solving and the decision making that will affect his child, whether this be in planning an early infant intervention program to be carried out at home or in a special school or other program setting. Fathers are vital resources, and they have not been sufficiently visible in the past.

One instance where health care professionals have fallen short is in the assessment process itself. For example, when a screening procedure is used, such as the Denver Developmental Screening Test (DDST), the Brazelton Neonatal Assessment Scale, the Developmental

Profile, Home Observation for Measurement of the Environment (HOME), or the Washington Guide for Promoting Development in the Young Child, it seems that the person who generally responds to the questionnaire or who gives answers about the child's behavior is the mother. The time has come in which professionals must take it upon themselves to see to it that fathers are included in the observational and screening procedures of a child. Both father and mother should be present together when any screening procedure is carried out and, particularly, should be together when the results of the screening procedures are shared. The father needs a chance, as well as the mother, to comment on his observations of the child; what strengths and weaknesses he sees in the child; what areas he thinks his child needs work or attention or help with; what each parent independently thinks the child needs to help him achieve and progress in his development; and what each parent thinks will work for him, has tried in the past, and thinks will work in the future. If the parents have an idea, and that idea does not work, what are their priorities and what do they plan to do? It is extremely important that this final question be asked to determine if parents are really aware of their child's situation, if both the mother and the father agree on the program being carried out, and if they both have realistic and compatible short- and long-term goals for their child.

CONSIDERING THE NEEDS OF SIBLINGS

Health care professionals must be able to respond to parents in their descriptions about how siblings are reacting to the birth or the presence of a retarded child in the family. Siblings also have feelings about children and particularly about children who are different. It is very important, for instance, that siblings learn from their own parents that something may be wrong with their young brother or sister rather than from a person in the neighborhood. Siblings may be fantasizing out of proportion what is wrong with the affected child. As soon as the parents can sense that the sibling is ready to explore what mental retardation means or that the sibling perceives something different or unusual about his brother or sister, the parents need to be encouraged to sit down with him and help him cope with the fact that his brother or sister might need extra help. Siblings, by and large, must be helped to develop

healthy and adaptive responses to their affected sibling rather than to hide their feelings. If they feel angry or neglected, this needs to be explored with the parents. The parents need to discuss how the sibling is responding to the handicapped child during infancy, the preschool period, the school years, and adolescence.

Counseling about the sibling should be an integral part of responding to the needs of parents who have a mentally retarded child in the home. Counseling is essential if the professional discovers an inappropriate or premature role revision or sex and age role revision.[9] For example, is the sibling taking on more responsibilities in the family and actually carrying out mothering or fathering responsibilities for the mentally retarded child? Is his time with his sibling depriving him of time he could spend with his peers in school? The nurse, social worker, or physician who is in a position to make home visits can also make school visits and find out if the sibling's peers are making fun of him or humiliating him about his retarded brother or sister and how he is coping with that. The strengths of the sibling in responding to pressures from others must be acknowledged, and the sibling must receive appropriate attention, love, and care as he expresses the need for it.

As Gayton[7] points out, the presence of a retarded child in a family may result in parents paying less attention to the other children or expecting older siblings to take on greater responsibility for the child's care. The siblings may respond by developing negative attitudes toward the child or by expressing anger in different forms. The child care professional can help by using anticipatory guidance, questioning the parents about what they feel is the best way to have siblings respond to the retarded child and if they have any concerns about the way they are assigning responsibility to older siblings. This questioning should take place before serious negative reactions occur.

Older siblings may experience embarrassment associated with the stigma of mental retardation. Parents are then faced with the difficulty of responding to this embarrassment in an understanding and appropriate manner without punishing the siblings for feeling the way they do. The child care professional should encourage parents to talk with the siblings about how they view their mentally retarded brother or sister. Siblings of a retarded child may express fears about their ability to bear normal children; adolescents, in particular, may not be able to discuss these vital issues with their parents and may prefer to consult with the child care professional. The professional should emphasize to parents that such behavior is natural for adolescence and should not be misconstrued as rebelliousness or as naughtiness.

Many parents express concern about when and how to inform the other children in the family about the birth or the presence of a child who is mentally retarded. The answer depends on each child's level of sophistication and understanding, but it is advisable to inform the siblings before a neighbor or other nonfamily member tells them. The child care professional can show by her behavior that she sees the parents as being capable in their own unique style of imparting information about mental retardation. However, the professional should make it clear that if they postpone informing the siblings, they run the risk of hindering the siblings' ability to develop a realistic understanding of the problem; uninformed siblings may fantasize or develop apprehensions that are out of proportion to the child's actual condition. Furthermore, if parents choose to be silent or deceptive about the issue, they are setting a negative precedent for the siblings to follow rather than encouraging them to cope with the experience in a healthy and nurturing way.

THE PROBLEM OF TELLING OTHERS

Parents commonly have difficulty telling other family members about the child's disabilities. Sometimes parents find this an extremely difficult issue. It seems that as the parents become more comfortable with the dilemma of mental retardation, they become more comfortable in sharing information with family members, friends, and neighbors. There is no formula for helping parents tell others about their child. One must consider the parents' readiness to tell others and the extent to which they agree that other family members should be told. It is also important to know if the parents agree about what information should be given and when and how this should be accomplished. It cannot be given haphazardly, and most families find their own ways of relating this tragic information to other family members.

RESPONDING TO OVERPROTECTIVE PARENTS

Gayton[7] points out that parents of a mentally retarded child are often unable to set limits on their child's behavior. They often do everything for him, thus making him a passive recipient of his environment rather than an active participant. Gayton[7] explains that parents are overprotective because they have built up frustrations about rearing a child who is retarded, they have feelings of rejection and anger toward the child, and they have developed a sense of guilt about their feelings toward their child. Overprotectiveness may also result from not having realistic expectations about the child's capabilities or from making up to the child for his being mentally retarded. Sometimes parents manifest overprotective behavior because it is simply easier for them to do something for the child than to wait and have him do it for himself or because if parents do something for the child, his failures may not be so conspicuous either to the child or to other people.

Professionals should take all of these explanations into consideration when responding to parents' overprotective behaviors. The nurse, social workers, or physician can best respond to parental uncertainty about a child's capabilities by listening to the parents describe their expectations, their views of the child's strengths, and what they think the child should be doing at various stages in his development. Once professionals understand what the parents think, they are in a better position to acknowledge parental behavior and concerns in an objective and systematic way. Parents who suffer guilt about mental retardation unnecessarily may need to participate in repeated discussions, receiving clarification about the causes of mental retardation and the fact that they were not the cause of their child's developmental status. Parents who have an "easier-to-do-it-myself" attitude can be encouraged to talk about what this means to them and what they think the long-term consequences of such behavior will be; they may be showing that they need more support, reassurance, guidance, and knowledge.

PROVIDING APPROPRIATE LITERATURE

It is important that the child care professional not simply warn the parents about archaic literature on mental retardation but provide them with current and appropriate literature that does justice to the kinds of questions and concerns parents continually bring up. Parents often describe how obsolete or destructive the literature is concerning mentally retarded children. It is the professional's responsibility to acknowledge that some literature is highly inappropriate and certainly outdated. Child care professionals should not become defensive about obsolete literature.

COMMITMENT OF PROFESSIONALS TO CHILDREN WITH MENTAL RETARDATION AND THEIR PARENTS

It is increasingly recognized that the job of the sensitive, dedicated, and committed professional in early child care who works with parents of handicapped children has some major responsibilities, which include the following:

1. Help take some of the mystery, confusion, and chaos out of parents' and children's lives; help reduce some of the struggles.

2. Make life easier for the parents by accepting their feelings of inadequacy, guilt, anger, and frustration. These are all normal manifestations at different times in a parent's life, and they are not present only at the diagnostic workup or when the child is first found to be lacking in a developmental skill but at other times as well. Professionals have belabored the issue that parents accept the child with mental retardation, but Olshansky[6] says that chronic sorrow is a normal manifestation to a catastrophe that occurs in a parent's life.

3. Communicate that life can be easier by helping parents develop effective observational skills and objective ways of interpreting the behavior of their children. Increasingly, professionals can model effective ways that parents can interact with their children, particularly when they have become so involved and are so subjective about what their child is doing and also what they are doing. It is vitally important that health care professionals help parents learn behavior modification, management skills, and ways to perceive, document, and record patterns of behavior. Parents must not only look at the child's behavior but examine their own behavior as well to see how they are contributing to the maintenance, acceleration, or termination of a specific behavior in their child.

4. Help parents learn principles of behavior modification; that is, help them reinforce behaviors they want repeated. They must learn that simply ignoring a child does not work. Before parents begin a program of behavioral intervention with a child, they must have documented data about the rates of behavior, what seems to reinforce it, and how the parents react. It is important that parents reinforce behavior they want repeated and ignore behavior

they do not wish repeated. For parents to be effective behavior modifiers with their children and to learn how to be future problem solvers rather than future health seekers, child care professionals must teach parents how to modify or reinforce desirable behavior rather than help parents change deviant behavior. Parents essentially need experiences encouraging normal, desirable behavior before they move on to working with deviant behavior.

5. Inject a hope for change because of the chronicity of problems that parents experience. Parents may lose sight of hope, and they may tend to see permanency of behavior with no relief in sight. Children with mental retardation tend to learn in increments; therefore change is not perceived as happening quickly, and parents can lose sight of the behavioral objective they had. It is important that parents be taught how to set both short-term and long-term realistic goals that are compatible with the child's developmental functioning. These goals can be planned only on the basis of systematic observations of what the child is currently doing. It is impossible to set up short- or long-term goals without impressive data about the child's current developmental functional levels within his environment. It is important, too, that parents learn that they cannot expect to change a number of behaviors at once.

6. Help parents see themselves as the greatest resources for change for their own children. Parents may regard professionals as resources for "fixing up" the child and returning him when he is ready. Parents need persons who can instill confidence in them as parents. They deserve the right to choose and reject alternatives of care and plan for their child as well as for themselves.

7. Support parents in their decision-making processes from the beginning to the time the objectives are accomplished. Parents must learn to state their goals in their own ways rather than relying on health care professionals to do so. Professionals must not usurp parental roles and state goals or make decisions for parents. Parents need to make and state the goals as they see them and become actively involved in the decision-making process. It is important that professionals help work out parental concerns *with* parents, *not* for them. As they take on more responsibility, parents become more accountable for the decisions that have been made for their children. This is not to say that child care professionals leave parents stranded but support them in appropriate problem solving

and decision making and help them become more objective in looking at the consequences of their own actions. It is important that professionals help parents become more responsible for their own behavior; thus they become controllers rather than victims. Parents need to know that they are basically in charge and that professionals have not usurped their roles. Often, parents in the past were awed and intimidated by professional persons. The real objectives of child care professionals should be to interact with parents in a mutually comfortable way that results in growth for the child, the parent, and the professional. It is also important that ultimately the professionals help parents understand their own feelings so that they can resolve them and move on to constructive problem solving instead of using their psychic energy on being angry at professionals or blaming themselves for things they have not done.

Professionals should also help parents identify and examine alternatives. They may forget that choices are actually available. For instance, they can learn to compare a foster home with a large institution. Child care professionals need to help parents see their strengths. Parents have made appropriate choices in the past, and professionals can point out specific abilities that can be transferred to other situations. This is particularly relevant when parents ask about what they will do about the child's future. Child care professionals should help parents examine their present actions and ask them how these affect the child's abilities as well as how they will affect the child's future behavior. Too often, parents do not give themselves credit for the excellent jobs that they are doing as parents. Professionals need to be able to reaffirm that parents are competent, resourceful, and essential to the successful outcomes of their child.

If a mother asks what she should do with the child when he grows up, professionals need to help the mother define what she is doing in the present and acknowledge her concerns for the future. One mother, for example, asked if people would reject the child. The nurse answered, "I can see that is a concern to you. I cannot tell you if people will reject her. What I need to know is, do they reject her now? If so, how did she respond to the rejection? How did you respond? Are you comfortable with what you did? Are you comfortable with what your daughter did? Is there a better way to respond to this behavior when it occurs?"

Child care professionals must help parents communicate their needs more effectively, encourage them consistently, and when they see parents over a period of time, help them make their needs known. It is important to see parents on a longitudinal rather than episodic basis and to check with parents as changes are occurring in their children. As children change their behaviors, parents change theirs. Professionals should know if parents are comfortable with the changes, if they see the changes in their children as positive, or if they wish to see other changes instituted. It is vital that child care professionals validate that parents are "good parents." They continually seek acknowledgment through their behavior and questions about whether they are good parents. Professionals need to be sensitive to the idea that parents may still be seeking an understanding of the cause of their child's handicap. They may be assuming too much if they think that parents have successfully dealt with the problem of mental retardation. Parents may still be questioning the role that they played in their child's handicap, and professionals need to check with them periodically about what they were told. Parents may need an understanding of the rationale for treatment or lack of a treatment plan. They may have been told repeatedly that something was wrong with their child, but what did it mean to them when they were told and what does it mean to them now? Whenever a parent of a child with mental retardation asks for advice, it is essential that child care professionals first find out what the parents have been told before planning a program of intervention. Professionals need to interact as openly with parents as they do with colleagues and respond to parents honestly.

What do parents need from health care professionals? They basically need a support system that meets their ongoing and changing needs. How can professionals do this?

1. By listing and confirming that the parents indeed are describing a valid concern
2. By letting parents know that they are accepted and that their feelings are accepted
3. By helping parents define their concerns. The professional can help the parents be more specific in their own descriptions of a child's behavior
4. By ascertaining what their concerns mean to the parents
5. By determining what the parents' priorities are for their child
6. By determining what the parents' priorities are for themselves

7. By investigating what the parents want to change, what they want to change first, and of all the changes that they want, what they want first

8. By determining how professionals can facilitate change in a healthy adaptive way

Parents need to be involved in an interaction model and not treated as passive recipients of the virtuoso model. They need to feel actively and essentially involved in achieving their child's welfare.

What do professionals need to be more confident in responding to parents' and children's needs. First, professionals must develop listening skills. Second, professionals in child care need to be more accepting of their own professional and personal feelings, behaviors, attitudes, and fears before they can respond to others and be nurturing and helpful to them when they need it the most. Health care professionals are working and interacting with others who are essentially in pain. They need to give themselves credit for their own strengths in responding to the needs of clients.

PARENTING BEHAVIORS THAT ASSIST CHILDREN IN LEARNING DEVELOPMENTAL TASKS

Parents in this culture help children to achieve competence in fine and gross motor control and coordination. Infants depend on their parents to help them learn to hold their heads up, to develop head support, to sit up, to stand alone, to walk forward and backward, to run and jump, and to be successful in tasks that require fine as well as large muscle coordination.

Children progressively learn to move from being dependent on their parents to learning to care for themselves. For example, parents teach children how to eat with a fork and spoon, to drink from a cup and glass, and to dress and undress. Children are taught to select their clothes and dress and undress without supervision. They gradually learn to take responsibility for putting away their own toys, to carry out simple requests of their parents, to imitate household tasks, and to become independent in their toileting behavior. They explore their environment, first with their parents present and gradually on a more independent basis.

Parents are expected to help children achieve a rhythm of living according to the culture in which the child lives. This means eating three meals a day, sleeping at regular hours, play-

ing at designated times, and learning at other regulated hours. Parents also help children learn the process of becoming a member of the family. This means that the child learns to share, give, take turns, wait, and contribute to and take from others. It means that the child learns a sense of responsibility to other members of the family and becomes an active part in the family routines.

As the child masters the tasks of relating to his family, he gradually learns the process of belonging to other social groups. This ordinarily begins with experiences at nursery school, day care center, preschool, and regular school. Parents also teach children to value themselves through the process of socialization. Parents are responsible for teaching children that they are valued, that they do belong, and that they are needed. Children learn to perceive themselves as acceptable, having positive traits and appealing behaviors. They learn the same values their parents teach them. Children also learn how to devalue themselves by the way others interact with them.

Parents in this culture are responsible for teaching children to give and receive affection. The best and nearest role models that children have early in their lives are parents. Children learn to share as they imitate adults sharing. Children also watch adult models give and receive affection in appropriate ways.

Parents are responsible for teaching communication to their children, a task which begins as early as the first week of life. Parents talk in front of their child, obtain (or at least try to obtain) eye contact, speak to him, label objects, help him identify body parts, and acknowledge him when he begins to coo or babble. An infant may learn that a certain coo brings mother near and she smiles at him, whereas a cry of distress brings mother near, but she has a different look on her face when she approaches. Thus children learn symbols of affection and rejection. Parents begin to stroke and caress their child, indicating approval and acceptance. As the child grows older, the parents may continue to demonstrate affection physically through touch, but they may substitute more verbal expressions such as, "I like the way you're doing that," or they may express disapproval, "Do it this way" or "No" or "I don't like that." Thus children learn the complexities of communication from their parents.

Parents also are responsible for providing

physical, social, and emotional stimuli when the child needs them. The child responds both to animate and inanimate stimuli, and it is the parents who mediate the amount, quality, duration, and appropriateness of the stimuli. Parents help children learn to differentiate between objects, to learn similarities, and to generalize from one situation to another. In this way, parents help children make judgments about situations and make personal choices. Parents help their children form concepts about numbers, space, timing, and other kinds of judgments. They help their children make judgments about subtle as well as conspicuous interactions that take place in their environment. Little by little children are taught by their parents how to solve problems, make choices, set priorities, make their wishes known, communicate their needs, and communicate their presence. In the beginning this may be by body language. As the child grows older, he uses words. Parents are responsible for socializing their children, helping them internalize rules of right and wrong, learn what is expected, and develop a conscience. From the beginning, the parent serves as a role model. The child learns from his parents what is and is not tolerated. As he grows older and achieves more autonomy, he is held to be responsible for a sense of right or wrong.

ADVICE TO PROFESSIONALS WHO WORK WITH MENTALLY RETARDED CHILDREN

Gorham and co-authors[10] suggest it is important for the child care professional to encourage parents to be involved in every step in the assessment process of the mentally retarded child. They stress that the dialogue which is developed and maintained with the parents may be the most important function the professional can accomplish. Gorham and co-authors suggest that if the parents' presence interferes with testing because the child will not cooperate, the assessment and diagnostic setup should include a complete review of the testing procedure with the parents. (Remote video viewing or one-way windows are excellent, but expensive, aids.)

Gorham and co-authors[10] urge the child care professional to develop a realistic management plan that is provided simultaneously with the assessment results. This plan should include suggestions for how to live with the problem of mental retardation on an hourly, daily,

monthly, and yearly basis. The child care professional needs to assess thoroughly the child's needs and strengths, the capacities and concerns of each family member, and the way that the family members view the child. The child care professional needs to know which community resources are available and should be able to recommend those which will meet the unique needs of each child and family member. It is important that the parents not interpret the management plan or the diagnostic results as absolute. They need to know that modifications can be made if any part of the plan proves ineffective.

Gorham and co-authors urge all child care professionals to inform themselves about community resources. It is important that the parents receive advice on the step-by-step process of going about and getting exactly what they need. Ideally, child care professionals should direct parents to local organizations that help parents meet and discuss common problems such as mental retardation. Professionals should know when there are openings in parent discussion groups and should let parents know when they might join, who will lead the meetings, and what the general objectives of the group are. Professionals should be able to tell parents about the advantages of these meetings. It is imperative that the parents be made active team members in all observations about the child, in each diagnostic step taken, and in planning, implementing, and evaluating any program designed for the child.

It is important that the child care professional always take advantage of observing how the parents and child interact in a variety of settings. In the past it seems that the professional focus has been mainly on observing the child and his behavior, and child care professionals have not always emphasized giving information and reports to both parents clearly and coherently.

Professionals must begin to use the strengths model after and during the assessment process, including both parents in the assessment process. For example, they should ask parents how they think their child will do in an assessment process. When the assessment procedure is finished, it is important that the parents be told systematically the child's strengths in each area assessed. The strengths should be presented before any weaknesses, and the weaknesses should be presented gently and with sensitivity.

In describing the child's weaknesses, the child care professional may pause and ask, "Do you agree with me?" If the parent says, "Yes, I do agree with you; however, did you see that he was able to do . . .?" In this case there is a dialogue. Information is being exchanged, and the parent feels very much a part of the assessment procedure. It is also important that, at the end of the assessment process, the professional says, "This is what I observed. Do you agree with me?" The parent might say, "No, I don't agree with you. At home he does it this way and this way and this way." If a parent describes the child's behavior as different at home, this is probably the case. The child care professional can then acknowledge this fact and may even say she would like to visit the home.

Parents need to know that their child is capable of performing, even though he has not completely mastered a task. The child care professional must be sensitive to the small, prerequisite behaviors that precede entire mastery of the task. Thus, even though the child is not spoon feeding himself, he might be focusing his attention on the spoon or the food. These discrete behaviors that precede mastery of the entire skill must be pointed out to the parents so that they understand that they have already made it possible for the child to make some developmental advances. Frequently, parents feel guilty about starting a task too late. Yet if one actually examines the small discrete behaviors the child can perform, the parents have probably been encouraging the child to prepare for the task that he is having trouble mastering. Emphasis should be placed on his beginning attempts, on the fact that he persevered, and that the professional observed his beginning the skill.

It is important that the child care professional become accustomed to sharing and writing clear, simple, and precise reports about the child that the parents can readily understand and discuss. Before giving a written report to the parents, it is wise to share the report with them verbally. Thus they can comment on what their understanding is at that time and any misunderstandings can be immediately corrected. All questions can be answered as they occur and at the time the report is given. The child care professional should realize that technical language and jargon are really barriers to parents' understanding. Parents naturally become frustrated and angry when trying to read difficult reports, and professionals should make it clear that they are available to answer any questions about the report.

As Gorham and co-authors[10] point out, child care professionals must remember that it is not they who must live and interact with the child daily, but the mother, father, and siblings. It is the family members who give assistance, reassurance, counseling, instructions, corrections, and approval throughout the day. And it is ultimately the parents whom the child must trust and seek for guidance and support. Thus the parents must be as well informed as the professional can possibly make them.

The real goal, as Gorham and co-authors see it, is to "produce" parents who understand their child well enough to help him handle his problems as he grows. He will face many. Therefore it becomes imperative that health care professionals be advocates for the child and individual family members as they experience the difficulties, delights, and tasks that parents and mentally retarded children experience.

It is essential that the parents receive the child care professional's written report. The parents will need all available information to begin to comprehend the assimilate the content in these reports. They will include not only the child's current developmental status but, between the lines, the implications of mental retardation for this child in the future. The parents are the ones who will have to give information to other people who will be interacting with the child. Therefore they must be very well informed to communicate effectively the child's needs, progress, short- and long-term goals, and a general comprehensive picture of the child and his situation. These comprehensive and clearly written reports can help parents avoid weeks and months of trying to get information and can help them avoid the time that it takes to process an application form to assure that the child will get into an appropriate program. Gorham and co-authors[10] point out that it is essential for child care professionals to make it extremely clear to the parents and siblings (as their age and maturity permits) that there is no final, unchanging diagnosis for the child. The family and child need to know that the child's development will be assessed periodically. As a child grows, his needs change. As he enters special programs, his behaviors may change and a new diagnosis may be made.

It is vitally important that parents clearly understand that a label is merely a device for communicating something about the child. Labels can communicate aspects of a child's behavior or development that may allow him to enter a special program because he must meet certain criteria. However, parents do need to know that negative implications are associated with labeling, that labels should be avoided if at all possible, that many labels are highly undesirable, and that once they are applied, it is difficult to undo the damage they can cause a child and family. Parents need to know that a label tells little about what a child can do in the present and even less about what he can do in the future. It is important to caution parents not to use labels when they are trying to describe or communicate the needs of their child. Parents should be encouraged to describe their children in terms of their behavior, their appealing traits, and their deficits. Parents sometimes feel they need permission to not discuss what is wrong with their child. They may feel the need to provide lengthy explanation of what mental retardation is or what syndrome their child has. Parents need to be encouraged to give as little information as they wish and to limit other people's questions. Parents can learn how to give only the information that they want to give and no more.

Parents need to know that they can be models for other people who interact with their child. In fact, others look to parents as examples of how to interact with or behave in front of the mentally retarded child because they have not had this experience. Therefore parents must know that they play a highly important part in the way that others interact with and convey acceptance of their child. If they show a positive, accepting, and wholesome view of their child, others will probably follow and demonstrate similar appropriate behavior. Conversely, if parents portray a negative approach, they are simply setting the stage for others to follow.

Gorham and co-authors[10] point out that child care professionals must assist parents to think in terms of life and experiences with their mentally retarded child in the same way as life with other children. In other words, if parents can see their child in the perspective of an ongoing, problem-solving process, they are miles ahead. It is important that parents be assured of the problem-solving abilities that they have demonstrated in the past. If problems that they do not feel adequate in coping with arise, they should know that the child care professional is accessible and available to solve problems with

them—not to make final decisions for them but to think about things together and to come up with the best answer that is possible for the child. Parents should consider life with their mentally retarded child as life is with any person—ups and downs, highs and lows, good days and days that are not as good. There will be times when the interactions between the child and the parent will not be absolutely positive, and there will be times when both the parent and the child will confront dilemmas that other parents and children face. It is not as if a particular dilemma will persist forever. Parents and children need to think of life in terms of a problem-solving framework so that they do not believe nothing will ever change.

At the same time, I would like to emphasize that parents need to know that they are capable of making highly astute observations about their child's behavior early in their child's life, and they can bring to the attention of child care professionals any concerns that they might have. If they suspect progress is not being made with their child, they should be encouraged to bring this concern to professional attention when the concern arises, not when too much time has passed to correct the situation.

It is vital that parents understand the child's strengths, appealing traits, and triumphs as well as his weaknesses and struggles. As Gorham and co-authors[10] say, what the child *can do* is far more significant than what the child cannot do. Therefore an appropriate goal of the parent becomes that of watching for small changes and new abilities, anticipating change, and welcoming with joy increments of change, no matter how slight they are.

It is also important to give parents permission, and encourage them to give themselves permission, to relax their continuous vigilance about everything that the child does. Sometimes parents become so involved in watching every detail that they overburden themselves and become fatigued and irritable. Child care professionals should encourage parents to relax and not to lose hope when behavioral changes do not occur rapidly. Parents need to learn to pace themselves and to give themselves permission to present challenges and appropriate learning experiences to the child. Sometimes parents need an objective outsider to help them see the changes that are occurring. Again, it is important that parents keep records and document carefully what their child is doing so that they can see progress as it occurs. A child may be holding his head up for only a second, and a second seems a very short period of time. But when parents begin to count 20 seconds, 30 seconds, 60 seconds, then 5 minutes, they begin to see changes that have occurred in a concrete way. This prevents them from giving up hope and from seeing only the child's deficits.

It is important that parents learn to be honest, first with themselves about their child and his behavior and, second, with their child, so that they present things to him on his level. Parents must speak clearly and simply to their child. As he learns to understand more and it is clear that his receptive abilities have improved, the parents can regulate their vocabulary and way of speaking accordingly. It is important that the parents not speak demeaningly in front of the child nor speak down to him. Parents need to be told repeatedly, both verbally and nonverbally (and professionals need to acknowledge this), that the most important aspect of the parents' responsibilities is to respect their child and to show others how to respect the child.

Next in importance, the parents must show and even say repeatedly that they love the child very much and approve of him. Through these demonstrations of feelings, the child learns to respect and approve of himself. A mentally retarded child may feel he has done something wrong for which he should punish himself because he is different and because of the subtle ways that others have mistreated him. The child needs to learn that some things he does are acceptable, that he does certain things very well, and that he is an important person. Parents need to watch for cues that the child accepts himself and behaves as if he likes and is proud of himself. When parents begin to hear the child make negative statements about himself or show self-destructive behavior, they must begin to solve the problem and work together on ways to improve the child's self-image. Parents must teach the child that self-blame is totally unacceptable. Mental retardation is nobody's fault. There still are many perplexing questions about mental retardation. It is one of the most misunderstood, mistreated, misdiagnosed, mishandled social and emotional problem that plagues the United States today.

It is important that child care professionals warn the parents about known service inefficiencies. Parents need advice and encouragement for their ways of making it through the system of the "helping services." Professionals should warn parents that some services will not always be helpful or appropriate to their needs. However, parents must know that they and their children are legally entitled to services and treatments. Professionals convey acceptance of parents when they view the parents as the primary helpers who monitor the child's behavior and progress, coordinate his activities and the services available to him, keep good and relevant records, and regard them as the major decision makers for their child. In this way health care professionals can treat parents appropriately—with dignity and as colleagues rather than as passive recipients, as has traditionally been the case with parents of mentally retarded children.

Parents should be encouraged to learn to keep records of their child's behaviors. It is essential that they start a notebook as soon as they know the child has a behavioral problem or a developmental delay. They should record the names, addresses, and telephone numbers of those persons who were present during the child's or parents' visits to the professional, the dates of the visits, and as much of what was said as possible. At the same time the parents should record their unanswered questions. If this is not done, the parents cannot be assertive or express what they want from child care professionals. Parents should write down the answers or any recommendations that the professionals gave. It is a good idea also for the parents to record the purpose and results of telephone calls to child care professionals or to agencies. Parents should record their feelings after making the telephone call. They should be encouraged to make important requests by writing letters and keeping copies of all correspondence in their notebook. Documentation of all of the parents' efforts to obtain services for their child can be extremely important in procuring appropriate solutions. Parents should be reminded to request copies of their child's records, particularly after informative conferences.

The parents should learn to maintain close contact with professionals who work with their child, whether this be the physician, the nurse, the social worker, or the teacher. It is helpful for the parents to observe their child in the classroom so that they can continue certain school programs at home and can discuss any difficulties with the teacher. Both the parent and the professional work best as a team. If they realize this, more successful outcomes are possible for the parent, the child, and the child care professional.

Finally, the child should be considered part

of the team whenever possible. His ideas should be taken into consideration. He should be actively invited and brought into conferences, even though he may not have language skills. Child care professionals should remember not to talk about a child in his presence. This is similar to gossiping about him. It is not certain what children can absorb and what they hear about themselves. If parents talk about the child as a problem and a cause of concern at home, the child begins to feel that he is indeed a burden rather than an asset to the family. Child care professionals should be sensitive to this kind of parental behavior. They should carefully observe how parents interact with children and even what names they call their mentally retarded child. The child should be addressed consistently by the same name. This should be a given, acceptable name and not a nickname such as "birdie," "feathers," "cutie," "sister," or a pronoun. The child needs to know that he has a name and that he is a person in his own right. He needs the dignity that comes with being addressed as a person.

Professionals need to encourage parents to be sensitive to their child by observing his behavior, watching for changes, and inviting him to discuss his needs or to somehow communicate or gesture when he is having problems. Children can learn appropriate ways to ask for help from their parents. Neither child care professionals nor parents have always been attuned to this. But parents need to become accustomed to listening to their child, both by hearing what he says and watching the way he acts. Parents can remember that the child's point of view is equally as important as that of the parents. The child is the expert regarding what is happening to him. This is especially important as the child grows up, develops more language skills, and becomes involved in decisions that affect his life, whether he is entering school, going through special programs, planning a vocation, or preparing to marry and have children of his own.

REFERENCES

1. Ehlers, Walter H., Krishef, Curtis H., and Prothero, Jon C.: An introduction to mental retardation: a programmed text, Columbus, Ohio, 1973, Charles E. Merrill Publishing Co.
2. Hobbs, Nicholas J.: Issues in the classification of children, San Francisco, 1975, Jossey-Bass, Inc., Publishers.
3. Grossman, Herbert J.: Manual on terminology and classification in mental retardation, American Association on Mental Deficiency, Special Publication Series No. 2, p. 11, 1973.
4. Wolfensberger, Wolf: Normalization: the principle of normalization in human services, Toronto, 1972, National Institute on Mental Retardation.
5. Benedek, Therese: Parenthood as a developmental phase, J. Am. Psychoanal. Assoc. **1:**389-417, 1959.
6. Olshansky, Simon: Chronic sorrow: a response for having a mentally defective child, Soc. Casework **43:**190-193, 1963.
7. Gayton, William F.: Management problems of mentally retarded children and their families, Symposium on Behavioral Pediatrics, Pediatr. Clin. North Am. **22:**561-570, 1975.
8. Caldwell, Bettye M.: Instruction manual inventory for infants (Home Observation for Measurement of the Environment), Little Rock, Ark., 1970.
9. Farber, Barnard, and Rykman, David B.: Effects of severely mentally retarded children on family relationships, Ment. Retard. Abs. **2:**1-17, Jan.-March, 1965.
10. Gorham, Kathryn A., Des Jardins, Charlotte, Page, Ruth, Pettis, Eugene, and Scheiber, Barbara: Effect on parents, vol. 2. In Hobbs, Nicholas, editor: Issues in the classification of children, San Francisco, 1975, Jossey-Bass, Inc., Publishers.

ADDITIONAL READINGS

Morgan, Sam B.: Team interpretation of MR 2 parents, Ment. Retard. **11:**10-13, June, 1973.
Stephens, Wyatt E.: Interpreting mental retardation to parents in a multidiscipline diagnostic clinic, Ment. Retard. pp. 57-59, Dec., 1969.
Wolfensberger, Wolf: Embarrassments in the diagnostic process, Ment. Retard. **3:**29-31, June, 1965.

20

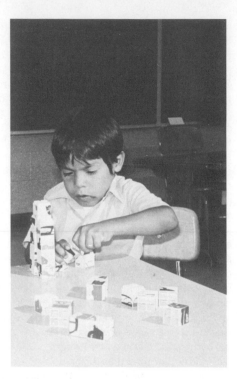

USE OF THE WASHINGTON GUIDE TO PROMOTING DEVELOPMENT IN THE YOUNG CHILD

Nurses and other child care professionals are playing a greater role in periodically assessing mentally retarded children as they attempt to ensure greater objectivity in collecting data about each child and his environment so that they can plan appropriate treatment and care. The assessment process consists of the following four phases:

1. Preparation of children and parents
2. Administration of screening test items
3. Interpretation and analysis of the results of a screening or assessment procedure
4. Communication of these findings to the parents and discussion of the parents' reaction to the assessment procedure before advice is given

To do a more thorough job of assessment, child care professionals are using a variety of standardized tools, placing greater emphasis on those screening tools which predict a child's future developmental and cognitive outcomes.

Each time a new assessment tool is used, the child care professional should prepare the parents by discussing the tool's purpose and limitations, how it was developed, and how the child

---

Above photograph from Gearheart, B. R.: Learning disabilities: educational strategies, ed. 2, St. Louis, 1977, The C. V. Mosby Co.

will be given credit. Before examining the child, the professional should ask the parents how well they think the child is doing in the areas to be tested and then ask them to observe as she assesses the child. At the end of the assessment procedure, the professional should (1) ask the parents how well they thought the child did; (2) present her observations of the child's strengths, attempts at tasks, attention to the tasks, ability to comply, and items passed; and (3) present those areas in which the child did not perform as well.

Nurses and other child care professionals who are working with mentally retarded children must recognize the great importance of making direct observations of the child while he is performing activities of daily living such as feeding, toilet training, and dressing. This is not to imply that the professional should discount parents' observations, which are also extremely important; however, her observations during a home visit can be more objective and will complement parental observations.

The child care professional is also in a favorable position to observe the child at play—what toys the child plays with, the pleasure he seems to derive from playing, the kinds of behaviors he initiates with a toy, whether or not he explores a variety of toys, his attention span to a given toy, and the availability of toys that are suitable for his functional behavior. The professional should also observe the child playing with other children. Does he initiate play activities? Does he imitate other play behavior? Can he follow rules? Is he able to take turns? Does he play with younger or older children? Does he lead or is he a follower? Is his appropriate play behavior reinforced by the parents? Does he respond appropriately in a play situation, or does he withdraw?

The child care professional can also observe the child's interactions with his parents. For example, regarding limit setting, how quickly does the child respond to a given request, and how do the parents respond to the child's behavior? Do parents give approval and show the child that he has carried out the request in an appropriate way or do they ignore his behavior? In general, do parents respond to the child when he is acting appropriately, or do they only attend to him and acknowledge his behavior when he is showing undesirable behaviors? Children with mental retardation may manifest a variety of behaviors that are difficult for family members, particularly parents, to interpret and respond to appropriately. With help from an objective outsider, such as a nurse or other professional person, parents are more capable of learning to interpret their child's behavior correctly and to respond in more appropriate ways.

In assessing speech, the child care professional can listen for the kinds of speech sounds the child can make, the actual words that he uses to indicate his needs, the ways that he makes his needs known, and whether or not his speech is appropriate for his needs.

A child who is mentally retarded is best assessed by a health care professional who can observe and encourage the child's best performance, no matter how difficult the task. This requires skills above and beyond those required to assess a "normal" child. The observational skills and ability of the child care professional to interpret objectively and accurately what the child can do are vitally important to both the child and his parents. The professional must strive to be continuously sensitive to the variety and number of cues the child emits in response to a request. These cues might include willingness to perform, ability to separate from a parent, attention to the task at hand, interest in participating, ability to ignore irrelevant stimuli, eagerness to please, desire to succeed, and ability to initiate and efforts to persist in the task.

Of course, an assessment of the child should begin only after he shows that he is comfortable and can perform optimally. The child care professional should encourage the child throughout the assessment procedure, obtaining the child's attention before she expects him to complete a task and being clear and concise in orienting the child to what is expected of him. She should concentrate on getting the child to respond to one request at a time and should reduce animate and inanimate extraneous stimuli. She also should be careful to present tasks in which the child has a chance for success before frustrating him with tasks that are beyond his ability to perform. The child should be allowed to perform at his own pace. Flexibility is necessary in attempting different observational approaches with a child, particularly one who might be showing unusual forms of behavior. If a child is exhibiting a variety of confusing behaviors, it is wise to plan for several observation sessions and to observe specific, discrete portions of selected behaviors at each session. The child care professional should be aware that all children are sensitive to the acceptance, approval, enthusiasm, or indifference which she shows during a developmental screening session.

The child care professional must also remain alert and tune in to the needs of the parents during an assessment procedure and should listen carefully to what they are saying about their child. It is essential to find out exactly what parents have been told about their child's condition, when and by whom they were told, and what it meant to them at the time. Any unresolved feelings they have about information they received earlier should be explored before further information is given about their child's performance. When the professional has to give feedback about a child's developmental delays or deficits, she should be prepared to make statements such as, "This may not be easy for you to observe or to talk about." She must be sure the parents are receptive to her comments rather than proceeding if they have, in essence, tuned her out.

ASSESSMENT TOOLS

A variety of developmental assessment or screening tools are available for use with children and their families. One of the most popular screening test is the Denver Developmental Screening Test (DDST), which helps screen a child's performance in four categories: personal-social skills, fine motor achievements, receptive and expressive language abilities, and gross motor tasks. The DDST is standardized—each child is asked to perform an item in the same way, using identical materials.

The Washington Guide to Promoting Development in the Young Child helps child care professionals to be more effective at assessing and preventing handicapping conditions in mentally retarded children. The Washington Guide is popular because it relies on direct observations of the child's activities in daily living and does not require elaborate testing equipment.

The DDST measures a child's physical abilities, self-help skills, social behavior, academic skills, and both receptive and expressive communication skills. The DDST relies somewhat on parents' verbal responses to questionnaire items, thus providing a structured way for the professional to listen to what parents are saying about their children. It has certain advantages over other tools that require direct observations: It can be used with children who are ill and cannot currently perform tasks in their usual and best ways or with parents of children who have acoustical impairments, sensory-motor disorders, emotional disturbance, and intellectual deficits.

DEVELOPMENTAL ASSESSMENT

It is necessary to observe children directly to assess functional levels and also to find out what is easy and what is not easy for children. Verbal reports are not sufficient but may be used in conjunction with watching a child being fed, eating, undressing, dressing, playing, responding to commands, practicing fine and gross motor skills, toileting, or preparing for bedtime.

The Washington Guide for Promoting Development in the Young Child provides one framework that can be used in making developmental assessments. This guide was specifically designed to assist nurses, physicians, social workers, psychologists and other child care professionals to do a better job in observing, assessing, case finding, and planning developmental interventions for infants and children. The guide helps a child care professional to be more objective about the information being obtained.

Using such a guide requires direct observations of a child's specific behaviors. This method helps reduce some of the inherent weaknesses of relying on others' reports of developmental tasks that they believe a child can or cannot ac-

complish. The organization of the Washington Guide is characterized by a distinct sequential format. Developmental items are arranged in an orderly way, giving a progressive guide of simple to complex tasks that are expected of a child in his development at different age periods. It is also characterized by the way in which it structures a one-to-one relationship; that is, information is derived from the child care professional interacting on a one-to-one basis with a child to elicit certain behaviors. It requires getting down to the child's level for closer observations and interactions.

This guide is used to observe well infants and children, those suspected of developmental delays, and those with known high-risk factors in their development. The guide is used in a variety of settings, such as well-child clinics, child development centers, maternal and infant projects, day care centers, institutions, pediatric floors in hospitals, physicians' offices, schools, and private homes.

The data gained from the guide are used as a basis for reassuring parents of their child's development, counseling them on expectations, offering anticipatory guidance, and giving suggestions in promoting development. The data can serve as guidelines for referral and a longitudinal record for ongoing developmental assessments.

As with any tool, both strengths and weaknesses are apparent. The Washington Guide has not been standardized on an adequate sample. The developmental items that comprise the expected tasks at various ages from newborn to 5 years are considered valid. The sources utilized as references in constructing the composite of items found in the Guide are listed at the end of the chapter.

Most screening tools, such as the DDST, primarily provide a means of identifying the significant variances in child development. The Washington Guide differs from these in that it is not specifically designed to be used as a screening tool; its primary purpose is to present a frame of reference about growth and development which will enable the child care professional to observe a child's abilities systematically and, on that basis, make recommendations regarding child-rearing practices which would capitalize on the child's present abilities and encourage further movement up the developmental ladder. In summary, the purpose of the Washington Guide is to provide a reference for the professional to use in observing development, giving parental counseling, or making appropriate referrals for evaluation.

The process of assessment is an expected and routine fact of child care today. Developmental assessment is the basis of case finding and prevention. The results of assessment are relied on to assist the family in promoting the optimal environment for the child's progression on the developmental continuum. The significant services given by child care professionals to parents who have children with developmental deviations consist essentially of assisting the family to learn to appraise a child's developmental status and thus guide parental expectations, discipline, and training to the functional level to promote the child's optimal development.

SUGGESTIONS FOR USING THE WASHINGTON GUIDE

A few suggestions regarding the structure and application of the guide will provide child care professionals with enough information to use it.

1. The guide follows the structure of the most common functional activities of the young child's daily life—feeding, sleep, play, language, motor activities, discipline, toilet training, and dressing. In each category of activity the developmental attainments that would be expected in accord with references on child development are grouped as "expected tasks" within a 3-month age range during the first 12 months of life, then at 6- to 12-month intervals until 5 years of age. Accompanying each category and age grouping of expected tasks is a listing of "suggested activities" that can serve as the basis of advice to the parents about enriching child-rearing practices.

2. No criteria have been established for the administration and scoring of items. The references that follow this chapter provide information of this nature.

3. There are no requirements for specific equipment or elaborate monitoring systems. The toys and equipment in the child's natural environment should be relied on.

4. In using the guide, it is suggested that you do the following:

   a. Familiarize yourself with the appropriate age grouping of the child to be observed.

   b. Start below the child's chronological age level so that success with tasks can be experienced from the beginning.

   c. Whenever possible, observe the child's performance.

   d. Ask the parents to relay information about the item when this is not possible.

   e. Carefully explain to the parents that you will be going from easy to difficult tasks.

   f. Ask the parent to refrain from prompting or interfering with the child's attempt to carry out a request.

   g. Cross out or note on a separate recording each item the child can do; this leaves you with listings of the target areas that represent possible points for making use of the suggested activities.

   h. List appropriate suggested activities and discuss them with the parents.

5. A precise numerical rating or score of the child's behavior is not sought. However, through directly observing the child in a series of activities, a functional age range can be established. It is recommended that a child be considered as functioning at a particular age range if he is doing a majority of the tasks in that grouping. The guide is arranged so that you have ready access to both the preceding and following age groupings. If a child is doing none of the tasks within an age range, refer to the previous ages; in instances in which the child has completed all activities in an age grouping, proceed to a more advanced grouping.

6. After the age-range skills that a child can perform are eliminated, the target areas of deficits in development that should be strengthened are automatically visible. The suggestions for activities that correspond to the identified target areas can then be used as a beginning point of teaching parents how they can specifically enhance the attainment of developmental skills.

The guide is presented in its entirety. It should be noted that *this tool is not expected to give precise information on the child's developmental level. The Washington Guide to Promoting Development in the Young Child will assist child care professionals in observing the child on a systematic basis, point out variations in development, and provide suggestions regarding appropriate child-rearing practices.*

Text continued on p. 314.

THE WASHINGTON GUIDE TO PROMOTING DEVELOPMENT IN THE YOUNG CHILD*

MOTOR SKILLS

Expected tasks	Suggested activities

1 to 3 months

Expected tasks	Suggested activities
1. Holds head up briefly when prone	1. Place infant in prone position
2. Head erect and bobbing when supported in sitting position	2. Support in sitting position with his head erect
3. Head erect and steady in sitting position	3. Pull infant to sitting position
4. Follows object through all planes	4. Provide with opportunity to observe people or activity
5. Palmar grasp	5. Hang bright-colored objects and mobiles within reach across crib
6. Moro reflex	6. Provide with opportunity to observe objects or people while in sitting position
	7. Use infant seat
	8. Alternate bright shiny objects with dark and light visual patterns

4 to 8 months

Expected tasks	Suggested activities
1. Sits with minimal support, with stable head and back	1. Pull up to sitting position
2. Sits alone steadily	2. Provide opportunity to sit supported or alone when head and trunk control are stabilized
3. Plays with hands, which are open most of time	3. Put bright-colored objects within reach
4. Grasps rattle or bottle with both hands	4. Give toys or household objects: rattles, teething ring, cloth animals or dolls, 1-inch cubes, plastic objects such as cups, rings, and balls
5. Picks up small objects, e.g., cube	5. Offer small objects such as cereal to improve grasp
6. Transfers toys from one hand to other	6. Offer a variety of patterns or textures to play with
7. Neck-righting reflex	7. Use squeak toys

9 to 12 months

Expected tasks	Suggested activities
1. Rises to sitting position	1. Provide playpen, allow child to pull himself to standing
2. Creeps or crawls, maybe backward at first	2. Give opportunity and space to practice creeping and crawling
3. Pulls to standing position	3. Have child practice moving on knees to improve balance prior to walking
4. Stands alone	4. Have child use walker or straddle toys
5. Cruises	5. Play airplane with child; have child practice catching himself while rolling on large ball
6. Uses index finger to poke	6. Provide with objects such as spoons, plastic bottles, cups, ball, cubes, finger foods, saucepans, and lids
7. Finger-thumb grasp	
8. Parachute reflex	
9. Landau reflex	

*The author wishes to thank Dr. Kathryn E. Barnard for granting permission to reproduce The Washington Guide to Promoting Development in the Young Child. In Barnard, Kathryn E., and Erickson, Marcene L.: Teaching children with developmental problems: a family care approach, ed. 2, St. Louis, 1976, The C. V. Mosby Co.

A. Paulus and Dr. Kathryn Barnard originally designed The Washington Guide to Promoting Development in the Young Child in 1966 at the University of Washington School of Nursing, Seattle, Wash. Dr. Barnard and Marcene Powell Erickson revised the Washington Guide in 1969 at the University of Washington School of Nursing.

THE WASHINGTON GUIDE TO PROMOTING DEVELOPMENT IN THE YOUNG CHILD

MOTOR SKILLS — cont'd

Expected tasks	Suggested activities
13 to 18 months	
1. Walks a few steps without support	1. Provide opportunity to practice walking, climbing stairs with help
2. Balanced when walking	
3. Walks upstairs with help, creeps downstairs	2. Give toys that can be pushed around
4. Turns pages of book	3. Supervise activity with paper and large crayons
	4. Provide toys such as cubes, cups, saucepans, lids, rag dolls, and other soft, cuddly toys
	5. Begin introducing child to swing
19 to 30 months	
1. Runs	1. Provide opportunity to practice and develop activities
2. Walks up and down stairs, one at a time (not alternating feet)	2. Provide pattern for child while he watches and then encourage him to try
3. Imitates vertical strokes	
4. Imitates building tower of four or more blocks	3. Provide tricycle or similar pedal toys; secure foot on pedal is necessary
5. Throws ball overhead	
6. Jumps in place	
7. Rides tricycle	
31 to 48 months	
1. Walks downstairs (alternating feet)	1. Continue with blocks, combining materials, toy cars, and trains
2. Hops on one foot	
3. Swings and climbs	2. Provide clay and other manipulating materials
4. Balances on one foot for 10 seconds	
5. Copies circle	3. Give opportunities to swing and climb
6. Copies cross	4. Provide with activities such as finger painting, chalk, and blackboard
7. Draws person with three parts	
49 to 52 months	
1. Balances well	1. Provide with music and games to synchronize hand and foot, tapping with music, skipping, hopping, and dancing rhythmically to improve coordination
2. Skips and jumps	
3. Can heel-toe walk	
4. Copies square	
5. Catches bounced ball	

FEEDING SKILLS

Expected tasks	Suggested activities
1 to 3 months	
1. Sucking reflex present	1. Consider a change in nipple or posturing if there is difficulty in swallowing
2. Rooting reflex present	
3. Ability to swallow pureed foods	2. Hold in comfortable relaxed position while feeding
4. Coordinates sucking, swallowing, and breathing	3. Pace feeding tempo to infant's needs

Continued.

THE WASHINGTON GUIDE TO PROMOTING DEVELOPMENT IN THE YOUNG CHILD

FEEDING SKILLS — cont'd

Expected tasks	Suggested activities

4 to 8 months

Expected tasks	Suggested activities
1. Tongue used in moving food in mouth	1. Give finger foods to develop chewing, stimulate gums, and encourage hand-to-mouth motion (cubes of cheese, bananas, dry toast, bread crust, cookies)
2. Hand-to-mouth motions	
3. Recognizes bottle on sight	
4. Gums or mouths solid foods	2. Encourage upright supported position for feeding
5. Feeds self cracker	3. Promote bottle holding
	4. Introduce solids, one kind at a time (use small spoon, place food well back on infant's tongue)

9 to 12 months

Expected tasks	Suggested activities
1. Holds own bottle	1. Bring child in highchair to table and include in part of or entire meal with family
2. Drinks from cup or glass with assistance	
3. Finger feeds	2. Have child in dry comfortable position with trunk and feet supported
4. Beginning to hold spoon	3. Encourage self-help in feeding; use of table foods
	4. Offer spoon when interest is indicated
	5. Introduce cup or glass with small amount of fluid

13 to 18 months

Expected tasks	Suggested activities
1. Holds cup and handle with digital grasp	1. Continue offering finger foods (wieners, sandwiches)
2. Lifts cup and drinks well	
3. Beginning to use spoon, may turn bowl down before reaching mouth	2. Use nontip dishes and cups; dishes should have sides to make filling of spoon easy
4. Difficulty in inserting spoon into mouth	3. Give opportunity for self-feeding
5. May refuse food	4. Provide fluids between meals rather than having child fill up on fluids at mealtime

19 to 30 months

Expected tasks	Suggested activities
1. Drinks without spilling	1. Encourage self-feeding with spoon
2. Holds small glass in one hand	2. Do not rush child
3. Inserts spoon in mouth correctly	3. Serve foods plainly but in attractive servings
4. Distinguishes between food and inedible material	4. Small servings of food will encourage eating more than large servings
5. Plays with food	

31 to 48 months

Expected tasks	Suggested activities
1. Pours well from pitcher	1. Encourage self-help
2. Serves self at table with little spilling	2. Give opportunity for pouring (give rice and pitcher to promote pouring skills)
3. Rarely needs assistance	
4. Interest in setting table	3. Encourage child to help set table
	4. Have well-defined rules about table manners

49 to 52 months

Expected tasks	Suggested activities
1. Feeds self well	1. Socialize with child at mealtime
2. Social and talkative during meal	2. Have child help with preparation, table setting, and serving
	3. Include child in conversation at mealtimes by planning special times for him to tell about events, situations, or what he did during day

THE WASHINGTON GUIDE TO PROMOTING DEVELOPMENT
IN THE YOUNG CHILD

SLEEP

Expected tasks	Suggested activities

1 to 3 months

1. Night: 4- to 10-hour intervals 2. Naps: frequent 3. Longer periods of wakefulness without crying	1. Provide separate sleeping arrangements away from parents' room 2. Reduce noise and light stimulation when placing in bed 3. Have room at comfortable temperature with no drafts or extremes in heat 4. Reverse position of crib occasionally 5. Place child in different positions from time to time for sleep 6. Alternate from back to side to stomach 7. Keep crib sides up

4 to 8 months

1. Night: 10 to 12 hours 2. Naps: 2 to 3 (1 to 4 hours in duration) 3. Night awakenings	1. Keep crib sides up 2. Refrain from taking child into parents' room if he awakens 3. Check to determine if there is cause for awakenings: hunger, teething, pain, cold, wet, noise, or illness 4. If a baby-sitter is used, attempt to find some person with whom infant is familiar. Explain bedtime and naptime arrangements

9 to 12 months

1. Night: 12 to 14 hours 2. Naps: 1 to 2 (1 to 4 hours in duration) 3. May begin refusing morning nap	1. Short crying periods may be source of tension release for child 2. Observe for signs of fatigue, irritability, or restlessness if naps are shorter. 3. Provide familiar person to baby-sit who knows sleep routines

13 to 18 months

1. Night: 10 to 12 hours 2. Naps: one in afternoon (1 to 3 hours in duration) 3. May awaken during night crying (associated with wetting bed) 4. As he becomes more able to move about, he may uncover himself, become cold, and awaken	1. Night terrors may be terminated by awakening infant and offering reassurance 2. Check to see that child is covered 3. Avoid hazardous devices to keep child covered, including blanket clips, pins, and garments that enclose child to neck

19 to 30 months

1. Night: 10 to 12 hours 2. Naps: one (1 to 3 hours in duration) 3. Doesn't go to sleep at once—keeps demanding things 4. May awaken crying if wet or soiled 5. May awaken because of environmental change of temperature, change of bed, change of sleeping room, addition of sibling to room, absence of parent from home, hospitalization, trip with family, or relatives visiting	1. Quiet period of socialization prior to bedtime—reading child book or telling story 2. Holding child—talking quietly with him 3. Ritualistic behavior may be present; allow child to carry out routine; helps him overcome fear of unexpected or fear of dark; for example, child may wish to arrange toys in certain way 4. Explain bedtime ritual to baby-sitter 5. Give more reassurance, spend more time before bedtime preparation

Continued.

THE WASHINGTON GUIDE TO PROMOTING DEVELOPMENT IN THE YOUNG CHILD

SLEEP—cont'd

Expected tasks	Suggested activities
	19 to 30 months
	6. Provide familiar bedtime toys or items
	7. Allow crying-out period if he is safe, comfortable, and tucked in
	8. Place in bed before he reaches excessive state of fatigue, excitement, or tiredness
	9. Eliminate sources of stimulation or fear
	10. Maintain consistent hour of bedtime
	31 to 48 months
1. Daily range: 10 to 15 hours	1. TV programs may affect ability to go to sleep; avoid violent TV programs
2. Naps: beginning to disappear	2. Anxiety about going to bed and desire to stay up with parents—requires limits
3. Prolongs process of going to bed	3. Regularity and consistency important to promote good sleeping habits
4. Less dependent on taking toys to bed	4. Reassurance—night light or leaving door ajar
5. May awaken crying from dreams	5. Don't use bedtime or naptime as punishment
6. May awaken if wet	6. Encourage naps if signs of fatigue or irritability are evidenced
	49 to 52 months
1. Daily range: 9 to 13 hours	1. Encourage napping if excessive or strenuous activity occurs and child is overly tired
2. Naps: rare	2. Explain to child if sitter will be there after child is asleep
3. Quieter during sleep	

PLAY

Expected tasks	Suggested activities
	1 to 3 months
1. Quieted when picked up	1. Encourage holding and touching of child by parents
2. Regards face of others	2. Provide with cradle gyms and mobiles, brightly colored, visually interesting objects within arm's distance
	4 to 8 months
1. Plays with own body	1. Begin patty-cake and peek-a-boo
2. Differentiates strangers from family	2. Provide for periods of solitary play (playpen)
3. Seeks out objects	3. Encourage holding and touching of child by parents
4. Grasps, holds, and manipulates objects	4. Provide variety of multicolored and multitextured objects that child can hold
5. Repeats activities he enjoys	5. Encourage exploration of body parts
6. Bangs toys or objects together	6. Provide floating toys for bath

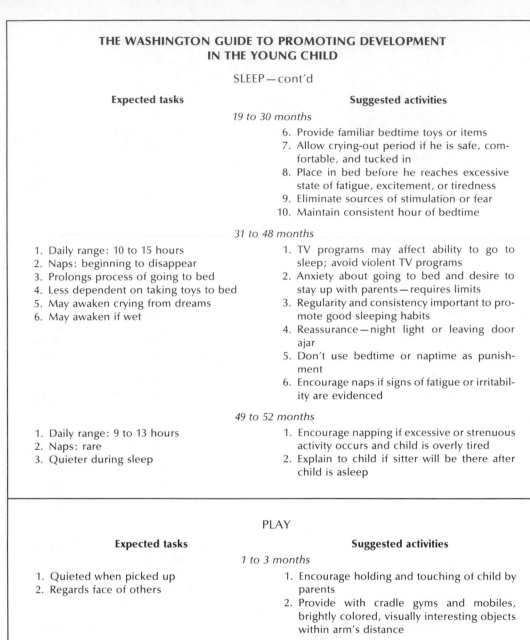

THE WASHINGTON GUIDE TO PROMOTING DEVELOPMENT IN THE YOUNG CHILD

PLAY—cont'd

Expected tasks	Suggested activities

9 to 12 months

Expected tasks	Suggested activities
1. Puts objects in and out of containers	1. Continue parent-infant games
2. Examines objects held in hand	2. Give opportunity to place objects in containers and pour out
3. Plays interactive games (peek-a-boo)	
4. Extends toy to other person without releasing	3. Provide large and small objects with which to play
5. Works to get toy out of reach	4. Encourage interactive play

13 to 18 months

Expected tasks	Suggested activities
1. Plays by himself—may play near others	1. Introduce to other children even though child may not play with them
2. Has preferred toys	
3. Enjoys walking activities, pulling toys	2. Provide music, books, magazines
4. Throws and picks up objects, throws again	3. Encourage imitative activities—helping with dusting, sweeping, stirring
5. Imitates, e.g., reading newspaper, sweeping	

19 to 30 months

Expected tasks	Suggested activities
1. Parallel play—not interactive but plays alongside another side	1. Provide with new materials for manipulating and feeling—finger paints, clay, sand, stones, water, and soap
2. Use both large and small toys	Wooden toys—cars and animals
3. Rough-and-tumble play	Building blocks of various sizes, crayons, and paper
4. Play periods longer than before—interested in manipulative and constructive toys	Rhythmical tunes and equipment—swing, rocking chair, rocking horse
5. Enjoys rhymes and singing (TV programs)	Children's books—short, simple stories with repetition and familiar objects; enjoys simple pictures, brightly colored
	2. Guide child's hand to actively participate with specific activities, e.g., using crayons, hammering

31 to 48 months

Expected tasks	Suggested activities
1. In playing with others, beginning to interact, sharing toys, taking turns	1. Encourage play with small groups of children
2. Dramatizes, expresses imagination in play	2. Encourage imaginative and dramatic play activities
3. Combining playthings; more use of constructive materials	3. Music: singing and experimenting with musical instruments
4. Prefers two or three children to play with; may have special friend	4. Group participation in rhymes, dancing by hopping or jumping
	5. Drawing and painting (seldom recognizable)

49 to 52 months

Expected tasks	Suggested activities
1. Dramatic play and interest in going on excursions	1. Painting and drawing (objects will be out of proportion; details that are most important to child are drawn largest)
2. Fond of cutting and pasting, creative materials	2. Encourage printing of numbers and letters
3. Completes most activities	3. Clay: making recognizable objects
	4. Cutting and pasting
	5. Provide with materials, e.g., boxes, chairs, barrels, for building sturdy structures

Continued.

THE WASHINGTON GUIDE TO PROMOTING DEVELOPMENT IN THE YOUNG CHILD

LANGUAGE

Expected tasks	**Suggested activities**

1 to 3 months

Receptive abilities

1. Movement of eyes, respiration rate, or body activity changes when bell is rung close to child's head
2. Smiles when socially stimulated
3. Has facial, vocal, and generalized bodily responses to faces
4. Reacts differentially to adult voices

Expressive abilities

1. Makes prelanguage vocalizations that consist of cooing, throaty sounds, e.g., gu
2. Makes "pleasure" sounds that consist of soft vowels
3. Makes "sucking" sounds
4. Crying can be differentiated for discomfort, pain, and hunger as reported by mother
5. An "A" sound as in cat is commonly heard in distress crying

Suggested activities (1 to 3 months):

1. Observe facial expressions, gestures, bodily postures, and movements when vocalizations are being produced
2. Smile and talk softly in pleasant tone while holding, touching, and handling infant
3. Hold, touch, and interact frequently with infant for pleasure
4. Refrain from letting infant engage in prolonged and incessant crying

4 to 8 months

Receptive abilities

1. Eyes locate source of sound
2. Responds to "hi, there" by looking up at face that is across and in front of him
3. Head turns to sound of cellophane held and crunched 2 feet away and at a 135-degree angle on either side of head
4. Will turn head to locate sound of "look here" when spoken at a 90-degree angle from head 2 feet away*
5. Turns head to sound of rattle
6. Responds differently to vacuum cleaner, phone, doorbell, or sound of dog barking: may cry, whimper, look toward sound, or parents may report change in body tension
7. Responds by raising arms when parents reach toward child and say "come up"

Expressive abilities

1. Uses different inflectional patterns:
   ah   ah
         uh
2. Laughs aloud when stimulated
3. Has differential patterns of crying when hungry, in pain, or angry
4. Produces vowel sounds and chained syllables (baba, gugu, didi)
5. Makes "talking sounds" in response to others talking to him
6. Babbles to produce consonant sounds: ba, da, m-m
7. Vocalizes to toys
8. Says "da-da" or "ma-ma" but not specific to presence of parents

Suggested activities (4 to 8 months):

1. Engage in smiling eye-to-eye contact while talking to infant
2. Vocalize in response to inflectional patterns and when infant is producing babbling sounds; echo the sounds he makes
3. Observe for subtle communication clues such as eye aversion, struggling to move away, flushing of skin, tension of body, or movement of arms
4. Vocalize with infant during handling, while feeding, bathing, dressing, diapering, bedtime preparation, and holding
5. Stimulate laughing by light tickling
6. Observe child's reactions to bells, whistles, horns, phones, laughing, singing, talking, music box, noisemaking toys, and common household noises
7. While talking to infant, hold in position so that he can see your face
8. Have infant placed at position of eye level while talking to him throughout day
9. If crying or laughing sounds are not discerned at this stage, report to family physician, pediatrician, public health nurse, or well-child clinic

---

*Do not test for localization of sound by producing sound directly behind infant's head.

THE WASHINGTON GUIDE TO PROMOTING DEVELOPMENT IN THE YOUNG CHILD

LANGUAGE—cont'd

Expected tasks	Suggested activities

9 to 12 months

Receptive abilities

1. Ceases activity when name is pronounced or "no-no" is said
2. Gives toys on request when accompanied by facial and bodily gestures
3. Attends to simple commands

Expressive abilities

1. Imitates definite speech sounds such as tongue clicking, lip smacking, or coughing
2. Should have two words that are *specific* for parents: "mama," "dada," or equivalents

1. Gain child's attention when giving simple commands
2. Accompany oral directions with gestures
3. Vocalize with child during feeding, bathing, and playtimes
4. Provide sounds that child can reproduce such as lip smacking and tongue clicking
5. Repeat direction frequently and have child participate in action: open and close the drawer; move arms and legs up and down
6. Have child respond to verbal directions: stand up, sit down, close door, open door, turn around, come here

13 to 18 months

Receptive abilities

1. Attends to person speaking to child
2. Finds "the baby" in picture when requested, e.g., on baby food jar, in magazine, or in storybooks
3. Indicates wants by gestures
4. Looks toward family members or pets when named

Expressive abilities

1. Uses three words other than mama and dada to denote *specific* objects, persons, or actions
2. Indicates wants by naming object such as cookie

1. Incorporate repetition into daily routine of home
   a. Feeding: name baby's food and eating utensils; ask if he is enjoying his dessert; concentrate on reviewing day's events in simple manner
   b. Household duties: mother names each item as she dusts; pronounces word while cooking and preparing foods
   c. Playing: Identify toys when using them; explain their function
2. Let child see mouthing of words
3. Encourage verbalization and expression of wants

19 to 30 months

Receptive abilities

1. Points to one named body part
2. Follows two or three verbal directions that are not accompanied by facial or body gestures, e.g., put ball on table, give it to mommy, or put toy in box

Expressive abilities

1. Combines two different words, e.g., "play ball," "want cookie"
2. Names object in picture, e.g., cat, bird, dog, horse, man
3. Refers to self by pronoun rather than by name

1. Continue to present concrete objects with words; talk about activities child is involved with
2. Include child in conversations during mealtimes
3. Encourage speech by having child express wants
4. Incorporate games into bathing routine by having child name and point to body parts
5. As child gains confidence in remembering and using words appropriately, encourage less use of gestures
6. Count and name articles of clothing as they are placed on child
7. Count and name silverware as it is placed on table
8. Sort, match, and name glassware, laundry, cans, vegetables, and fruit with child
9. Have child keep scrapbook and add new picture every day to increase recognition of vocabulary words

Continued.

THE WASHINGTON GUIDE TO PROMOTING DEVELOPMENT
IN THE YOUNG CHILD

LANGUAGE — cont'd

Expected tasks	Suggested activities

19 to 30 months

10. Spend 15 to 20 minutes per day going through booklets and naming pictures; have child point to pictures as objects are named
11. Help child develop functional core vocabulary to express safety needs and information about neighborhood
12. Whenever possible, use word (e.g., paper), show object, have child handle and use it, encourage him to watch your face while you say the words, and suggest that he repeat it; refrain from undue pressure

31 to 36 months

Receptive abilities
1. Takes turns when asked while playing, eating
2. Attends longer to stories and TV programs
3. Demonstrates understanding of two prepositions by carrying out two commands one at a time, e.g., "put the block under the chair"
4. Can follow commands asking for two objects or two actions
5. Demonstrates understanding of concepts of big and little, e.g., selects larger of two balls when asked for big one
6. Points to additional body parts

Expressive abilities
1. Uses regular plurals, e.g., adds "s" to apple, box, orange (does not use irregular plurals, e.g., mouse to mice)
2. Gives first and last name
3. Names what he has drawn after scribbling
4. On request, tells you his sex, e.g., are you a little boy or a little girl?
5. Can repeat a few rhymes or songs
6. On request, tells what action is going on in picture, e.g., the kitten is eating

1. Read stories with familiar content but with more detail: nonsense rhymes, humorous stories
2. Expect child to follow simple commands
3. Give child opportunity to hear and repeat his full name
4. Listen to child's explanation about pictures he draws
5. Encourage child to repeat nursery rhymes by himself and with others
6. Address child by his first name

37 to 48 months

1. Expresses appropriate responses when asked what child does when tired, cold, or hungry
2. Tells stories
3. Common expression: I don't know
4. Repeats sentence composed of twelve to thirteen syllables, e.g., "I am going when daddy and I are finished playing"
5. Has mastered phonetic sounds of p, k, g, v, tf, d, z, lr, hw, j, kw, l, e, w, qe, and o

1. Provide visual stimuli while reading stories
2. Have child repeat story
3. Arrange trips to zoo, farms, seashore, stores, and movies and discuss with child
4. Give simple explanations in answering questions

THE WASHINGTON GUIDE TO PROMOTING DEVELOPMENT IN THE YOUNG CHILD

LANGUAGE — cont'd

Expected tasks	**Suggested activities**

49 to 52 months

Receptive abilities

1. Points to penny, nickel, or dime on request
2. Carries out in order command containing three parts, e.g., "pick up the block, put it on the table, and bring the book to me"

Expressive abilities

1. Names penny, nickel, or dime on request
2. Replies appropriately to questions such as "What do you do when you are asleep?"
3. Counts three objects, pointing to each in turn
4. Defines simple words, e.g., hat, ball
5. Asks questions
6. Can identify or name four colors

Suggested activities

1. Play games in which child names colors
2. Encourage use of please and thank you
3. Encourage social-verbal interactions with other children
4. Encourage correct usage of words
5. Provide puppets or toys with movable parts that child can converse about
6. Provide group activity for child; children may stimulate each other by taking turns naming pictures
7. Allow child to make choices about games, stories, and activities
8. Have child dramatize simple stories
9. Provide child with piggy bank and encourage naming coins as they are handled or dropped into bank

DISCIPLINE

Expected tasks	**Suggested activities**

1 to 3 months

1. Draws attention by crying

   1. a. Needs should be identified and met as promptly as possible
      b. Every bit of fussing should not be interpreted as emergency requiring immediate attention
      c. Infant should not be ignored and permitted to cry for exhaustive periods

2. Infant desires whatever is pleasant and wishes to avoid unpleasant situations

   2. Begin to present limit of having to wait so that infant can learn that tension and discomfort are bearable for short periods

3. Beginning to "wiggle" around

   3. Place infant on surfaces that have sides to protect him from falling off

4 to 8 months

1. Begins to respond to "no-no"

   1. a. Reserve "no-no" for times when it is really needed
      b. Be consistent with word "no-no" for same activity and event that requires it; be friendly and firm with verbal control of limit setting

2. Infant who is left alone for long periods of time may become bored or fretful; learns that crying and whining result in attention

   2. Make special efforts to attend to infant when he is quiet and amusing himself

3. Beginning to show signs of timidity and fretfulness and may whimper and cry when mother separates from him or when strangers pick him up

   3. a. Gradually introduce strangers into infant's environment
      b. Refrain from promoting frightening situations with strangers during this stage
      c. Play hiding games like peek-a-boo in which mother disappears and reappears

Continued.

THE WASHINGTON GUIDE TO PROMOTING DEVELOPMENT IN THE YOUNG CHILD

DISCIPLINE—cont'd

Expected tasks	Suggested activities

4 to 8 months

	d. Allow infant to cling to mother and get used to unfamiliar persons a little at a time
	e. If baby-sitter is used, find person familiar to infant or introduce for brief periods before mother leaves infant in her care
	f. Encourage gentle handling by mother, father, and siblings. Discourage rough handling, particularly by strangers
4. Beginning to grasp objects and bring to mouth, but unable to differentiate safe from hazardous items	4. a. Provide toys that do not have small detachable parts b. Check frequently for small objects in his line of reach
	5. When traveling in car, place in crib or seat with safety belts securely fastened

9 to 12 months

1. Beginning to respond to simple commands, e.g., "pick up the ball, put the toy in the box"	1. a. Avoid setting unreasonable number of limits b. Give simple commands one at a time c. Once limit is set, adhere to it firmly each time and connect it immediately with misbehavior d. Respond with consistency in enforcing rule e. Allow time to conform to request f. Gain child's attention
2. Ready to go places on his own and is trying out newly developing motor capacities (not to be confused with naughtiness, "spoiled," or stubbornness)	2. a. Begin setting and enforcing limits on where child is allowed to travel and explore b. Remove tempting objects c. Remove sources of danger such as light sockets, protruding pot handles, hanging table covers, sharp objects, and hanging cords d. Keep child away from fans, heaters, and certain drawers and don't place vaporizer close to infant's crib e. Keep highchair at least 2 feet away from working and cooking surfaces in kitchen f. Use gate to keep child out of kitchen when it is being used g. Be certain that pans, basins, and tubs of hot water are never left unattended h. Remove all possible poisons or substances that are not food that can be eaten or drunk off floor, low-level cabinets, and under sink i. Keep child from objects or surfaces that he may chew, e.g., porch rails, windowsills, *repainted* toys or cribs that may contain lead j. Instruct baby-sitter on all safety items

THE WASHINGTON GUIDE TO PROMOTING DEVELOPMENT IN THE YOUNG CHILD

DISCIPLINE—cont'd

Expected tasks	Suggested activities
9 to 12 months	
3. Has emerging desires to look at, handle, and touch objects	3. a. Experiment with diversionary measures b. Provide child with own play objects
4. Explores objects by sucking, chewing, and biting	4. a. Remove household poisons, cosmetics, pins, and buttons that he could put in his mouth b. Be certain that objects that go into mouth are hygienic c. Check toys for detachable small parts
5. Beginning to test reactions to certain parental responses during feeding and may become choosy about food	5. a. Once problem behaviors are defined, plan to work on changing only one behavior at a time until child behaves or conforms to expectations b. Be certain that child understands old rules before adding new ones c. Respond with consistency in enforcing old rules: enforce each time, don't ignore next time d. Provide regular pattern of mealtimes e. Refrain from feeding throughout day f. Allow child to decide what he will eat and how much g. Introduce new foods gradually over period of time h. Continue to offer foods that may have been rejected first time i. Don't force food j. Refrain from physically punishing child for changes in eating habits
6. Beginning to test reactions to parental responses at bedtime preparation	6. a. Provide regular time for naps and bedtime b. Avoid excessive stimulation at bedtime or naptime c. Ignoring fussing and crying once safety and physical needs are satisfied and usual ritual is carried out d. Keep child in own room e. Refrain from picking up and rocking and holding if needs seem satisfied
13 to 18 months	
1. Understands simple commands and requests	1. a. Begin with one rule; add new ones as appropriate b. In selecting new rules, choose on the basis of being able to clearly define it to self and child, having it reasonable and enforceable at all times; demand no more than fulfillment of defined expectations c. Plan decisive limits and plan to give consistent attention to them
2. In learning mastery over impulses and self-control, child begins testing out limit setting	2. a. Immediately correct errors in behavior as they occur

Continued.

THE WASHINGTON GUIDE TO PROMOTING DEVELOPMENT IN THE YOUNG CHILD

DISCIPLINE—cont'd

Expected tasks	Suggested activities

13 to 18 months

	b. Use consistent enforcement of short-term rules (which are given as verbal commands) and long-term rules (which pertain to chores and family routines)
	c. Ignore temper tantrums
	d. Show child when you approve of his behavior and praise for obedience throughout day
3. With increasing fine motor control, child can manipulate objects that may be hazardous	3. a. Set limits regarding play with doorknobs and car door handles
	b. Keep away from open windows; latch screens
	c. Supervise around pools and ponds or drain or fence them
	d. Lock cabinets
	e. Keep open jars and bottles out of reach
	f. Use gate to protect child from falling down stairs

19 to 30 months

1. Attention span increasing	1. a. Gain attention before giving simple commands, one at a time; praise for success
	b. Add new rules as child conforms to old ones
	c. Refrain from expecting *immediate* obedience
2. Begins simple reasoning—asks question why; may be repetitive	2. Make special efforts to answer questions; give simple explanations; gauge need for simplicity by number of times act is repeated or question asked
3. Interested in further exploration of environment; may lack physical control	3. a. Supervise on stair rails and waxed floors
	b. Set rules about crossing streets and carrying knives, sharp objects, or glass objects
	c. Have outdoor play area securely fenced or supervised
	d. When riding in car, secure child safely by seat belt or insist on his sitting in back seat; do not permit standing on car seats
	e. Keep matches out of reach
	f. Shield adult tools such as knives, lawn mowers, sharp tools
4. Negativistic behavior is expected; respond more frequently with word "no"; may show more resistance at bedtime preparation and during mealtime	4. a. Practice consistency in responding to behavior
	b. Allow more time to conform to expectation
5. Behavior may change if new sibling is introduced into family unit	5. a. Explain verbally or through play that new child is expected
	b. Exercise more patience with child
	c. Set special times aside for parental attention to child
	d. Allow child to help with special care tasks of new sibling

THE WASHINGTON GUIDE TO PROMOTING DEVELOPMENT IN THE YOUNG CHILD

DISCIPLINE — cont'd

Expected tasks	Suggested activities

31 to 48 months

1. Displays more interest in conforming

  1. a. Exercise consistency in parental demands; enforce each time and avoid ignoring behavior next time
    b. Show concrete approval and give immediate recognition for acceptable behavior
    c. Refrain from use of threats that produce fearfulness

2. Shows greater understanding when simple reasoning is communicated

  2. a. Give simple explanations; allow child chance to demonstrate understanding by talking about event, situation, or rule
    b. Eliminate unnecessary and impractical rules
    c. Refrain from constant verbal reprimands
    d. Denial of privileges should not be excessive or prolonged

3. Will respond to simple commands such as putting toys away

  3. a. Assign simple household tasks that child can carry out each day; show approval for performance and success
    b. Decide if child is capable of doing what is asked by observing him
    c. Determine how much time is necessary to complete a chore or activity before expecting maximum performance

4. Displays a greater independence in general activities

  4. a. Be extra cautious about supervising riding tricycles in streets and watching for cars in driveways
    b. Don't permit dashing into street while playing
    c. Don't allow child to follow ball into street
    d. Areas under swings and slides should not be paved
    e. Provide an imitative model that child can copy, e.g., don't jaywalk
    f. Provide scissors that are blunt tipped

49 to 52 months

1. Can be given two or three assignments at one time; will carry out in order
2. Complies readily with reasonable, well-defined, and consistent requirements
3. Understands reasoning

  1. Give more opportunities to be independent
  2. Use simple explanations and reasoning
  3. Ask child to define role if he disobeys
  4. Have child correct mistakes as they occur
  5. Don't use punishment without warnings
  6. Praise for successful performance
  7. Use gold stars on chart for rewards
  8. If leaving for social obligation, vacation, or visiting away from home, let child know
  9. Avoid making promises that can't be kept
  10. Avoid bribing, ridicule, shaming, teasing, inflicting pain, using unfavorable comparison with other children, and exhibition of behavior by parents they are trying to stop in child

Continued.

THE WASHINGTON GUIDE TO PROMOTING DEVELOPMENT IN THE YOUNG CHILD

DISCIPLINE—cont'd

Expected tasks	Suggested activities
	49 to 52 months
	11. Remember that child may be imitating models of behavior set up by parents, brothers, sisters, a neighborhood child, or maybe a TV hero
	12. Recognize that there are stress periods in family or child's life that may result in changes in child's behavior including accidents, illness, moving into new neighborhood, separation from friends, death, divorce, and hospitalization of child or parents (be more patient with child's behavior, give more time to conform, show more approval for mastery of tasks, and exercise consistency in handling problems as they occur)

TOILET TRAINING

Expected tasks	Suggested activities
	9 to 12 months
1. Beginning to show regular patterns in bladder and bowel elimination	1. Watch for clues that indicate child is wet or soiled
2. Has one to two stools daily	2. Be sure to change diapers when wet or soiled so that child begins to experience contrast between wetness and dryness
3. Interval of dryness does not exceed 1 to 2 hours	
	13 to 18 months
1. Will have bowel movement if put on toilet at approximate time	1. Sit child on toilet or potty chair at regular intervals for short periods of time throughout day
2. Indicates wet pants	2. Praise child for success
	3. If potty chair is used, it should be located in bathroom
	4. Training should be started when social disruptions are at minimum
	5. Respond promptly to signals and clues of child by taking him to bathroom or changing pants
	6. Use training pants, once toilet training is commenced
	7. Plan to begin training when disruptions in regular routine are minimized, i.e., don't begin on vacation
	19 to 30 months
1. Anticipates need to eliminate	1. Continue regular intervals of toileting
2. Same word for both functions	2. Reward success
3. Daytime control (occasional accident)	3. Dress in simple clothing that child can manage
4. Requires assistance (reminding, dressing, wiping)	4. Remind occasionally, particularly after mealtime, juicetime, naptime, and playtime
	5. Take to bathroom before bedtime
	6. Bathroom should be convenient to use, easy to open door

THE WASHINGTON GUIDE TO PROMOTING DEVELOPMENT IN THE YOUNG CHILD

TOILET TRAINING—cont'd

Expected tasks	Suggested activities

31 to 48 months

Expected tasks	Suggested activities
1. Takes responsibility for toilet if clothes are simple 2. Continues to verbalize need to go; apt to hold out too long 3. May have occasional accident 4. Needs help with wiping	1. May still need reminding 2. Dress in simple clothing that child can manage 3. Ignore accidents; refrain from shame or ridicule

49 to 52 months

Expected tasks	Suggested activities
1. General independence (anticipates needs, undresses, goes, wipes, washes hands)	1. Praise child for his accomplishment

DRESSING

Expected tasks	Suggested activities

13 to 18 months

Expected tasks	Suggested activities
1. Cooperates in dressing by extending arm or leg 2. Removes socks, hat, mittens, shoes 3. Can unzip zippers 4. Tries to put shoes on	1. Encourage child to remove socks, etc., after task is initiated for him 2. Do not rush child 3. Have him practice with large buttons and with zippers

19 to 30 months

Expected tasks	Suggested activities
1. Can undress 2. Can remove shoes if laces are untied 3. Helps dress 4. Tries to unbutton 5. Pulls on simple clothes	1. Provide opportunities to button with extra-large–sized buttons 2. Encourage and allow opportunity for self-help in getting drink, removing clothes with help, hand washing, unbuttoning, etc. 3. Simple clothing 4. Provide mirror at height child can observe himself for brushing teeth, etc.

31 to 48 months

Expected tasks	Suggested activities
1. Greater interest and ability in dressing 2. Intent on lacing shoes (usually does incorrectly) 3. Does not know back from front 4. Washes and dries hands, brushes teeth 5. Can button	1. Provide with own dresser drawer 2. Simple garments encourage self-help; do not rush child 3. Provide large buttons, zippers, slipover clothing 4. Self hand washing but help with brushing teeth 5. Provide regular routine for dressing, either in bathroom or bedroom

49 to 52 months

Expected tasks	Suggested activities
1. Dresses and undresses with care except for tying shoes and buckling belts 2. May learn to tie shoes 3. Combs hair with assistance	1. Assign regular task of placing clothes in hamper or basket 2. Continue to use simple clothing 3. Encourage self-help in dressing and undressing 4. Allow child to select clothes he will wear

CASE ILLUSTRATION

The following case illustration represents an approach to summarizing significant observations about the child, his functioning, and the parents' practices. This format has been helpful to child care professionals in reporting their findings when using the Washington Guide.

Clinical record

Date: 12/3   Sam Smith
               Chronological age: 5 years 8 months

Nursing assessment

This follow-up home visit was made for the purpose of determining Sam's current levels of functioning in self-help skills and play.

An application of the Washington Guide revealed the following profile:

Assessment of functional abilities

Motor development. Motor tasks fall within the range of 9 to 12 months of age (able to stand momentarily, walk with support [holding onto furniture], and pick up a raisin with right thumb and finger).

Language. Receptive and expressive abilities appear to be at the low end of the 4- to 8-month scale. His head turns when a bell is rung and when others talk to him. He responds by raising arms when parents request him to come near or up. Expressive abilities include laughing aloud and emitting vowel sounds. No words were elicited.

Play behaviors. Play activities range within a 4- to 8-month level of development. He amuses himself for short intervals. He presently lacks initiative in spontaneously exploring his play environment; that is, toys are selected and presented to him. Play objects are held momentarily and released. The majority of toys presented to him are explored by mouth. Transparent objects are characteristically licked with lips and tongue, raised to eye level, and lowered again in stereotyped fashion, to be explored with mouthing movements. He engaged in sitting and pushing a musical ball back and forth with his father. Pushing, rather than holding, releasing, and tossing are characteristics of this particular activity. Imitative behaviors for scribbling with a crayon, dialing a toy phone, or hitting a pounding block with a toy hammer could not be elicited. Samples of problem-solving behaviors are absent.

Discipline. Responses are characteristic of a 4- to 8-month-old level of development. He occasionally responds to no-no.

Feeding skills. Presently he is functioning within a range of 9 to 12 months of age. He drinks from a cup with assistance, finger feeds, and is beginning to progress in independent feeding with a spoon.

Dressing skills. He falls below the 16-month norm for independently removing a garment. He does anticipate dressing by extending arms and legs, a 13-month-old task.

Toileting. He does not indicate needs, a 13- to 18-month-old developmental task.

This informal assessment provided the opportunity for acknowledging the parents' past and present efforts for giving Sam an appropriate environment for his present level of functional abilities; that is, their expectations for performance correspond readily to his abilities rather than his chronological age. He is provided with varied sources of sensory stimulation and opportunities to move about freely, and his parents are attempting to fulfill his emotional and social needs.

Behavioral observations. It has become more apparent that Sam has developed some effective behavioral patterns to gain parental attention. The parents responded immediately to a number of Sam's attention-seeking behaviors; for example, they responded to his arm waving and frequent whining by putting records on for Sam's benefit, turning the TV on, taking him downstairs to swing, walking him back and forth across the living room, and placing him in a rocker.

Chief concern expressed by mother

Mrs. Smith asserted herself, in the absence of Mr. Smith, as wishing to meet and communicate with another mother who is confronted with the needs of a handicapped child. Appropriate arrangements for this request will be explored further in future contacts with the mother.

Recommendations

In consideration of this random sample of parent-child interactions and the lack of consistent and systematic limit setting by both parents, it would appear that the Smiths might benefit from exploring a method to modify their responses to these constant attention-seeking behaviors. Another priority to consider is the need for consistently gaining Sam's attention for any task or performance expected of him.

Specific programs for developmental stimulation will be suggested after further observations are collected. Additional observations should be made to determine the frequency of the child's attention-getting behaviors and the parents' responses to them.

Sara Dippity, R.N.

SUMMARY

Increased emphasis is being placed on sharing the results of a developmental assessment with parents. It is important to first share the child's developmental assets, positive features, and attractive behavioral traits. Less attractive traits and weaknesses should be considered last, since parents usually know about these.

In addition, it is important that the child care professional check with the parents to validate observations of what the parents perceive as strengths or weaknesses. There is increasing evidence that parents are more accurate in their assessment and interpretation of their children's behaviors than they have traditionally been given credit for. Parents deserve greater recognition for this.

REFERENCE

1. Barnard, Kathryn E., and Erickson, Marcene L.: Teaching children with developmental problems: a family care approach, ed. 2, St. Louis, 1976, The C. V. Mosby Co.

ADDITIONAL READINGS

Campbell, M. M., and Ramsey, O. E.: Developmental screening scales (composite of the Cattell Infant Scale, the Gesell Scales, the Composite Scale by B. M. Caldwell and R. H. Drachman's Scale, and the Vineland Social Maturity Scale), Seattle, 1965, Clinic for Child Study, University of Washington (mimeographed).

Dittman, L. L.: The nurse in home training programs for the retarded child, Social Security Administration and Children's Bureau, U.S. Department of Health, Education, and Welfare, Washington, D.C., 1961, U.S. Government Printing Office.

Dittmann, L. L.: The mentally retarded child at home: a manual for parents, Welfare Administration and Children's Bureau, U.S. Department of Health, Education, and Welfare, Washington, D.C., 1964, U.S. Government Printing Office.

Doll, E. A.: Vineland social maturity scale: manual of directions, Minneapolis, 1947, Educational Test Bureau, Educational Publishers, Inc.

Frankenburg, W. K., and Dodds, J. B.: Denver Developmental Screening Test, Denver, 1967, Ladoca Project and Publishing Foundation.

Gesell, A., and Ilg, F. L.: Feeding behavior of infants, Philadelphia, 1937, J. B. Lippincott Co.

Gesell, A.: The first five years of life: a guide to the study of the pre-school child, New York, 1940, Harper Brothers, Publishers.

Ginott, H. G.: Between parent and child: new solutions to old problems, New York, 1969, Avon Books.

Hedrick, D., and Prather, E., chief investigators: Washington language scale, Seattle, 1970, University of Washington Child Development and Mental Retardation Center.

Holtgrewe, M. M.: A guide for public health nurses working with mentally retarded children, Welfare Administration and Children's Bureau, U.S. Department of Health, Education, and Welfare, Washington, D.C., 1964, U.S. Government Printing Office.

Illingworth, R. S.: The normal child: some problems of the first five years and their treatment, Boston, 1964, Little, Brown & Co.

Jensen, G. D.: The well child's problems: management in the first six years, Chicago, 1962, Year Book Medical Publishers, Inc.

Paulus, A. C.: A tool for the assessment of the retarded child at home, Nursing Clinics of North America, Philadelphia, Dec., 1966, W. B. Saunders Co.

Spock, B.: Baby and child care, New York, 1976, Pocket Books, Inc.

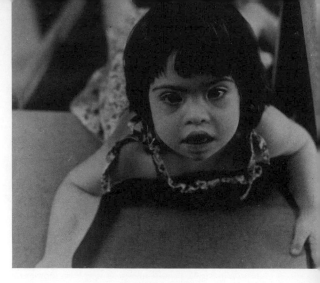

21

MANAGEMENT OF MENTALLY RETARDED INFANTS AND CHILDREN

Parents may experience frustration and have difficulty responding to an infant who presents a variety of needs. They need support to enable them to describe their concerns about this behavior and what it means to them. For example, when a parent describes listlessness, the child care professional needs to acknowledge that the parent has a legitimate concern, but she can also point out that the parents can describe periods when the infant is alert and is processing information. If parents describe their infant as having poor muscle tone, the professional can acknowledge their concern and discuss comfortable ways to posture the infant. If parents report sleep disturbances, they can be asked to document the actual amount of time that the infant is asleep and awake. Using this documented record, the child care professional can offer reassurance and guidance and can help the parents promote longer periods of sleep or encourage less sleeping. Together, they can explore the different causes of sleep disturbances—the environment, medications, ways the parents are interacting with the infant, an immature nervous system, or a disturbance in the central nervous system.

Similarly, if parents are complaining about eating problems, the professional should ob-

serve the infant during feeding time. She should note the child's posture, the way the parent holds the child while preparing him for eating, and the interactions between the parent and infant during feeding. Difficulties in feeding can be serious and are often signals of disturbances in the basic parent-child relationship. If a parent is concerned that the infant is not receiving enough food or not growing enough, the child care professional can take objective measurements (height and weight) and share them with the parents. She can also encourage parents to keep records of the infant's intake and consumption of foods and fluid for a 7-day period before offering reassurance and advice.

If parents are concerned that the infant is not visually tracking, does not seem to notice them, or does not look at the mother's face while she is talking, the professional should objectively assess the infant's ability to look at and follow inanimate as well as animate objects. If the infant is under 1 month of age, items from the Brazelton Neonatal Behavioral Assessment Scale can be used; if the infant is over 1 month of age a number of items from the Denver Developmental Screening Test (DDST) can be tried to elicit visual behavior. If parents complain about their infant's ability to cuddle, the professional should have them describe what they perceive as a "cuddly" infant and ask if there are times when the infant does cuddle.

Above photograph from Chinn, P. C., Drew, C. J., and Logan, D. R.: Mental retardation: a life cycle approach, ed. 2, St. Louis, 1979, The C. V. Mosby Co.

If parents mention repetitive behavior that their infant or child exhibits, the professional must listen carefully to what parents are saying. Reports about repetitive behavior are extremely serious, and the child care professional should prepare to observe and monitor the infant's behavior to determine the frequency of the behavior in question, when it occurs, and what consequences it produces. The professional should especially consider whether the parents reinforce the behavior.

If parents describe the infant as having a limited attention span, this report also merits careful study. The child care professional should gather data on when the infant does attend; how long he attends to objects, events, or people; and the actual length of his longest and shortest attention spans. The parents can help by documenting the infant's behavior in his home setting. The professional and the parents can then discuss the implications of the data and how best to get and maintain the infant's attention.

MANAGEMENT OF MENTALLY RETARDED PRESCHOOLERS

Preschoolers present a wide range of problematic behaviors such as having a short attention span, being distracted easily, having toilet training accidents, having difficulties with self-help skills, manifesting excessive activity, showing repetitive movements, exhibiting impulsive behavior, whining, showing a lack of language, showing inability to carry out commands by adults, having problems with motor coordination, and manifesting excessive dependency on others. Additional parental concern during the preschool period may be that the child shows no interest in toys, is unable to entertain himself, or exhibits peculiar behavior.

The first step for the child care professional toward effective intervention in any of these cases is to have the parents define their exact concern and give specific examples of behavior. Data collection is the next essential—the frequency and duration of the behavior, the events that occurred in the environment before the behavior was manifested, and what happened after this child exhibited the behavior. In other words, the professional must determine whether the parents inadvertently reinforced the behavior or appropriately ignored it. The child care professional can then begin a mutual problem-solving process with the parents. During this process, the professional should remember that it is extremely easy for parents to get caught up in a negative cycle, whereby they describe only the negative traits of a child; therefore they should also be asked to describe the strengths they are seeing in the child.

APPLICATION OF PRINCIPLES OF NORMALIZATION AND HUMANIZATION

By applying principles of normalization, health care professionals can humanize the environment for the individual with mental retardation. Adherence to the normalization principle means establishing a normal rhythm to a day, a year, and to life itself. Normalization affects all aspects of daily living. Most people in this society live in one place, work or attend school somewhere else, and have leisure-time activities in a variety of places. All activities do not occur in the same room, as has been customary for the person with mental retardation.

One example of applying the principles of normalization, advanced by Wolfensberger,[1] concerns sleeping. The mentally retarded person should not be put to bed earlier than his siblings or peers simply because he is handicapped. He should sleep in a regular bed, not be restrained in a crib. He should not have a light burning all night just for him. He should be freed from the routines of the day and should not be awakened at 4 A.M. to accommodate the staff of an institution or the caregivers in his environment.

Another example of normalization pertains to eating. Persons with mental retardation are entitled to an eating environment appropriate for their individual needs. They should be able to eat in a place different from the room where they sleep, and they should eat with an appropriate number of other people. For example, if a person eats rapidly because he is anxious that others will take his food, he needs the opportunity to be by himself while eating. Persons with mental retardation should learn to obtain and eat food according to their caloric needs. If they are more active, they may need more calories per day. They should learn to distinguish both hunger and satiety; cold foods, not just cold or lukewarm foods; and be able to eat when they are hungry, not just every 4 hours at the convenience of others. Health care professionals and parents or other care givers should learn how to respond to children's cues when they are full or when they are hungry. Professionals can encourage caregivers to help children with mental retardation express their feeding needs because they may have difficulty with language. The child may be thirsty but yet have difficulty expressing it. Significant people around this child should be able to learn how to interpret a child's behavior and cues and to respond to his need for water or food more appropriately.

Feeding, ideally, should be thought of as a learning experience just like any other developmental task such as playing. It should proceed from the simple to the complex. The person with mental retardation should have a variety of foods to experiment with from the time he is an infant, no matter how physically impaired he is. He should be offered food with a wide variety of textures and food that he can chew and move around in his mouth, not just food that slides down the throat or food that has already been cut up or pureed. The mentally retarded child needs to experiment and even play with his food without fear of punishment, just like other children, and needs to see the food that he is eating. Food should be labeled and talked about in front of the child. It should be attractively arranged, esthetically appealing, and separated into different sections, not just heaped into one big mess of a serving.

Children need both to smell and to taste food. They sometimes need help in learning to discriminate the differences in food; for example, food has different shapes, sizes, fragrances, tastes, and textures. Children need to be able to smell spicy foods, fruits, vegetables, meats, breads, cookies, cheeses, and drinks. They need to experience feeling, touching, holding, and exploring their food; to learn that food is hard and soft, crunchy and smooth, thick and thin, wet and dry, sweet and sour, round, square, green, white, and yellow; and to experiment with big and little bites of food. Children need freedom from a monotonous menu that is offered day after day and have novelty in sensory experiences with feeding. They need to move food from one side of their mouth to the other and from front to back and to learn that they can control food and where it goes. They need to learn how their lips, tongue, mouth, and teeth work. The more severely handicapped child should have food presented on parts of his lips, or if he cannot reach it himself, it can be placed inside his mouth.

A child with mental retardation in particular deserves the right to learn how to eat and drink so that when he is older, he does not have to unlearn so many inappropriate habits like gulp-ing down a glass of milk, stuffing his mouth full of food, or snatching foods from the plates of others. If a person develops obnoxious or repulsive feeding habits, this behavior helps set him apart from others and makes him less acceptable. Most inappropriate habits that children learn are reinforced and then need to be unlearned. Mentally retarded children should be given choices about food and participate and select food that they are going to eat. If they have language, they can be asked what they would like for lunch or dinner. They can be helped to identify food with language or behavioral gestures. They can also be encouraged to critique the food offered to them. They can become good judges about their food, just like other children, but they need the opportunity.

In the past, feeding may have been a highly aversive and stressful experience for some children with mental retardation. Children can develop phobias and anxieties that center around eating.

If a mentally retarded person has been given only pureed foods or has been tube fed, he is being deprived of the normal experiences of eating. If a child is being "bird-fed," meaning that the food is forced into him while he is lying in a supine position, then he is in a feeding environment in which his rights to an appropriate and individualized program of care are being abused. This approach to feeding is an obsolete institutional practice that is no longer acceptable either in an institutional or a home setting. If a child has to be tube fed, it is a serious last-resort approach. The child care professional needs to question whether there might not be time for another method. If an infant, child, or adult is being tube fed, he deserves the opportunity at least to sit up and have an optimal eating environment created for him on a gradual basis. The professional can prepare him by talking about feeding, observing his reactions and responses, and making every effort to help him advance to more optimal adaptive eating patterns.

Ideally, the goal of child care professionals is to help the mentally retarded person function independently within his environment. As he becomes more adaptive and functional, he actually becomes more accountable for his own behavior. He has more choices available to him, and ultimately he is less dependent on others. His more appropriate behavior, in turn, generates more appropriate responses from others, and experiencing more positive interactions with others reinforces a new set of desirable and acceptable behaviors. Child care professionals should recognize that there is no single correct way to help mentally retarded persons achieve greater levels of independence. An interdisciplinary, problem-solving approach is best— nurses and child care professionals consulting with psychologists, nutritionists, speech and hearing clinicians, pediatricians, social workers, occupational therapists, physical therapists, dentists, and special educators.

BEHAVIOR MODIFICATION

Most child management problems possess common features that are conducive to behavioral programming. Generally, the behaviors emitted by the child occur at a rate that is either too high or too low. Parents can learn to identify their child's problematic behavioral manifestations and keep accurate records before intervention begins. The child care professional should remind them not to interact differently with their child while they are documenting behavioral occurrences and not to try out behavioral modification techniques such as ignoring or using positive reinforcement until adequate data are available to plan a management program. Once they have systematically identified a problem that requires intervention and have begun to apply principles of behavioral modification, they can effectively evaluate the success of an intervention program. As behavior changes occur in children, parents can keep records of their own feelings, reactions, thoughts, and responses to the changes.

Behavioral approaches to promoting self-feeding

Self-feeding is recognized as the first major self-help skill that children learn. It actually involves the integration of fine motor skills, visual perception, and gross motor skills. Most parents take for granted that they will automatically be successful in teaching their children to feed themselves. Therefore child care professionals must also be especially sensitive to the needs of the parent as well as the child when they offer assistance.

Before beginning a self-feeding program, the child care professional should do a task analysis, breaking the process of feeding into its smallest component parts. For example, the child orients to the food by looking at it, looks at the spoon, reaches for the spoon, touches the spoon, grasps the spoon, lifts the spoon, delivers the spoon to the bowl, lowers the spoon into the food, scoops the food onto the spoon, lifts the spoon, delivers the spoon to his mouth, opens his mouth, inserts the spoon into his mouth, moves his tongue and mouth to receive the food, closes his lips, swallows the food, and returns the spoon to the bowl. It is important that the professional observe the child eating to determine whether he has mastered any of these small steps that make up the entire task of self-feeding. If he has, she should comment positively to the mother.

In addition to doing a task analysis, the child care professional must assess a number of other factors. She should examine the child's mouth; its shape; his control of mouth movements; lip movements; and tongue movements, including whether the tongue moves forward and backward, from side to side, and with rotary motions. The professional should also look for the presence of teeth, which will determine the textures and consistencies of food that may be offered to the child. She must observe the child's ability to maintain head and trunk support; his ability to sit without support; his eye-hand coordination; the firmness of his hand grasp; and his ability to reach for, hold, and release an object. It must be determined whether the child has any dietary deficiencies, as revealed by a 7-day dietary history kept by the mother, whether there have been any changes in the child's eating habits, and whether he is being given a metabolic diet. The professional should also assess neurological factors, such as whether the child has seizures, is receiving medications that control seizures, chokes often, or has difficulty swallowing or a history of such difficulties.

The child care professional should next obtain further data from the mother by interviewing her, specifically about the family's approach to teaching.[2] For example, who feeds the child regularly? Does the child eat at regularly scheduled times? Is the child fed when he is hungry or according to someone else's convenience? What are the child's appetite patterns? Does the mother know when the child is full? What foods does the child like? How long does feeding take? A short eating time like 10 or 20 minutes might indicate that the child is being deprived of sensory experiences or appropriate interactions; a long time might indicate frustration and fatigue on the mother's part. Does the mother describe the feeding environment as quiet and nondistracting? What is the best time for the mother to begin teaching this new task? (If the family is going on vacation, if someone is visiting, or if there has been major family stress, this may not be the ideal time to begin a teaching program.) The professional must also determine whether the mother is really asking for help; her questions, comments, and ability to keep records are good clues. Does the child have models to imitate? What are the mother's expectations about the child's performance?

The child care professional should take time to discuss various principles of learning with the mother before beginning a feeding program. The mother needs to know that the behavior she reinforces is the behavior which will be repeated and that it is vitally important to get and maintain the child's attention and to give him specific cues regarding what is expected of him. The mother must understand the technique of fading: physically taking the child through each sequence of feeding and gradually fading out her physical assistance to the child so that he becomes more independent. She should also be familiar with the technique of shaping[2]—waiting for the child to give a response that approximates the desired behavior, then reinforcing him by social approval or by touching or talking to him. She should understand that it is crucial not only to reinforce desirable behavior continuously but also to ignore undesirable behavior consistently. Ignoring the child is particularly difficult for many mothers, since they may equate it with being a "bad mother"; therefore the child care professional should be especially supportive as the mother attempts it. The mother should realize that repetition plays an important part in her child's learning. As the child gains mastery, the mother will be encouraged to thin out the social or physical reinforcement she has been offering her child. She should understand that if the feeding program does not move forward successfully, she and the professional will re-evaluate the last sequence the child mastered to determine if she is expecting too much too soon.

Once the feeding program begins, the professional is in an important position to give parents supportive feedback.[2] She should call attention to the mother's observational skills and ability to share observations, to keep records of the child's progress, and to establish a goal that is appropriate and realistic for both the child and the mother. The child care professional can give support and encouragement for the mother's willingness to try a feeding program *now* rather than waiting. She can also acknowledge the mother's creativity and resourcefulness, the appropriate speed or frequency with which she gives reinforcement to the child, her beginning success, her continued efforts when behavioral change seems slow, and her ability to withhold reinforcement (i.e., ignore the child, remove the food, and wait until the child is exhibiting desirable behavior before proceeding). By acknowledging all of these aspects of the mother's continued efforts, the professional promotes mastery of a task that is extremely important to the child who is mentally retarded.

The following outline summarizes the factors of readiness that influence a child's independent feeding skills.

Motor development *(fine and gross motor skills)*

1. Head support
2. Trunk support
3. Eye-hand coordination
4. Sits without support
5. Firm hand grasp
6. Reaches for objects
7. Holds objects
8. Releases objects
9. Brings hand to mouth

Task analysis of feeding

1. Orients to food by looking at it
2. Looks at spoon
3. Reaches for spoon
4. Touches spoon
5. Grasps spoon
6. Lifts spoon
7. Delivers spoon to bowl
8. Lowers spoon into food
9. Scoops food onto spoon
10. Lifts spoon
11. Delivers spoon to mouth
12. Opens mouth
13. Inserts spoon into mouth
14. Moves tongue and mouth to receive food
15. Closes lips
16. Swallows food
17. Returns spoon to bowl

Self-feeding interview information from mother

1. Consistency of her approach:
   Who feeds child regularly?
   Are there regularly scheduled times?
2. Does child have imitative models?
3. Mothers' expectations of child's performance?
4. Child's patterns of feeding?
   Frequency of meals and time?
5. Child's characteristic pattern of appetite?
6. Child's likes and dislikes?
7. What has mother tried?
   Has it worked?
   Has it failed?
   Has she thought of other methods?
8. How long does feeding take?
9. Mother's description of teaching environment:
   Quiet?
   Nondistracting?

10. Mother's daily routine?
    What is best time for her to begin teaching?
11. Are there differences in family's schedule?
12. Is mother asking for help (e.g., questions, verbal clues, keeping records)?
13. Is mother teaching other tasks to child?

Behavioral approaches to toilet training

Independent toileting is another major self-help skill that can be taught using behavioral modification principles.

The nurse must begin by assessing the child's readiness for a toilet-training program.[2] Can the child reach a toilet or will a potty chair be more suitable? Can he sit comfortably by himself? Can he stand alone? Does he balance well, walk backward and forward, and climb onto a chair, his bed, or the couch? Can he undress? Does he ride a tricycle? All of these skills require coordinated movement, posture, and balance and suggest that the child is physically and neurologically ready for toilet training.

It is also important that records kept by the parents for 7 days indicate that the child can retain urine for at least 2 hours. If the child is physically ready for toilet training, is he also exhibiting behavioral signs of readiness? Can the parents describe differences in his behavior that signal his need to urinate or defecate or the fact that he has wet or soiled clothing? For example, does he become quieter or verbally seek attention? Does he shift his weight? Does the color of his face change? Does he cry? Does he fuss or become more dependent and clinging? Has he developed a word, gesture, or symbol indicating that he needs to eliminate? Does he associate the bathroom with eliminating? The child care professional should interview the parents regarding their readiness to pursue a toilet-training program that is characterized by a positive, consistent, individualized, nonpunitive, nonpressured style of teaching. It is important to explore the parents' willingness to participate, the time they have to invest in the program, the advantages they see, the inconveniences that toilet training may cause them, the reason they wish to start, and whether this is the best time for both the parents and the child to begin a program.

The professional should ask the parents about any past attempts at toilet training the child. When did the parents start training? Was training their idea or were they pressured by others? What methods did they use? Did they experience feelings of frustration, indifference, or discomfort?[2] How long did they attempt training, and what were their reasons for discontinuing training efforts? Looking back, how did they view the experience for themselves and the child? Were their efforts consistent? What did they do most consistently? Do they think that it is important to try again?

If the parents are presently attempting to train the child, do they regret having started? How do they react when a child is wet or soiled? Are they so eager for him to succeed that they display anxiety or tenseness when he fails? Do they comment on negative or angry feelings?[2] If the parents admit to using punishment in any form, including spanking, scolding, withholding privileges, using suppositories, withholding fluid, getting the child up in the middle of the night, or making the child wash his sheets or clothes, the professional should appeal to them to discontinue these unnecessary and ineffective methods. Do they stay with the child in the bathroom? Can they describe his behavior? Is it a pleasant time—do they talk with, look at, smile at, touch, or play special games with the child? Does the child indicate listlessness or boredom, cry, or attempt to get off the toilet? Does the child stay in the bathroom longer than 10 minutes? What is the longest the child has ever had to sit or stand at the toilet? How often has the child gone successfully in the last 3 days? How did the parents know when the child eliminated? How did they respond? How soon? What specifically did they do to show disapproval, disappointment, or approval? Where do the parents teach the child to eliminate? (Encourage them to keep the potty chair in the bathroom, not in the kitchen, bedroom, or living room.) Is the child usually dressed in simple clothes that he could remove if he needed to go to the bathroom and no one was available to help? Does he have imitative models to copy in the bathroom? Are the parents relying on verbal cues alone to teach him? If so, what are their usual comments? Do they consistently use the same words for potty, defecation, and urination?

If the present method of toilet training is not progressively successful, what else have the parents thought of?[2] What would they like to try next? If the child is not complying, what worries them or bothers them the most? What is the least of their worries? Can the parents accept the concept that the child will learn according to his own individual readiness? Do they expect him to master the entire role of independent toileting behavior within a short period of time?

Can they relax and take it easier on themselves? Can they reduce some of their own expectations to succeed immediately and be satisfied in learning how to systematically observe the child first?

As part of their procedure for determining the readiness of both parents and child to become involved in a successful toilet-training program, the child care professional should ask parents to keep detailed records for a period of 7 days. They should be cautioned to discontinue record keeping if the child becomes ill or if fluid intake is changed. Parents must record the exact time that the following events occur:

- The child ate or drank, no matter how little he consumed
- The child's behavior was suddenly distinctly different (e.g., when the child was noticeably quiet or louder, started fussing or tugging at his clothes, pointed toward the bathroom, cried, or squirmed)
- Parents gave the child positive attention related to toileting behaviors only, in the form of praise, concrete rewards, affection, or approval
- Parents gave attention in the form of scolding, threatening, or spanking if the child had wet or soiled his underclothes or did not tell them before eliminating
- The child indicated his need to go to the toilet either by gestures or words
- The child was noted to have dry underclothes
- The child was noted to have wet underclothes

It is crucial to refrain from beginning any toilet-training program until such records are completed because they show how parents are responding to the child's behavior and at what times the child is most likely to eliminate. After the records are completed to the parents' expressed satisfaction, the professional should acknowledge their efforts to keep accurate records, their diligence in making observations, and their ability to follow through.

The goal of any toilet-training program is to help the child achieve small goals and experience comfort and success and simultaneously to help the parents experience feelings of adequacy, minimal tension, and success. Parents should understand that they will be capitalizing on the times the child is most likely to eliminate and that they should respond immediately to any cues indicating this need. They must be cautioned to ignore accidents.[2]

A task analysis of toileting reveals the following steps, which parents must systematically reinforce in positive, natural, spontaneous ways:[2]

- Sitting on the toilet or potty and playing there without fussing, crying, or attempting to get off
- Eliminating into the toilet on a regular basis when sitting on it
- Waiting to eliminate before being placed on the toilet
- Indicating the need to eliminate before going into the bathroom
- Asking to go to the toilet or just going to it
- Remaining dry for longer periods of time
- Climbing onto the toilet independently
- Helping undress himself before getting on the toilet
- Independently undressing himself before getting onto the toilet
- Wiping independently
- Flushing the toilet
- Dressing
- Washing his hands with soap in a correct manner
- Drying his hands with a towel

A positive and relaxed attitude toward toilet training is important. The parents should begin by leading the child gently into the bathroom, staying with him, and showing approval for each aspect of his cooperative behavior. If the child has had no success after 5 minutes, he should be wiped, praised for sitting quietly and appropriately, and asked to get off the potty seat. Children associate diapers with their old habits of elimination; therefore parents should begin substituting training pants during the toilet-training program. Ideally, parents should place the child on the potty for voiding when he first gets up in the morning, just before breakfast, midmorning, after snacks, after lunch, midafternoon, before and after dinner, and before bedtime. They cannot expect the child to have a regular pattern of elimination unless they feed him at approximately the same times each day. Parents should also remember to help the child only when he needs it; this may take longer but is the best way for a child to really learn.

The following list contains the objective data needed before commencing any intervention with parents and children in a toilet-training program:

Major points of helping mothers in toilet training

1. Ascertain motivation of mother:
   What does she do when child is wet?
   Where does she teach him?
   Is child in diapers?
   Is she relying on verbal cues alone?
   Has she tried before? Did it work? Has she thought of ways to go about toilet training?
   When does she want him trained and why?

2. Record pertinent information
3. Structure environment for learning
4. Dress child in appropriate clothing
5. Break task down into small steps
6. Ascertain child's readiness (motor and physical)
7. Use appropriate and meaningful rewards
8. Acknowledge mastery of small gains of child
9. Repeat trials
10. Be consistent
11. Provide models for imitation

Task analysis of independent toileting

1. Exhibits signs of discomfort
2. Looks at bathroom area
3. Walks toward bathroom
4. Opens and enters
5. Looks at toilet
6. Walks toward toilet
7. Reaches for clothing
8. Removes clothing
9. Climbs onto toilet
10. Sits
11. Eliminates
12. Wipes self
13. Climbs down
14. Rearranges clothing
15. Walks toward sink
16. Washes hands
17. Dries hands
18. Exits bathroom

Signs of readiness for a mother to begin and complete toilet training

1. Keeps records of child's physiological patterns (7 days):
   Time of wetting and soiling
   Child's response and mother's response
   Time and intake of food and fluids
2. Keeps records in convenient place in bathroom
3. Shares records
4. Observes child for indications of needing to eliminate
5. Mother stays with child in bathroom during initial attempts to regularize schedule
6. Plans for bathroom to be accessible to child (easy to open door—not locked)
7. Arranges bathroom facilities according to child's needs (footstool)
8. Starts training when social disruptions are at a minimum
9. Takes child to bathroom at regular times (on arising, after meals, midmorning, midafternoon, before bed)
10. Substitutes training pants for diapers
11. Praises child for success; ignores failures
12. If progress is not consistent, questions should be raised:
    Is mother applying rewards immediately?
    Is mother consistent in applying rewards?

Is training being carried out step by step?
Is mother expecting too much, too soon?

Factors of readiness that influence a child's independent toileting

1. Retains urine for about 2 hours and is having one or two bowel movements a day
2. Balances well, stands alone, can walk, can climb onto a chair, can undress
3. Shows some sign of awareness of elimination such as following:
   Changing facial expression
   Quietness
   Pulling at clothes
   Making different sounds
   Engaging in attention-getting devices
   Squirming
   Irritability
4. Feeds self
5. Is not sick
6. Can climb onto toilet
7. Dressed in clothes that are easy to manage
8. Beginning to indicate needs

Behavioral approaches to dressing and undressing

Undressing and dressing consist of many small, discrete tasks. Fine discrimination and coordination are involved in tasks such as tying, buttoning, snapping, placing shoes on the correct feet, and getting garments right side out and in the correct order. Before effective skills in dressing can be mastered, the child must attain a level of motor development that permits arm and leg extension, balance, finger dexterity, and other fine motor adaptive skills. The following outline summarizes the factors of readiness that influence a child's independent dressing skills:

Major points of helping mothers with dressing skills

1. What is mother's daily schedule?
2. Does she have time to invest in teaching dressing?
3. Has she tried to teach these skills before? What worked? What did not work? Why is it important for her to begin teaching?
4. Can she rearrange her schedule for teaching?
5. What does she expect of child?
6. Has she selected clothes that are not complicated to put on and take off?
7. Has she thought of dressing aids? Is she intending to incorporate dressing into a daily routine?
8. Does she anticipate success in teaching?

Task analysis of undressing and dressing skills

1. Removal of undershirt:
   a. Pulls undershirt up to shoulders

    b. Pulls one arm out of sleeve
    c. Pulls other arm out of sleeve
    d. Pulls undershirt over head
    e. Gets head out of neckhole
2. Put on undershirt:
    a. Place neckhole on top of head
    b. Pull shirt down over head
    c. Put one arm into sleeve
    d. Put other arm into sleeve
    e. Pull shirt down to waist level
3. Removal of blouse:
    a. Put button halfway through buttonhole
    b. Complete unbuttoning
    c. Pull blouse off one shoulder
    d. Pull one arm from sleeve
    e. Pull other arm from sleeve
4. Put on blouse:
    a. Put one arm in correct sleeve
    b. Put other armhole up to other arm
    c. Put other arm in sleeve
    d. Put button halfway through buttonhole and complete
    e. Proceed with other buttons
5. Take off pants:
    a. Unfasten belt
    b. Take belt out of one belt loop
    c. Take belt out of remaining belt loops
    d. Unzip pants
    e. Unfasten pants
    f. Pull pants down to knees
    g. Pull pants down completely
    h. Pull pants off feet
6. Put on pants:
    a. Put feet into pants
    b. Pull pants up to knees
    c. Pull pants up near waist
    d. Pull pants up completely
    e. Fasten pants
    f. Zip up pants
    g. Put belt through first belt loop; put belt through remaining belt loops
    h. Fasten belt
7. Take off shoes:
    a. Push shoe partway off heel
    b. Push completely off heel
    c. Remove shoe from foot
8. Put on shoes:
    a. Put toes into shoes
    b. Push shoe onto heel
    c. Push shoe onto foot
9. Tie laces:
    a. Put hands on laces
    b. Cross laces
    c. Tighten laces
    d. Make bow
    e. Tighten bow
10. Untie laces:
    a. Grasp laces
    b. Tug at laces
    c. Pull one lace
    d. Untie completely
11. Tighten laces:
    a. Place hands on laces
    b. Tighten partially
    c. Tighten completely

HELPING PARENTS TEACH THEIR CHILD A DEVELOPMENTAL TASK

In teaching a child independent skills, it is important for parents to be successful, first in teaching their child parts of a task rather than expecting him to complete the task in its entirety. The child care professional should observe how the mother or father customarily teaches the child. Do they obtain the child's attention, explain or show what should be done, permit him to respond at his own rate, and give him feedback?

Parents must first draw the child's attention to the task and then maintain this attention while the task is being taught. Once the child loses attention, his chances for learning are greatly reduced. Parents should become accustomed to analyzing a task, reducing the learning situation into its smallest parts, and helping the child put the discrete parts of the task together for eventual success. The parents should always start at the last discrete part of the task that the child mastered rather than introducing a new part of the skill.

Parents must let the child try on his own and become sensitive to their attempts to intrude or take over while the child is trying to learn. The child must be given ample time, and the parents must proceed in a calm, relaxed way. It is important that they not rush the child or punish him for accidents. They must not add new rules until the child masters the old rules that accompanied learning a task. The child needs to become accustomed to doing things in a routine way and with a regular timetable. This enables him to predict what is expected of him.

As the child gains more control and independence, the parent must be able to allow the child to be on his own. This is extremely important because although parents may not be able to admit it, they may have difficulty allowing the child new independence. It was gratifying for them to be able to help the child do something. Attention may need to shift to the parents' needs rather than to the child's success in learning a task. Before the task or learning begins, the child care professional should have the parents describe how they see the child's behavior at the moment, what this behavior means to them, how much of it they will be able to tolerate, what worries them the most, what worries them the least, and if they are willing to keep records of the child's behavior. Not only does the child need feedback on his success but the parents must also receive reinforcement for their efforts at teaching.

HELPING PARENTS LEARN HOW CHILDREN LEARN

One of the first principles that the child care professional must share with the parents is that the child learns best by progressing from the simple to the more complex. This applies whether the parent is teaching a developmental task or new behavior or teaching the elimination of an old behavior. The child needs ample opportunities to practice what he is learning. He requires praise and acknowledgment as soon as he produces the proper behavioral response, and, in the beginning, he needs continuous praise and reinforcement for correct behavior. Parents encounter problems by thinking that they can simply ignore behavior and the child will improve. This is not so. If parents choose to reinforce certain behaviors, they must also choose behaviors that they will not reinforce. However, ignoring in itself does not work. It is important for parents to reinforce repeatedly those behaviors which they wish to see again and not inadvertently reinforce the behavior they do not want repeated. This must be discussed and clarified with the parents before any approach to behavioral modification is even considered.

Parents should also discuss the importance of repetition and providing opportunities for the child to practice a skill over and over again. If a parent is not comfortable watching a child repetitiously perform a task, this needs to be explored with the parent. Perhaps the parent is not the most suitable person to be conducting a teaching program with the child. It is important for the child care professional to be sensitive to the parents' cues indicating whether they do or do not want to become involved in a teaching-learning task. Parents often need permission from the child care professional not to be involved in every teaching task. They need to give themselves permission not to have to teach the child. Maybe they can let someone else teach the child a particular task while they critique it or acknowledge the person teaching the child.

It is important, however, that no matter who does the teaching, the parent acknowledge the child's success. Children are highly sensitive to approval. They need it in abundance from whomever is teaching and from their parents.

Parents should learn that it is not enough to *tell* the child what to do or what not to do. They must *show* the child what to do, in other words, model the behavior and be prepared to model it more than once. Parents need to be able to approach a teaching task at a convenient time when they feel comfortable about it themselves and its importance. They need to set realistic goals so that they and the child can succeed in the teaching-learning venture. A parent who begins to feel tense or irritable needs to stop and think: "Is this the best time to proceed?" "Am I expecting too much too soon?" "Am I hurrying the child too much?" "Is he ready to master this part of the skill?" The child may not be ready to progress to a more advanced step, and the parent must be willing to go back to the last step mastered to help the child learn.

During the teaching-learning process it is important for the child care professional to check with the parents to find out how they are reacting to the changes in the child's behavior; what are their observations of the child's behavior; what is different from, and similar to, old behavior; whether they are essentially pleased with the responses that are occurring; what pleases them most about the behavior; what may worry them about the behavior, if anything; and what they wish to see the child accomplish. For example, a child may be gaining more control or may be showing more independent behavior. In this case the parents need to be able to express their feelings about these changes. Health care professionals have arrived at the point where they know it is essential not to bypass parents in the teaching process. The best laid plan for a child's success might go astray if the parents are, in fact, not ready for the change in the child's behavior.

ADVISING AND REASSURING PARENTS

As parents learn more about growth and development, they can become more relaxed with their children and may cease to regard them as naughty. Most mentally retarded children become autonomous and independent to different degrees just as other children do. Parents often need anticipatory guidance about the fact that their child will try to explore his environment, will become more mobile, and will be more independent. Parents need to know that this is not naughty behavior but simply a good sign that the child is progressing.

As parents come to understand that their child cannot learn an activity simply by being told how to do it, they learn the importance of a child's discovering things on his own. Parents can learn when not to help the child or force him into learning. As they learn more about growth and development from child care professionals, they begin to offer more choices to their child. In the past I think that parents were led to believe that their child would be unable to make a choice; therefore they did not offer choices. As they begin to see learning as a continuous process, they tend to be less likely to overreact to the moment-to-moment, day-by-day experiences, and they learn the importance of providing a consistently supportive learning and developmental environment.

It is important for child care professionals to learn the goals and values that the parents have for their child, let the parents state them in their own way, and be careful not to state them for the parents. That is, the professional must learn to assist the parents in a consultant capacity rather than to usurp their role and direct them in their child-rearing activities. The professional should assist parents to become creative teachers and helpers for their children. Too often the child care professional assumes that parents have no goals for their children, but if the professional listens to the parents, she finds that they not only have short-term goals but may also have highly realistic long-term goals. The child care professional must refrain from allowing parents to feel that they are somehow inadequate to a parental task and need to submit to the "outside experts" who know it all.

When parents ask for help with a problem or a concern, the child care professional should ask them how often and when the problem behavior occurs, when it occurred last, how the parents generally tend to respond to it, and how they think they would like to change that behavior. It is important for the child care professional to remember that parents know that child care professionals cannot change a whole host of behaviors at once. They need to start with something that is important to the parents and to the child. Once the parents have determined the behavior they want to change, it may be appropriate to suggest that they keep records of how often the behavior occurs at home and to obtain the necessary documented data before intervention is attempted. The parents and the professional then can observe and plan together the best ways to reduce or eliminate the behavior. It is far better for the professional to have parents participate in collecting data and recording behavior than for the professional to respond

immediately to the parents with instant advice or many different recommendations. The child care professional should find out why the parents are asking for help and when they want to implement a program of care. She should then stress that she plans to meet with the parents again to review the information the parents have collected and to plan together to meet the child's needs in the best way possible.

It simply is not enough to tell the parents what to do and say that she will see them in another month. Again, the child care professional needs to check with the parents: "Does this seem appropriate to you?" "Is it convenient for you to keep records?" "Do you think it is important for you to record this information?" "Are you willing to observe his behavior now?" "Am I asking too much of you?" "Is there a better time when you would like to keep records of your child's behavior?" "Is there a better time when we could plan something for your child?" The idea is to accustom parents to being actively involved in a problem-solving process and to discourage them from becoming dependent. When parents begin to engage in too much help-seeking behavior, the professional needs to examine their feelings of adequacy and the implications of directing the parents too often rather than asking them to participate in a plan of care.

Videotapes can be especially useful to parents and child care professionals. Tapes of the child's behavior, mother-child interactions, father-child interactions, and mother-father interactions are all helpful. By viewing the videotape with a skilled child care professional, parents can gain impressive insight. They can see their own behavior much more objectively and can learn the value of observing their child rather than guessing how the child is doing or how they are responding to their child. It is important for parents to learn that there are different ways to collect data about a child's development and behavior. The use of a videotape is just one more way of gathering information systematically and objectively so that the child's care can be planned on a solid foundation. It is important for parents to be invited to critique the videotapes that are made of themselves or their children. They should be asked to state what they saw on the videotape and if they observed patterns or consistency in their behavior toward their child. The child care professional should invite the parents to give their descriptions first, and then she can comment on the videotape. This is an appropriate way for the parents and the professional to interact and is more likely to produce successful interactions in the future.

As widespread as mental retardation is, it is still underdiagnosed at an early age. Even at older ages, it is undertreated once it is discovered, and even then it remains one of the most misunderstood afflictions of newborns, infants, children, adolescents, and adults. The term "mental retardation" is global. It is essential for child care professionals—nurses, physicians, and social workers—to recognize the behaviors, or lack of them, that signal mental retardation and to learn to distinguish the degrees and ranges with which it occurs.

GENERAL ORIENTATION TO HELP PARENTS TEACH THEIR CHILDREN SUCCESSFULLY

Certain factors of readiness are necessary for the parents to have success with teaching and the child to have success with learning. It is important that the parents be able to observe certain behaviors that signal the child is ready for a task. The child care professional should be available to help parents decide if the child is ready to begin tasks such as learning to play, undress, dress, feed himself, or toilet train or to respond more effectively to the parents' requests for compliance.

At the same time it is important that the parents themselves exhibit behavior indicating that they are ready to assume teaching a task. The child's readiness to learn does not guarantee that the parent will be successful in teaching. Therefore it becomes essential that the parents' readiness for the teaching task be examined. Does parents' behavior indicate they have a relaxed attitude about their child's learning? When are they relaxed? When do they become tense? Do they become anxious before, during, or after teaching? These are questions that can be explored with the parents before, during, and after a teaching session with their child. If they appear to be tense, irritable, or indifferent to the child, perhaps their feelings can be explored so that they can have a more successful outcome with their child.

Once the parents are committed to teaching a task and at a time convenient for them, it is important that they be firm but gentle with their child. Before teaching even begins, a discussion should occur concerning the requisites of successful teaching and learning. Parents need to be patient and not hurry the child along and be able to persevere with the task and not give up

easily. During the teaching session, the parents should feel comfortable and good about what they are doing with their child and spontaneously express love and acceptance toward him. The child, at the same time, learns that he is valued, loved, cared for, and a vital part of what the family is doing. Children are highly responsive when their parents use affectionate gestures, smile, or express approval for what he is doing.

The parents should also be prepared for repetition. They may need to have the term defined, since it is so important to the child's success in learning. Repetition is one way by which the child acquires the skills that he is attempting to master. Parents must be prepared to give praise, to give it abundantly, and to give it when it is appropriate. They should think about terms that they will use with the child as he goes about a learning task and be prepared to say things such as, "You ate so well." "I like what you are doing." "I love you." "You are a good girl." "You held your spoon very well." "You did not spill your food." "You drank from your cup." "You put your little shoes on." "You did that so well." It is important that parents learn that they do not have to give praise for every little behavior but that it should be given spontaneously when the child is manifesting the behavior that the parent wishes to see repeated.

When first learning a task, the child responds readily to approval and the affectionate praise that parents give, and it should be given so that the child distinguishes it from the parents' usual ways of talking to him. In other words, intonation and inflection should change and praise should be given enthusiastically and in a manner that lets the child know the parents are pleased. The child usually looks at his parents' facial expressions as praise is given. Their eyes should be shining and bright, and they should be smiling. Definite and different behavior should be apparent when they are giving praise. The child care professional should discuss with the parents the fact that children are highly perceptive and sensitive to praise and whether it is given genuinely and spontaneously.

If the parents are going to give a concrete reward, they should determine and plan in advance what rewards would be best for the child and what kinds of rewards he might like so that he can choose them in advance. It is important that they not satiate the child with great amounts of chocolates, sweets, or high-calorie foods but give appropriate rewards. If they do give food rewards, they should be selective about the times they are given. A bunch of little snacks just before the child eats dinner is undesirable. Sometimes children respond more favorably and quickly to social approval than to concrete rewards such as food, candy, money or stars on a chart. However, brightly colored charts with colored stars or stickers may help the child reach his developmental goal.

Parents should avoid the habit of praising the child for something that is not well done but should simply ignore it and look for improved behavior in the next session. Parents should also avoid making statements such as, "Well that's not so good, but you will do better the next time around." That can be confusing to a child. It is desirable for him to quickly learn those behaviors which the parents like and dislike.

It is important that parents make a habit of teaching only one thing at a time. Just before parents begin teaching a task, they need to get the child's attention, establish eye contact, ensure that he is listening, and watch for behavior such as turning his head.

The parents need to remain calm, relaxed, and pleasant regardless of the number of accidents or incorrect trials that the child may have. The parents should plan for short practice sessions, yet they should allow plenty of time for the child to master a task. It is important that the parents do not rush the child but, at the same time, they need to make it clear that they will not tolerate the child's playing around. The child may have played around in the past to attract the parents' attention, and they need to ignore this kind of behavior.

Parents should make it a habit to name objects as a child eats, dresses, or toilet trains. For example, the parents can say, "These are your red socks, these are your black shoes, this is your spoon, this is your glass, this is your hat." At the same time the parents refer to the objects that the child is using they can also reinforce the child's speech. When he makes a sound, the parents can reinforce the speech while the child is learning a task. Parents should realize that if the child learns a skill in one situation, he will not automatically transfer it to another situation. For example, if he learns about a hot match, he will not necessarily know about a hot iron.

One of the most successful approaches and attitudes that parents must internalize is to *help the child only when he actually needs help*. The parents may have become accustomed to doing things for the child, but they must learn and probably should discuss the difficulty of not helping the child when he is trying. However, only by insisting that the child do more of a task himself will he learn what is expected of him.

It is important that parents learn the value of being consistent in their behavior with their child. Once they have established a pattern reinforcing his behavior and speaking and showing enthusiasm in a certain way, they need to continue their way of interacting. The routine becomes important for the child and is a way for him to learn that his environment is predictable. The parents should arrange for the child to learn the task in the same place at about the same time each day, particularly when he is beginning to learn.

Teaching anything in a distracting situation must be avoided. A child sometimes has difficulty sorting out stimuli that are not relevant to his learning needs, and therefore he cannot concentrate on the task at hand. It is therefore important that the parents choose an area where there will be no interruptions, where the child will not be distracted, and where the child will feel comfortable, safe, and not pressured.

The child should finish parts of any task that he has started, even though he may not have successfully mastered the entire task. He should not be allowed to do things halfway. The parents need to consider the child's learning needs and attention span, presenting tasks that are appropriate for his developmental functioning and that will hold his interest until he is finished. Therefore it becomes essential for the parents to have baseline information about their child's behavior and know his abilities to concentrate and sustain interest.

Parents should become accustomed to demonstrating tasks in front of the child after they have gotten his attention. The child learns by the examples the parents set and by imitating others. He learns social skills such as being polite, how to greet other persons, how to say goodbye, and other socially acceptable behavior. It is far better to take the time to teach a child to do something correctly rather than spend a great amount of time later teaching him to unlearn an undesirable way of interacting.

As far as teaching the child to respond to discipline, there are some basic concepts that can be taught by other caregivers. The child definitely needs to know the difference between what is right and what is not right. He needs to learn from the outset which behaviors are acceptable and which will not be tolerated. Parents will need experience in learning how to respond to both appropriate and inappropriate behavior. They key to success is for the parents to show abundant reinforcement when the child shows acceptable behavior and to ignore him when he is exhibiting unacceptable behavior. The child soon learns the difference. Parents are responsible for praising the child when he is cooperative, trying, attempting a task, attempting to correct his mistakes, and initiating something on his own rather than having somebody initiate it for him. The parents need to learn to accept calmly any mistakes that the child makes and to offer reinforcement, approval, and acceptance until he learns what he is expected to do. The child may need frequent reminders from his parents, which they must be prepared to give. It is extremely important in setting limits for a child that the parents decide together how they will enforce certain rules, how they will respond to the child so that he learns what is acceptable, and how much they will and will not tolerate. They must be prepared not to deviate from these decisions.

In planning a limit-setting program, parents must know that their expectations are realistic. They must learn to be flexible and change their approach if it becomes too harsh, overwhelming, or incomprehensible to the child. The parents should remain consistent, however, so that once the child has responded successfully to their behavior, they continue to use the same approaches. Thus the child knows exactly what is expected of him and what will and will not be tolerated. Parents must use words consistently. If they are going to punish the child, they need to plan this in advance. They should not impulsively punish the child because they suddenly become angry.

The parents must be prepared to teach by example, be comfortable in the way they are teaching, and be proud of the examples they are setting. Parents should not teach something in which they do not believe. The child care professional sometimes can establish a dialogue with parents if they are showing the child how to do something in which they really do not believe. The parents must show the child what to do, how to do it, and when to do it. Again, they need to allow the child to practice the task that they want the child to accomplish. In the final analysis, the child must feel that what he is learning is important to himself, to his mother, and to his father. In addition, the parents must

believe it is important to learn the task or change the behavior.

If parents are going to correct a child, it is imperative that they correct the child as soon as the behavior occurs. When the child is corrected, he should be approached firmly. Parents should not correct the child and should avoid teaching or making changes when they are angry. Parents may learn that isolating the child from persons or his favorite toys or activities for short periods of time may be effective in reducing inappropriate behavior. If the child becomes excited, uncontrollable, or difficult in a group, he should be removed quickly and placed where he can quiet down and become more comfortable. Parents should be discouraged from slapping the hands or spanking if it is too hard or if it frightens the child. On the other hand, parents can discuss how they feel about using physical punishment, whether or not they think this is an effective solution, and how they think it is effective. Sometimes slapping the child or hitting him very lightly only reinforces his behavior. They should be asked if they have thought of other ways to set limits with the child.

It is also important for parents to learn that threatening the child is not successful, since the child's memory may be short, he may confuse what he is being told with something else, and he may even forget why he was threatened. Parents simply drain themselves by making a habit of threatening a child. They develop a pattern of inconsistently following through with what they said they intended to do. If the parents agree that they should punish the child by putting him to bed, they need to examine if this is an appropriate method for limiting certain kinds of behavior. Putting the child to bed may have an undesirable consequence. Parents may face the dilemma of trying to put the child to bed at night and he resists because he is afraid. As a discipline measure, putting the child to bed may confuse him because at night he goes to sleep, hopefully, under calm circumstances and during the day he is put to bed when things are not at all calm.

Parents should not make a habit of telling their child they will not love him anymore if he continues to do something. Not only is this ineffective but it also makes the parent feel guilty. Parents need to remember that children, by and large, respond much better if they know that they are loved, cared for, and valued as shown by their parents' loving behavior. Parents need to discuss scolding or nagging as a way of changing the child's behavior. Usually this results only in noise and anger coming from the parents. There is little evidence that nagging or scolding is useful in terminating unacceptable behavior in a child or adult. Parents might learn to record when a child's behavior is unacceptable. Scolding or screaming at the child only results in the parent's feeling guilty and useless and he still fails to gain the child's cooperation. Sometimes a child will benefit from a simple warning and from being told how much time will be allowed before the child will be asked to carry out a request. This gives the child an opportunity to stop what he is doing and to orient himself to the task that needs to be done. If parents are going to reason with the child or give explanations, they need to discuss if this is the best way to set limits for the child. Long verbal explanations may need to be modified or eliminated, since they might confuse the child rather than help him learn to do something better.

It is important that the child understand exactly what is expected of him. Telling him is often not enough. He must be shown and asked to repeat what he is shown. Otherwise, how can the parents know whether the child knows what is expected? The child care professional should ask the parents how they know when their child understands a request. Does the child act differently toward one parent than he does toward the other? The parents need to tell the child what to do rather than what not to do. For example, the parents should say, "Put your foot in your shoe" rather than, "Don't put your sock on the floor." Sometimes self-fulfilling prophecies come about, and a child will act as if the parent expects him to obey. If the parent conveys the attitude that the child cannot learn, chances are he will not learn. Thus it is important for parents to expect certain behavior from their child and not to show surprise or make negative statements when he does succeed.

It is necessary for the child to receive one direction at a time after his attention has been gained and for commands to be kept simple. The parents need to be asked how they give directions to the child and how they judge these directions—are they too simple, too complex? How does their child usually respond? Parents also may be helped by exploring the causes for the child's failure to comply with requests. Are the parents expecting more than the child is capable of performing? Are they setting their expectations too high? Have the parents been told and do they realize his current capabilities

of functioning within the environment? If the child seems to be naughty, stubborn, or provoking the parents, they need to discuss reasons for this behavior. There may be another more appropriate explanation. For example, the child may be uncomfortable, tired, hungry, overwhelmed, or confused as to what is expected of him. There may be too many distractions or too many rules to follow, or the child may be becoming ill. Most children delight in pleasing their parents. This is equally true of a mentally retarded child. The child may be failing to comply so that he will get attention from his parents. If this seems to be the case, the parents need to think of ways to give the child attention when he is behaving well.

With any teaching task it is important that parents keep their expectations at the proper level. They should know on a serial basis or over a period of time what their child is capable of doing and what he cannot do. At the same time, parents should not underestimate his abilities. In this case they often do too much for the child. This is a common practice for parents of mentally retarded children, particularly those parents who do not know the child's functional levels. Parents must be reinforced for encouraging the child to develop independence and when he begins to show capabilities in unexpected new areas. Parents will be most successful when they break the learning task down into small, discrete steps that the child can successfully master one by one, when they allow the child to repeat a task over and over again. The parents must be willing to demonstrate expected performance. They need to keep explanations to a minimum and use simple words. For the best outcome they must be willing to praise the child, give approval, and show enthusiasm for any improvements in behavior and for any performance well done. They must acknowledge the child when he does a job well, no matter how minor it might seem. It is a major accomplishment for the child. It is also important that the parents do not praise the child when he has done something poorly, yet learn not to make him feel he has failed. Furthermore, once the child begins to respond to praise and efforts by others on a one-to-one basis, the parents should begin to consider giving the child experiences within a group situation.

Although mental retardation presents numerous significant problems, child care professionals such as social workers, nurses, pediatricians, psychologists, nutritionists, physical therapists, speech pathologists, and child psychiatrists continue to seek improved and better ways to respond to the vast and perplexing problems of children and their parents. It is possible to ensure maximal progress for children with mental retardation and their families. The one key to successful approaches seems to be based in sound assessment, screening, and objective and systematic planning for the management problems that continue to be encountered by professionals from all child health care disciplines.

SUMMARY

The roles of child care professionals in screening, assessment, and management of children who are well and those who have mental retardation are changing, as can be seen in the following table, which lists changing practices in assessment and management of children with developmental changes and problems in development.

Nurses and other child care professionals are assuming new and changing roles and responsibilities in the care and management of children who are well and those who have handicapping conditions such as mental retardation. A major difference in child care practices today is that all child care professionals are exchanging responsibilities in becoming the "care manager" for parents and children. Without question, this role was once relegated solely to the physician. Now the nurse as well as other child care professionals are coordinating, planning, and evaluating care; more importantly, however, other child care professionals along with the nurse are being held accountable for providing appropriate services and care to infants, children, parents, and their families.

REFERENCES

1. Wolfensberger, Wolf: Normalization: the principle of normalization in human services, Toronto, 1972, National Institute on Mental Retardation.
2. Barnard, Kathryn E., and Erickson, Marcene L.: Teaching the child with developmental problems: a family care approach, ed. 2, St. Louis, 1976, The C. V. Mosby Co.
3. Erickson, Marcene: Developmental assessment. In Curry, Judith B., and Peppe, Kathryn K., editors: Mental retardation: nursing approaches to care, St. Louis, 1978, The C. V. Mosby Co.

ADDITIONAL READINGS
General

Baker, Amanda S., and Barton, Pauline H.: The mentally retarded child. In Scripien, Gladys, et al., editors: Comprehensive pediatric nursing, New York, 1975, McGraw-Hill Book Co.

Barnard, Kathryn E.: Developmental disabilities, Am. J. Nurs. **75:**1700-1708, 1975.

Baumeister, Alfred A., editor: Mental retardation: appraisal, education and rehabilitation, Chicago, 1967, Aldine Publishing Co.

Bean, Margaret R., and Bell, Betty Jo.: Nursing intervention in the care of the physically handicapped, severely retarded child, Nurs. Clin. North Am. **10:** 353-359, 1975.

Bensberg, Gerard J., editor: Teaching the mentally retarded: a handbook for ward personnel, Atlanta, 1965, Southern Regional Education Board.

Bijou, S. W.: Theory and research in mental (developmental) retardation, Psychol. Rec. **13:**95-110, 1963.

Bijou, S. W.: A functional analysis of retarded development. In Ellis, N. R., editor: International review of research in mental retardation, vol. 1, New York, 1966, Academic Press, Inc.

Bowley, Agatha H., and Gardner, Leslie: The handicapped child: educational and psychological guidance for the organically handicapped, Baltimore, 1972, The Williams & Wilkins Co.

Bumbalo, Judith A., and Seidel, Mary A.: Identifying and serving a multiply handicapped population, Nurs. Clin. North Am. **10:**341-352, 1975.

Curry, Judith B., and Peppe, Kathryn K., editors: Mental retardation: nursing approaches to care, St. Louis, 1978, The C. V. Mosby Co.

Drotar, Dennis, Baskiewiez, Ann, Irvin, Nancy, Kennell, John, and Klaus, Marshall: The adaptation of parents to the birth of an infant with a congenital malformation: a hypothetical model, Pediatrics **56:** 710-717, 1975.

Dybwad, Gunnar: Who are the mentally retarded? Children **15:**43-48, March-April, 1968.

Ehlers, Walter H., Krishef, Curtis H., and Prothero, Jon C.: An introduction to mental retardation: a programmed text, Columbus, Ohio, 1973, Charles E. Merrill Publishing Co.

Erickson, Marcene: Talking with fathers of children with Down's syndrome, Child. Today **3:**22-25, Nov.-Dec., 1974.

Fairburn, Sandra J.: Comparative child rearing attitudes and practices of mothers considered to be mentally retarded and non-retarded mothers, unpublished Master's thesis, University of Washington School of Nursing, Seattle, 1973.

Farber, Bernard, and Ryckman, David: Effects of severely mentally retarded children on family relationships, Ment. Retard. Abs. **2:**1-17, Jan.-March, 1965.

Gorham, Kathryn A.: A lost generation of parents, Except. Child. **41:**521-525, May, 1975.

Haring, N. G., Hayden, A. H., and Beck, R.: General principles and guidelines in programming for severely handicapped children and young adults, Focus Except. Child. **8:**1-14, 1976.

Kauffman, James M., and Payne, James S.: Mental retardation: introduction and personal perspectives, Columbus, Ohio, 1975, Bell & Howell Co.

Kluss, Kathryn: Training the mentally retarded child in self-help skills. In Brandt, Patricia A., Chinn,

Peggy L., and Smith, Mary E., editors: Current practice in pediatric nursing, vol. 2, St. Louis, 1978, The C. V. Mosby Co.

Kugel, R. B.: Combatting retardation in infants with Down's syndrome, Children **17:**188-192, 1970.

Norris, Geraldine J.: National concerns for children with handicaps, Nurs. Clin. North Am. **10:**309-318, June, 1975.

Pipes, Peggy L.: Nutrition and feeding of children with developmental delays and related problems. In Pipes, Peggy L.: Nutrition in infants and children, St. Louis, 1977, The C. V. Mosby Co.

Powell, Marcene: An interpretation of effective management and discipline of the mentally retarded child, Nurs. Clin. North Am. **1:**689-702, 1966.

Powell, Marcene: An analysis of behaviors to promote independent feeding skills. In Nursing in mental retardation programs, Proceedings of 4th National Workshop for Nurses in Mental Retardation, University of Miami, Miami, 1967.

Robinson, Nancy M., and Robinson, Halbert: The mentally retarded child, New York, 1976, McGraw-Hill Book Co.

Russell, F.: Interdisciplinary early intervention program, Phys. Ther. **56:**155-158, 1976.

Seidel, Mary: Nursing care of children with mental retardation and other developmental disabilities: career development in the health professions, Washington, D.C., 1976, Bureau of Community Health Services, U.S. Department of Health, Education, and Welfare.

Smith, David W., and Wilson, Ann A.: The child with Down's syndrome: causes, characteristics and acceptance, Philadelphia, 1973, W. B. Saunders Co.

Whitney, Linda: Operant learning theory: a framework deserving nursing investigation, Nurs. Res. **15**(3):229-235, 1966.

Whitney, Linda, and Barnard, Kathryn E.: Implications of operant learning theory for nursing care of the retarded child, Ment. Retard. **3:**26-29, June, 1966.

Wolfensberger, Wolf: Counseling the parents of the retarded. In Baumeister, Alfred A., editor: Mental retardation: appraisal, education and rehabilitation, Chicago, 1967, Aldine Publishing Co.

Zelle, Raeone: A study to determine the need for a conceptual guide to assess the effect of a retarded child on family relations and life, unpublished Master's thesis, University of Washington School of Nursing, Seattle, 1969.

The family

Ainsworth, Mary: The development of infant-mother attachment, In Caldwell, Bettye M., and Riccuiti, Henry, editors: Review of child development research, Chicago, 1966, University of Chicago Press.

Anthony, E. James, and Benedek, Therese, editors: Parenthood: its psychology and psychopathology, Boston, 1970, Little, Brown, & Co., Inc.

Anthony, E. James, and Koupernik, C.: The child in his family. I. New York, 1970, John Wiley & Sons, Inc.

Anthony, E. James, and Koupernik, C.: The child in his family. II. New York, 1973, John Wiley & Sons, Inc.

Barnard, Kathryn E., editor: Symposium on mental retardation, Nurs. Clin. North Am. **4:**629-723, 1966.

Barnard, Kathryn E., and Powell, Marcene: Family considerations. In Barnard, Kathryn E., and Erickson, Marcene. Teaching children with developmental problems: a family care approach, ed. 2, St. Louis, 1976, The C. V. Mosby Co.

Barsch, Ray H.: The parent of the handicapped child, Springfield, Ill., 1968, Charles C Thomas, Publisher.

Baumeister, Alfred A., editor: Mental retardation: appraisal, education, and rehabilitation, Chicago, 1967, Aldine Publishing Co.

Becker, Wesley C.: Parents are teachers, Champaign, Ill., 1971, Research Press Co.

Bell, Norman W., and Vogel, Ezra F.: A modern introduction to the family, Glencoe, Ill., 1962, The Free Press.

Bell, Richard Q.: Contributions of human infants to caregiving and social interaction. In Lewis, Michael, and Rosenblum, Leonard A., editors: The effect of the infant on its caregiver, New York, 1974, John Wiley & Sons, Inc.

Bell, Robert R.: The impact of illness on family roles. In Folton, Jeanette R., and Deck, Edith S., editors: A sociological framework for patient care, New York, 1966, John Wiley & Sons, Inc.

Benedek, Therese: Parenthood as a developmental phase, J. Am. Psychoanal. Assoc. **1:**389-417, 1959.

Berado, Felix: The anthropological approach to the study of the family. In Nye, F. I., and Berado, Felix M.: Emerging conceptual framework in family analysis, New York, 1966, The Macmillan Co.

Brazelton, T. Berry, Koslowski, Barbara, and Main, Mary: The origins of reciprocity: the early mother-infant interaction. In Lewis, Michael, and Rosenblum, Leonard A., editors: The effect of the infant on its caregiver, New York, 1974, John Wiley & Sons, Inc.

Caplan, Gerald: Support systems and community mental health, New York, 1974, Human Sciences Press, Inc.

Cone, John D., and Sloop, E. Wayne: Parents as agents of change. In Jacobs, A., and Spradlin, W. W., editors: Group as agent of change, New York, 1974, Human Sciences Press, Inc.

Coopersmith, Stanley: Parent-child relationships. I. Acceptance. In Coopersmith, Stanley, editor: The antecedents of self esteem, San Francisco, 1967, W. H. Freeman & Co., Publishers.

Coopersmith, Stanley, editor: The antecedents of self esteem, San Francisco, 1967, W. H. Freeman & Co., Publishers.

Davis, D. R.: Family processes in mental retardation, Am. J. Psychiatry **124:**340-350, 1967.

Disbrow, Mildred A.: Changing roles and self-concepts of people. In Clausen, Joy, et al., editors: Maternity nursing today, New York, 1973, McGraw-Hill Book Co.

Duvall, Evelyn M.: Family development, ed. 4, Philadelphia, 1971, J. B. Lippincott Co.

Dybwad, Gunnar: Who are the mentally retarded? Children **15:**43-48, March-April, 1968.

Edwards, John N.: The family and change, New York, 1969, Alfred A. Knopf, Inc.

Ehlers, Walter H.: Mothers of retarded children, Springfield, Ill., 1966, Charles C Thomas, Publisher.

Farber, Barnard: Mental retardation, Boston, 1968, Houghton-Mifflin Co.

Gough, Kathleen: The origin of the family. In Winch, Robert, and Spaner, Graham B., editors: Selected studies in marriage and the family, New York, 1974, Holt, Rinehart & Winston, Inc.

Gordon, Thomas: Parent effectiveness training, New York, 1970, Peter H. Wyden, Inc.

Grossman, Herbert J., editor: Symposium on mental retardation, Pediatr. Clin. North Am. **15:**819-1110, 1968.

Handel, Gerald: Sociological aspects of parenthood. In Anthony, E. James, and Benedek, Therese, editors: Parenthood: its psychology and psychopathology, Boston, 1970, Little, Brown & Co., Inc.

Hess, R. D., and Shipman, V. C.: Early experiences and the socialization of cognitive modes in children, Child Devel. **36:**860-866, 1965.

Hess, R. D., and Shipman, V. C.: Maternal influences upon early learning; the cognitive environments of urban pre-school children. In Hess, R. D., and Bear, R. M., editors: Early education, Chicago, 1968, Aldine Publishing Co.

Hill, Reuban: Generic features of families under stress. In Parad, Howard J., editor: Crisis intervention: selected readings, New York, 1965, Family Service Association of America.

Holt, D. S.: The influence of a retarded child upon family limitations, J. Ment. Defic. **2:**28-34, 1958.

Kirk, S. A., Karnes, M. B., and Kirk, W. D.: You and your retarded child, New York, 1955, The Macmillan Co.

Klaus, Marshall J.: Maternal attachment: significance of the first postpartum days, New Engl. J. Med. **286:**460, 1972.

Koch, Richard, and Dobson, James, editors: The mentally retarded child and his family, New York, 1971, Brunner/Mazel, Inc.

Kogan, Kate: Specificity and stability of mother-child interaction styles, Child Psychiatry Hum. Dev. **2:**160-168, 1972.

Leik, R. K., and Northwood, L. K.: The classification of family interaction problems for treatment purposes, J. Marriage Fam. **26:**288-294, 1964.

Matarazzo, J. D.: Some national developments in the utilization of nontraditional mental health power, Am. Psychol. **26:**363-372, 1971.

Nursing in mental retardation programs, Children's Bureau, Department of Health, Education, and Welfare and Child Development Center, University of Miami, Coral Gables, April, 1967, pp. 1-161.

O'Neill, Sally M., Newcomer McLaughlin, Barbara, and Knapp, Mary Beth, editors: Behavioral approaches to children with developmental delays, St. Louis, 1977, The C. V. Mosby Co.

Parad, Howard J., and Caplan, Gerald: A framework for studying families in crisis. In Parad, Howard J., editor: Crisis intervention: selected readings, New York, 1966, Family Service Association of America.

Parsons, Talcott, and Bales, Robert F.: Family socialization and interaction process, Glencoe, Ill., 1955, The Free Press.

Patterson, E. Gene, and Rowland, G. Thomas: Toward a theory of mental retardation nursing: an educational mold, Am. J. Nurs. **70:**531-535, 1970.

Patterson, G. R.: Families: applications of social learning to family life, Champaign, Ill., 1971, Research Press Co.

Patterson, G. R., and Gullion, M. E.: Living with children, Champaign, Ill., 1968, Research Press Co.

Rosen, B., and D'Anlrade, R.: The psychosocial origins of achievement motivation, Sociometry **22:**185-218, 1959.

Rossi, A. S.: Transition to parenthood, J. Marriage Fam. **30:**26-39, 1968.

Rubin, Reva: Attainment of the maternal role. I and II. Nurs. Res. **13**(3, 4), Summer, Fall, 1967.

Satir, Virginia: Conjoint family therapy, Palo Alto, Calif., 1967, Science & Behavior Books, Inc.

Satir, Virginia: Peoplemaking, Palo Alto, Calif., 1972, Science & Behavior Books, Inc.

Schaefer, Earl S.: Parents as educators: evidence from cross-sectional longitudinal, and intervention research. In Hartup, W. W., editor: The young child: reviews of research, vol. 2, Washington, D.C., 1972, National Association for the Education of Young Children.

Scheinfeld, D. R., et al.: Parents' values, family networks, and family development: working with disadvantaged families, Am. J. Orthopsychiatry **39:**323-324, 1969.

Streissguth, Ann, and Bee, Helen L.: Mother-child interactions and cognitive development in children. In Hartup, W. W., editor: The young child: reviews of research, Washington, D.C., 1972, National Association for the Education of Young Children.

Szasz, Thomas S., and Hollender, Marc H.: A contribution to the philosophy of medicine, Arch. of Intern. Med. **97:**585-592, 1956.

Terrill, James M., and Terrill, Ruth E.: A method of studying family communication, Fam. Process **4:**259-290, 1965.

Winch, Robert F.: The modern family, New York, 1964, Holt, Rinehart & Winston, Inc.

Winch, Robert F.: Theorizing about the family. In Winch, Robert, and Spanier, Graham B., editors: Selected studies in marriage and the family, New York, 1974, Holt, Rinehart & Winston, Inc.

Worby, Cyril M.: The family life cycle: an orienting concept for the family practice specialist, J. Med. Educ. **46:**198-203, 1973.

Wolfensberger, Wolf, and Kentz, Richard A.: Management of the family of the mentally retarded, Chicago, 1969, Follett Publishing Co.

Yarrow, Leon J., and Pedersen, Frank A.: Attachment: its origins and course, In Hartup, W. W., editor: The young child: reviews of research, Washington, D.C., 1972, National Association for the Education of Young Children.

York, Eileenamy G.: The evolution of the parent-child relationship: focused on developmental tasks. In Parent-Child relationships: role of the nurse. Presented at Rutgers University, New Brunswick, N.J., Nov., 1963, S & S Printing.

Responding to parental needs: the supportive processes

Bakwin, H.: Psychologic aspects of pediatrics, informing the parents of the mentally retarded child, J. Pediatr. **49:**486-498, 1956.

Beck, Helen L.: Casework with parents of mentally retarded children, Am. J. Orthopsychiatry **32:**970-977, 1962.

Boyd, D.: The three stages in the growth of a parent of a mentally retarded child, Am. J. Ment. Defic. **55:**608-611, 1951.

Cohen, Pauline: The impact of the handicapped child on the family, Soc. Casework **43:**137-142, 1962.

Dalton, Juanita, and Epstein, Helene: Counseling parents of mildly retarded children, Soc. Casework **44:**523-530, 1963.

Fackler, Eleanor: The crisis of institutionalizing a retarded child, Am. J. Nurs. **68:**1508-1512, 1968.

Gianninni, Ngr, and Goodman, Lawrence: Counseling family during the crisis reaction to mongolism, Am. J. Ment. Defic. **67:**740-747, 1963.

Golden, Deborah A., and Davis, Jessica G.: Counseling parents after the birth of an infant with Down's syndrome, Child. Today **3:**7-11, 36, March-April, 1974.

Gordon, E. W., and Ullman, M.: Reactions of parents to problems of mental retardation in children, Am. J. Ment. Defic. **61:**158-163, 1956.

Hawley, Eleanor F.: The importance of extending public health nursing services to retarded children living at home, Ment. Retard. **1:**243-247, 1965.

Kaplan, D. M., and Mason, E. A.: Maternal reactions to premature birth viewed as an acute emotional disorder, Am. J. Orthopsychiatry **30:**539-552, 1960.

Kaplan, S., and Williams, M. J.: Confrontation counseling: a new dimension in group counseling, Am. J. Orthopsychiatry **42:**114-118, 1972.

Klaus, Marshall, and Kennell, John: Mothers separated from their newborn infants, Pediatr. Clin. North Am. **17:**1015-1037, 1970.

Klaus, Marshall, and Kennell, John: Maternal-infant bonding: the impact of early separation or loss on family development, St. Louis, 1976, The C. V. Mosby Co.

Lageay, Camile, and Keogh, Barbara: Impact of mental retardation on family life, Am. J. Nurs. **66:**1062-1065, 1966.

Layman, William A.: Grief and grieving. In parent-child relationships: role of the nurse. Presented at Rutgers University, New Brunswick, N.J., Nov., 1968, S & S Printing.

Lindemann, Eric: Symptomatology and management of acute grief. In Parad, Howard J., editor: Crisis intervention: selected readings, New York, 1966, Family Service Association of America.

Mandelbaum, Arthur, and Wheller, Mary E.: The meaning of a defective child to parents, Soc. Casework **42:**78-83, 1961.

Miller, Lee: Towards a greater understanding of the parents of the mentally retarded child, J. Pediatr. **73:**699-705, 1968.

Milligan, G. E.: Counseling parents of the mentally retarded, Ment. Retard. Abs. **2**(3):1-9, July-Sept., 1965.

Morris, Marian G.: Maternal claiming–identification processes: their meaning for mother-infant mental health. In Parent-child relationships: role of the nurse, New Brunswick, N.J. Presented at Rutgers University, New Brunswick, N.J., Nov., 1968, S & S Printing.

Olshansky, Simon: Chronic sorrow: a response for having a mentally defective child, Soc. Casework **43:**190-193, 1963.

Ownby, Ralph: From the interpretative conference with parents of a mentally retarded child. In Wolfensberger, Wolf, and Kurtz, Richard, editors: Management of the family of the mentally retarded, Chicago, 1969, Follett Publishing Co.

Patterson, Letha L.: Some pointers for professions, Children **3:**13-17, Jan.-Feb. 1956.

Rheingold, Harriet L.: Feedback phase: interpreting mental retardation to parents. In Wolfensberger, Wolf, and Kurtz, Richard, editors: Management of the family of the mentally retarded, Chicago, 1969, Follett Publishing Co.

Roos, Phillip: Psychological counseling with parents of retarded children. In Wolfensberger, Wolf, and Kurtz, Richard A., editors: Management of the family of the mentally retarded, 1969, Follett Education Corp.

Sarason, Seymour B.: From interpretation of mental deficiency to parents. In Wolfensberger, Wolf, and Kurtz, Richard A., editors: Follett Education Corp.

Solnit, Albert J., and Stark, Mary H.: Mourning and the birth of a defective child, Soc. Casework **43:**190-193, 1963.

Warrick, L. H.: Family centered care in the premature nursery, Am. J. Nurs. **71:**2134-2138, 1971.

Watts, Evadean M.: Family therapy: its use in mental retardation, Ment. Retard. **7:**41-44, Oct., 1969.

Wolfensberger, Wolf: Counseling the parents of the retarded. In Baumeister, Alfred A., editor: Mental retardation: appraisal, education and rehabilitation, Chicago, 1967, Aldine Publishing Co.

Zelle, Raeone: A study to determine the need for a conceptual guide to assess the effect of a retarded child on family relations and life, unpublished Master's thesis, University of Washington School of Nursing, Seattle, 1969.

Zuk, G. H., et al.: Maternal acceptance of retarded children: a questionnaire study of attitudes and religious background, Child Dev. **32:**525-540, 1961.

Parent-centered approaches to meeting the needs of children

Baldwin, Victor, et al.: A training program for parents of retarded children, Springfield, Ill., 1973, Charles C Thomas, Publisher.

Bee, Helen L., Van Egereu, Lawrence F., Streissguth, Ann P., Nyman, Barry A., and Leckie, Maxine S.: Social class differences in maternal teaching strategies and speech patterns, Dev. Psychol. **1:**726-734, 1969.

Bernal, M. E.: Behavioral feedback in the modification of brat behaviors, J. Nerv. Ment. Dis. **148:**375 385, 1969.

Caldwell, Bettye M.: What is the optimal learning environment for the young child? In Frost, Joe L., editor: Early childhood education rediscovered, New York, 1968, Holt, Rinehart & Winston, Inc.

Carkhuff, R. R., and Bierman, R.: Training as a preferred mode of treatment of parents of emotionally disturbed children, J. Counsel. Psychol. **17:**157-161, 1970.

Ginott, H.: The therapist as a parent, Ment. Hyg. **57:** 11-12, Spring, 1973.

Gordon, Ira: The young child: a new look. In Frost, Joe L., editor: Early childhood education rediscovered, New York, 1968, Holt, Rinehart & Winston, Inc.

Gordon, Ira J.: Reaching the young child through parent education. In Spodek, Bernard, editor: Early childhood education, Englewood Cliffs, N.J., 1973, Prentice-Hall, Inc.

Johnson, Claudia, and Katz, Roger: Using parents as change agents for their children: a review, J. Child Psychol. Psychiatry **14:**181-200, Sept., 1973.

Johnson, S. M., and Brown, R. A.: Producing behavior change in parents of disturbed children, J. Child Psychol. Psychiatry **10:**107-121, Sept., 1969.

Kamii, Constance: A sketch of the Piaget-derived preschool curriculum developed by the Ypsilanti early education program. In Spodek, Bernard, editor: Early Childhood education, Englewood Cliffs, N.J., 1973, Prentice-Hall, Inc.

Karnes, M. B., Feska, J. A., Hodgins, A. S., and Badger, E. D.: Educational intervention at home by mothers of disadvantaged infants, Child Dev. **41:** 925-935, 1970.

Karnes, M. B., Studkey, W. M., Wright, W. R., and Hodgins, A. S.: An approach for working with mothers of disadvantaged preschool children, Merrill-Palmer Q. Behav. Dev. **14:**174-184, 1968.

Kogan, Kate L., and Wimberger, Herbert C.: An approach to defining mother-child interaction styles, Percept. Mot. Skills **23:**1171-1177, 1966.

Kogan, Kate L., and Wimberger, Herbert C.: Behavior transactions between disturbed children and their mothers, Psychol. Rep. **28:**395-404, 1971.

Kogan, Kate L., Gordon, Betty N., and Wimberger,

Herbert C.: Teaching mothers to alter interactions with their children: implications for those who work with children and parents, Child. Educ. (reprint) **3:**107-110, Nov., 1972.

Kogan, Kate L., and Tyler, Nancy: Mother-child interaction in young physically handicapped children, Am. J. Ment. Defic. **77:**492-497, 1973.

Kogan, Kate L., et al.: Analysis of mother-child interaction in young mental retardates, Child Dev. **40:** 799-812, 1969.

Lambie, Dolores Z., and Weikart, David P.: Ypsilanti Carnegie infant education project. In Hellmuth, Jerome, editor: Disadvantaged child, New York, 1970, Brunner/Mazel, Inc.

Levenstein, Phyllis: Cognitive growth in preschoolers through verbal interactions with mothers, Am. J. Orthopsychiatry **40:**426-432, 1970.

Levenstein, Phyllis, and Sunley, Robert: Stimulation of verbal interaction between disadvantaged mothers and children, Am. J. Orthopsychiatry **38:**116-121, 1968.

Lytton, H.: Observation studies of parent-child interaction: a methodological review, Child Dev. **42:**651-684, 1971.

Mash, Eric J., and Terdal, Leif: Modification of mother-child interactions: playing with children, Ment. Retard. **4:**44-49, Oct., 1973.

Mash, E. J., Lazere, R. L., Terdal, L. G., and Garner, A. M.: Modification of mother-child interactions: a modeling approach for groups, Child Study J. **4:**165-168, 1973.

Mash, E. J., Terdal, L. G., and Anderson, K.: The response-class matrix: a procedure for recording parent-child interactions, J. Consult. Clin. Psychol. **40:** 1-19; 163-164, 1973.

Patterson, G. R., and Gullion, M. E.: Living with children: new methods for parents and teachers, Champaign, Ill., 1968, Research Press, Co.

Rose, S. D.: A behavioral approach to the group treatment of parents, Soc. Work **14:**21-29, 1969.

Schaefer, Earl S.: Need for early and continuing education. In Denenberg, Victor H., editor: Education of the infant and young child, New York, 1970, Academic Press, Inc.

Seitz, Sue, and Terdal, Leif: A modeling approach to changing parent-child interactions, Ment. Retard. **10:**39-43, June, 1972.

Shearer, Marsha S., and Shearer, David S.: The Portage Project: a model for early childhood education, Except. Child. **28:**210-217, 1972.

Steward, Margaret, and Steward, David: The observation of Anglo, Mexican, and Chinese-American mothers teaching their young sons, Child Dev. **44:** 329-337, 1973.

Terdal, Leif, Jackson, Russell H., and Garner, Ann M.: Mother-child interactions: a comparison between normal and developmentally delayed groups, unpublished manuscript, March, 1975.

Weikart, David P.: Symposium on parent-centered education, Child. Educ. **9:**135-137, Dec., 1971.

Weikart, David P., and Lambie, Dolores Z.: Early enrichment in infants. In Denenberg, Victor H., editor: Education of the young child, New York, 1970, Academic Press, Inc.

Zeihberger, J., Sampen, S. E., and Sloane, H. N.: Modification of a child's problem behaviors in the home with the mother as therapist, J. Appl. Behav. Anal. **1**:47-53, 1968.

Parental perceptions of children's behaviors and development

Alpern, Gerald D., and Boll, Thomas J.: Development profile, Indianapolis, 1972, Psychological Development Publications.

Barclay, A., and Vaught, G.: Maternal estimates of future achievement in cerebral palsy children, Am. J. Ment. Defic. **68**:62-65, 1964.

Broussard, E. R., and Hartner, M.: Further considerations regarding maternal perceptions of the firstborn. In Hellmuth, Jerome, editor: Exceptional infant: studies in abnormalities, New York, 1971, Brunner/Mazel, Inc.

Capobianco, R. J., and Knox, S.: I.Q. estimates and the index of marital integrations, Am. J. Ment. Defic. **68**:718-721, 1964.

Ehler, W. H.: The moderately and severely retarded child: maternal perceptions of retardation and subsequent seeking and using services rendered by a community agency, Am. J. Ment. Defic. **68**:660-668, 1964.

Ewert, J. D., and Green, M. W.: Conditions associated with the mother's estimates of the ability of her retarded child, Am. J. Ment. Defic. **62**:621-633, 1957.

Kurtz, Richard A.: Comparative evaluations of suspected retardates, Am. J. Dis. Child. **109**:58-65, 1965.

Meyerowitz, J. H.: Parental awareness of retardation, Am. J. Ment. Defic. **71**:637-643, 1967.

Wolfensberger, Wolf, and Kurtz, Richard A.: Measurements of parents' perceptions of their children's development, Genet. Psychol. Monogr. **83**:3-92, 1971.

Worchel, T., and Worchel, P.: The parental concept of the mentally retarded child, Am. J. Ment. Defic. **65**:782-788, 1961.

Zuk, G. H.: Autistic distortion in parents of retarded children, J. Consult. Psychol. **23**:171-176, 1959.

General references on parents

Appell, Louise S., and McKeen, Ronald L.: Parents and professionals rate SMR and PMR adults on developmental tasks: a comparison study, Ment. Retard. **5**:14-16, Oct., 1974.

Gorham, Kathryn A., Des Jardins, Charlotte, Page, Ruth, Pettis, Eugene, and Schreiber, Barbara: Effect on parents. In Hobbs, Nicholas, editor: Issues in the classification of children, vol. 2, San Francisco, 1975, Jossey-Bass, Inc., Publishers.

Heisler, Verda: A handicapped child in the family: a guide for parents, New York, 1972, Grune & Stratton, Inc.

Holyroyd, Jean, and McArthur, David: Mental retardation and stress on the parents: a contrast between

Down's syndrome and childhood autism, Am. J. Ment. Defic. **80**:431-436, 1976.

Luckey, Robert E., and Neman, Ronald S.: The President's panel recommendations today, Ment. Retard. **13**:32-34, Aug., 1975.

McDonald, Eugene T.: Understand those feelings, Pittsburgh, 1962, Stanwix House, Inc.

Sternlicht, Manny, and Sullivan, Ina: Group counseling with parents of the MR: leadership selection and functioning, Ment. Retard. **4**:11-13, Oct., 1974.

Stewart, J. C.: Counseling parents of exceptional children, New York, 1974, MSS Information Corp.

Wolfensberger, Wolf: How to exclude mentally retarded children from school, Ment. Retard. **13**:30-31, Dec., 1975.

Interdisciplinary concepts in the care of children with handicaps

Albee, George W.: Needed—a revolution in caring for the retarded, Transaction **5**:37-42, Jan.-Feb., 1968.

Anderson, Edith H.: Nursing education in the university-affiliated center of the mentally retarded. In Nursing in mental retardation programs, Children's Bureau, Department of Health, Education, and Welfare and Child Development Center, University of Miami, Coral Gables, April, 1967.

Barclay, A., Goulet, L. R., Holtgrewe, M. M., and Sharp, A. R.: Parental evaluation of clinical services for retarded children, Am. J. Ment. Defic. **67**:232-237, 1962.

Baumstein, David S.: Improving communication between team members of a mental retardation diagnostic clinic. Presented at Mental Retardation Workshop, Washington Health Department, Seattle, Sept. 30, 1965.

Bax, Martin: The case conference (editorial), Dev. Med. Child Neurol. **14**:281-282, 1972.

Beck, Helen L.: The advantages of a multi-purpose clinic for the mentally retarded, Am. J. Ment. Defic. **66**:789-794, 1962.

Bobath, Bertha, and Finnie, Nancie P.: Problems of communication between parents and staff in the treatment and management of children with cerebral palsy, Dev. Med. Child Neurol. **12**:629-635, Oct., 1970.

Bolian, George C.: The child psychiatrist and the mental retardation team: a problem of role definition, Arch. Gen. Psychiatry **18**:360-366, 1968.

Caccamo, James M.: Consumer oriented evaluation, Ment. Retard. **12**:48-49, April, 1974.

Caldwell, B. M., Manley, E. J., and Nissan, Y.: Reactions of community agencies and parents to services provided in a clinic for retarded children, Am. J. Ment. Defic. **65**:582-589, 1961.

Caldwell, B. M., Manley, E. J., and Seelye, B. J.: Factors associated with parental reaction to a clinic for retarded children, Am. J. Ment. Defic. **65**:590-594, 1961.

Close, Kathryn: Promoting child health through comprehensive care, Children **16**:130-137, July-Aug., 1969.

Garfunkel, F.: Interdisciplinary diagnosis of mental retardation: a demonstration of professional interaction, Ment. Retard. 1:158-168, June, 1964.

Gordon, Neil: Parent counseling, Dev. Med. Child Neurol. 14:657-659, 1972.

Grass, Constance, and Umansky, Richard: Problems in promoting the growth of multidisciplinary diagnostic and counselling clinics for mentally retarded children in non-metropolitan areas, Am. J. Public Health 61:698-710, 1971.

Heiss, Ann M.: The multidisciplinary or the interdisciplinary approach to professional education. In Proceedings from national workshop on teaching nutrition to professionals of various disciplines at university-affiliated centers for the care of mentally retarded and handicapped children, Seattle, May, 1970, University of Washington and Maternal and Child Health Service, Health Services and Mental Health Administration, U.S. D.H.E.W.

Hersey, William S.: Restoring the balance, Pediatr. Clin. North Am. 20:221-231, 1973.

Hormuth, R. P.: Community clinics for the mentally retarded, Children 4:181-185, Sept.-Oct., 1957.

Howell, Sarah E.: Psychiatric aspects of habilitation, Pediatr. Clin. North Am. 20:203-219, 1973.

Justice, R. S., Campbell, M., O'Connor, G., and Sabotta, E.: A look at the population served by a university clinic for retarded children, Ment. Retard. 3: 43-47, June, 1970.

Kaplan, M. M., and Hingeley, H.: A study of the outpatient clinic services for the mentally retarded at the Muscatatuck State School, Am. J. Ment. Defic. 63:517-523, 1958.

Koch, Richard: The multidiscipline approach to mental retardation. In Baumeister, Alfred A., editor: Mental retardation: appraisal, education, and rehabilitation, Chicago, 1967, Aldine Publishing Co.

Koch, Richard, and Dobson, James C.: The multidisciplinary team: a comprehensive program for diagnosis and treatment of the retarded. In Koch, Robert, and Dobson, James C., editors: The mentally retarded child and his family: a multidisciplinary handbook, New York, 1971, Brunner-Mazel, Inc.

Koch, Richard, et al.: The child development traveling clinic project in Southern California, Ment. Retard. 7:46-52, April, 1969.

Kunze, LuVerne, Campbell, Mary M., and McBain, Kenneth: Interdisciplinary student training in mental retardation, Ment. Retard. 7:15-19, Feb., 1969.

Leininger, Madeleine: This I believe . . . about interdisciplinary health education for the future, Nurs. Outlook 19:787-791, 1971.

Livingstone, John B., Portnoi, Tikuah, Sherry, Norman, Resenheim, Eliyahu, and Onesti, Silvio, Jr.: Comprehensive child psychiatry through a team approach, Children 16:181-186, Sept.-Oct., 1969.

McGraw, Richard M.: Components and organization of interdisciplinary teamwork in the provision of high quality health care. Presented at National Health Forum on Quality in Health Care, Los Angeles, March, 1968.

McIntire, M. S., and Kiehhacher, T. C.: Parental reaction to a clinic for the evaluation of the mentally retarded, Nebr. Med. J. 118:69-73, 1969.

Morgan, Sam B.: Team interpretation of MR to Parents, Ment. Retard. 11:10-13, June, 1973.

Philips, Irving: Problems of training and professional in the field of mental retardation: a review of a training program, J. Am. Acad. Child Psychiatry 5:693-705, 1966.

Pinkerton, P.: Parental acceptance of the handicapped child, Dev. Med. Child Neurol. 12:207-212, 1970.

Pinkerton, P.: Pitfalls in interpretative procedure within the diagnostic clinic, Dev. Med. Child Neurol 12: 516-517, 1970.

Rubenstein, Jack H.: Role of the diagnostic clinic in the care of the mentally retarded child, Am. J. Ment. Defic. 66:544-550, 1962.

Scheerenberger, R. C.: Generic services for the mentally retarded and their families, Ment. Retard. 8:10-16, Dec., 1970.

Sherrard, W. J. W.: Assessment and action (editorial), Dev. Med. Child Neurol. 13:561-562, 1971.

Sherif, Musafer, and Sherif, Carolyn W.: Interdisciplinary relationships in the social sciences, Chicago, 1969, Aldine Publishing Co.

Slobody, L. M. J., Giannini, J. B., Scanlan, H. R., and Kelman, H.: An interdisciplinary personnel training program in a specialized clinic for retarded children, Am. J. Ment. Defic. 62:866-869, 1958.

Stephens, Wyatt E.: Interpreting mental retardation to parents in a multidiscipline diagnostic clinic, Ment. Retard. 7:57-59, Dec., 1969.

Stickler, G. B.: Take it easy when evaluating the mentally retarded child, Clin. Pediatr. 11:373-374, 1972.

Symposium on interdisciplinary training, Proceedings on University-Affiliated Training Center Conference, 93rd Annual Meeting of the American Association on Mental Deficiency, Memphis, May, 1969, University of Tennessee.

Terdal, Leif, and Buell, Joan: Parent education in managing retarded children with behavior deficits and inappropriate behaviors, Ment. Retard. 7:10-13, June, 1969.

Van Antwerp, Malin: An interdisciplinary approach to functional mental retardation, Ment. Retard. 8: 24-26, Feb., 1970.

Walker, J. H., Thomas, M., and Russell, I. T.: Spina bifida—and the parents, Dev. Med. Child Neurol. 13:462-476, 1971.

Watts, Evadean M.: Family therapy: it suse in mental retardation, Ment. Retard. 7:41-44, Oct., 1969.

Wolfensberger, Wolf: Diagnosis diagnosed, J. Ment. Subnorm. 11:62-70, 1965.

Wolfensberger, Wolf: Embarrassments in the diagnostic process, Ment. Retard. 3:29-31, June, 1965.

Wortis, Joseph: Introduction: the role of education in mental retardation work. In Wortis, Joseph, editor: Mental retardation and developmental disabilities: an annual review, vol. J, New York, 1973, Brunner/Mazel, Inc.

INDEX